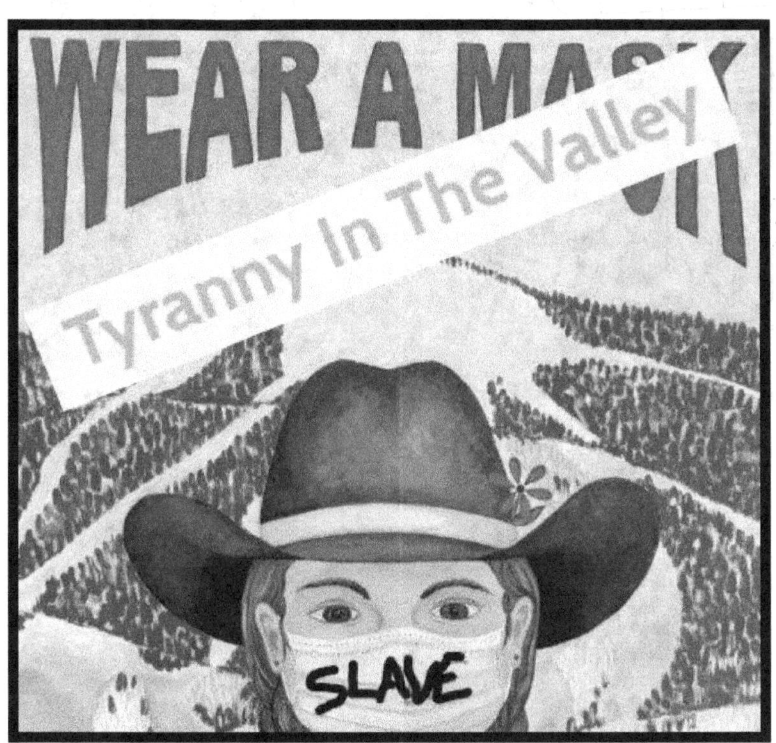

Tyranny In The Valley

Second Edition

© 2022 David Caddell

Introduction:

I am writing with an alert that the entire country may very likely soon experience an approximately 10-day shutdown that could also be accompanied by a media and Internet blackout.

This is likely to result from the consequence of the Executive Order signed by President Trump on September 12, 2018:

Significant within this Executive Order is this statement, **"I hereby declare a national emergency to deal with this threat."**

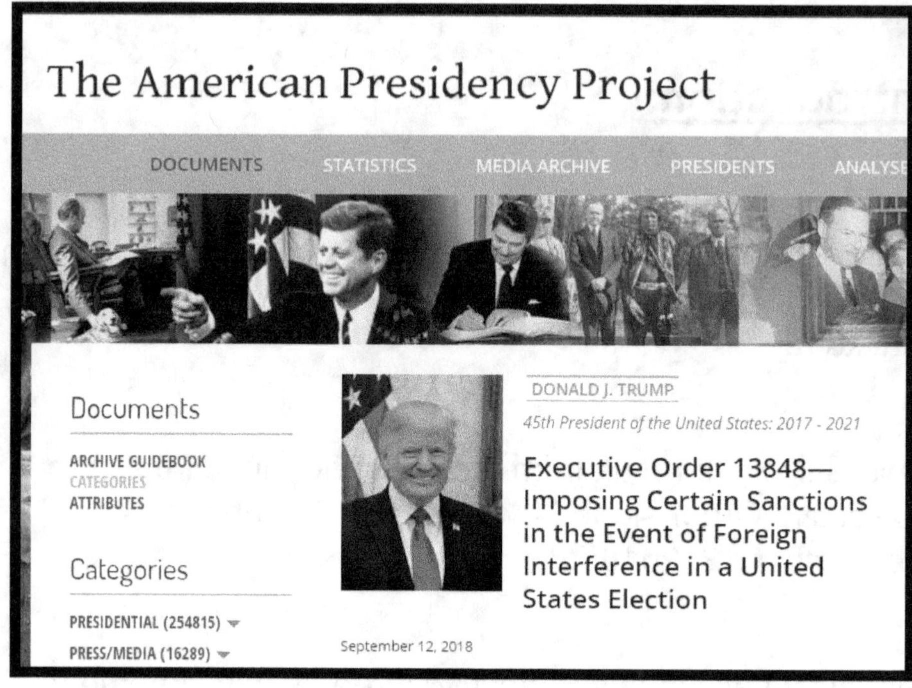

You may know that a state of "national emergency" provides the Executive Branch special powers in order to protect the Constitution of the United States.

Now this story recently broke revealing a hack into the "Solarwinds" software system that was used in the vote – A hack by foreign actors – Considering the Executive Order above, consider what this means:

3

"The Cybersecurity and Infrastructure Security Agency (CISA) tonight issued Emergency Directive 21-01, in response to a known compromise involving SolarWinds Orion products that are currently being exploited by malicious actors. This Emergency Directive calls on all federal civilian agencies to review their networks for indicators of compromise and disconnect or power down SolarWinds Orion products immediately."

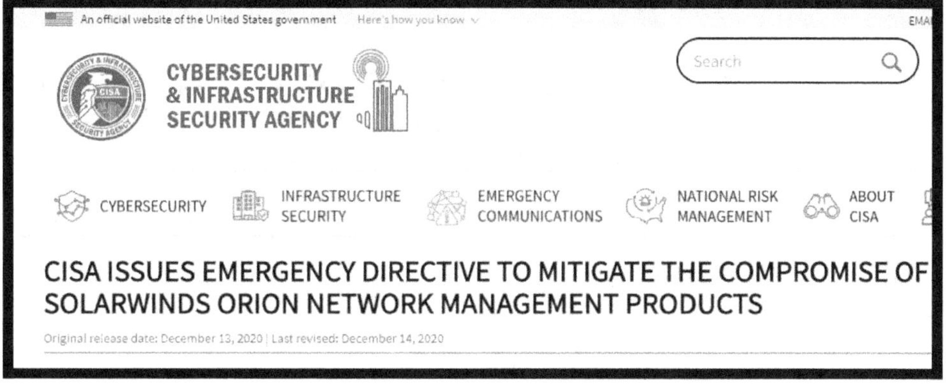

The "Solarwinds" offices were just recently raided by the FBI.

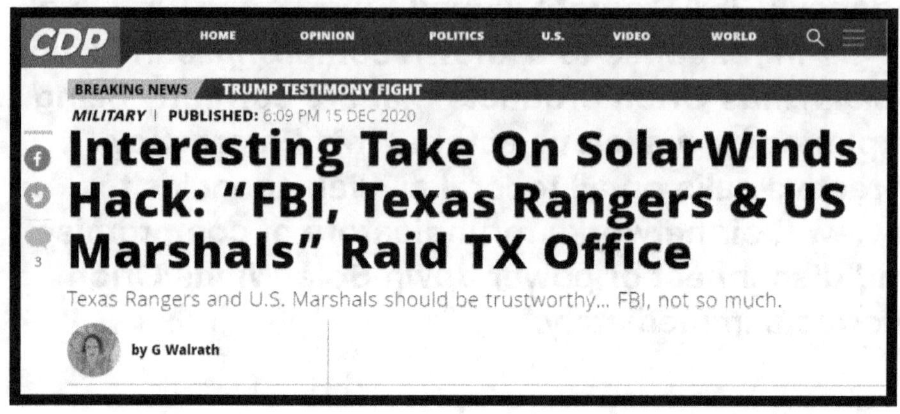

What I am sharing with you is a sliver of the big picture of what is currently happening, however these significant developments may very likely trigger the event that researchers have been anticipating for over the past 10 years.

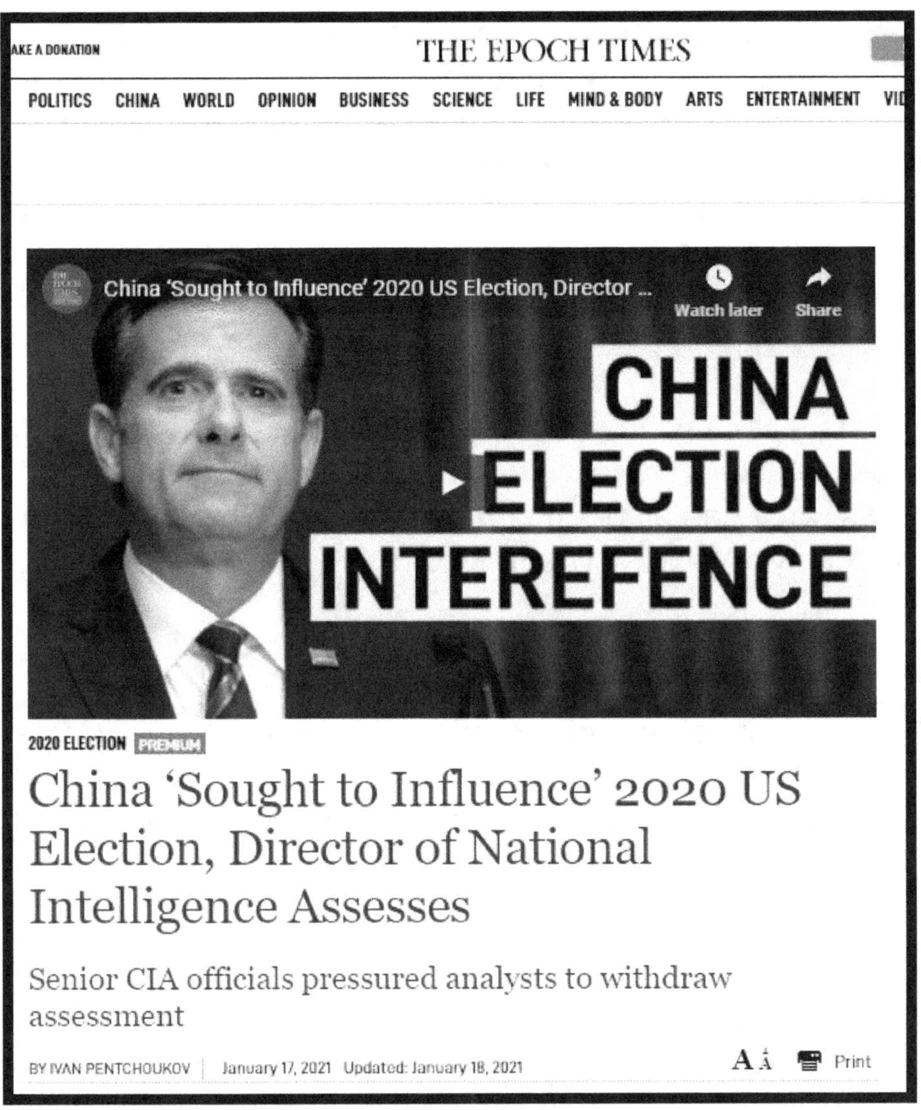

China 'Sought to Influence' 2020 US Election, Director of National Intelligence Assesses

Senior CIA officials pressured analysts to withdraw assessment

BY IVAN PENTCHOUKOV | January 17, 2021 Updated: January 18, 2021   A A   Print

Additionally, it is significant to recognize that the intelligence agencies are consolidating against this threat:

"Over the course of the past several days, the FBI, CISA, and ODNI have become aware of a significant and ongoing cybersecurity campaign. Pursuant to Presidential Policy Directive (PPD) 41, the FBI, CISA, and ODNI have formed a Cyber Unified Coordination Group (UCG) to coordinate a whole-of-government response to this significant cyber incident."

This is all to say, in short, really big things are happening – Do not expect to learn anything from the "mainstream news" as it has all been compromised to China – You might say, "No way, you're kidding!" I wish I were.

I do not intend to convince anyone of anything, however I hope to inspire enough interest and provide the resources that you might decide to learn for yourself because only your own reason will ever convince you of anything, but you need to be aware.

It has recently been revealed that 2 million communist Chinese operative spies have infiltrated all levels of government and society all the way to local School Board and, yes, County Commissioners and City Council – I am not making any accusations, however it is true that what is coming during the upcoming "shutdown" will be mass arrests that will include corrupted officials from US

Senators, Congressmen, Governors all the way to County representatives.

It is being reported that there are over 200,000 sealed indictments currently being held by the Federal Department of Justice that have been collected over the past four years.

In similar fashion to "taking down the mob," all of the corrupt officials will be arrested in one swoop.

The state of "National Emergency" triggered by the Executive Order due to foreign interference in the election with the "Solarwinds" hack will empower the US Military to operate with domestic powers to arrest these hundreds of thousands of corrupt government officials nationwide all at once – Now you might find it a coincidence that the US military is being deployed nationwide to distribute the vaccine… Get it?

Have you ever heard President Trump call the "coronavirus" the "hidden enemy?" Well, it appears that the US military is likely to be the "vaccine" for the "hidden enemy" in the name of the "deep state," or the "shadow government" that has been coordinating with communist China to stage an insurrectionist coup against the United States and I am not being hyperbolic when I say that Chinese troops are staged and ready to make a land invasion into the United States and completely take us over – Yep, "Red Dawn" – But it's not just a movie.

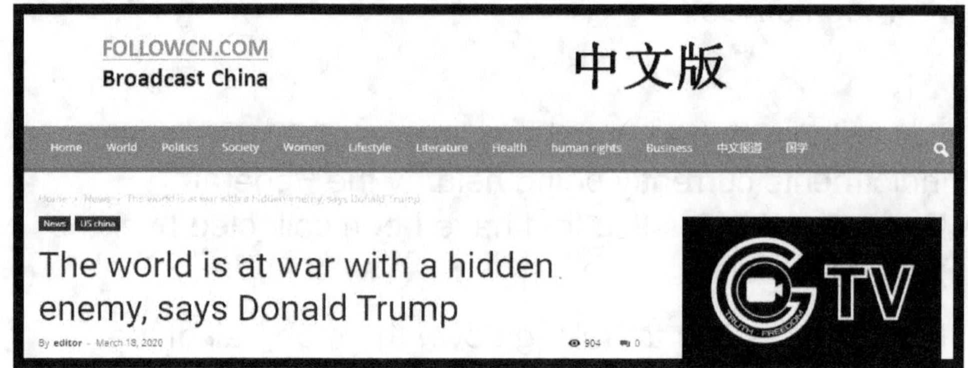

Upcoming will be such an undeniable revelation of the truth that it will be indisputable – It will be shocking and traumatizing to many to learn that those that we had most revered will be exposed to have sold us out.

You may not be aware of the widespread ballot fraud that occurred during the 2020 Presidential Election because the "mainstream media" continues the mantra that "there is no evidence" – However, that is a trick because evidence cannot be disclosed if it will compromise a court proceeding and there are many now happening and many more on the way – Many, many more – Here is a source, and this is just for Arizona:

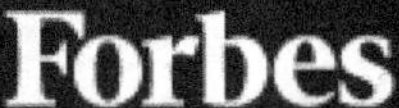

For those who have been watching closely, it is obvious that President Trump overwhelmingly won the 2020 Presidential Election, and now Maria Bartiromo is the first "mainstream media" anchorperson brave enough to speak the truth – The others are afraid both for their contracts and for the safety of their families:

"Maria Bartiromo Says Her 'Intel Source' Told Her President Trump Actually Won"

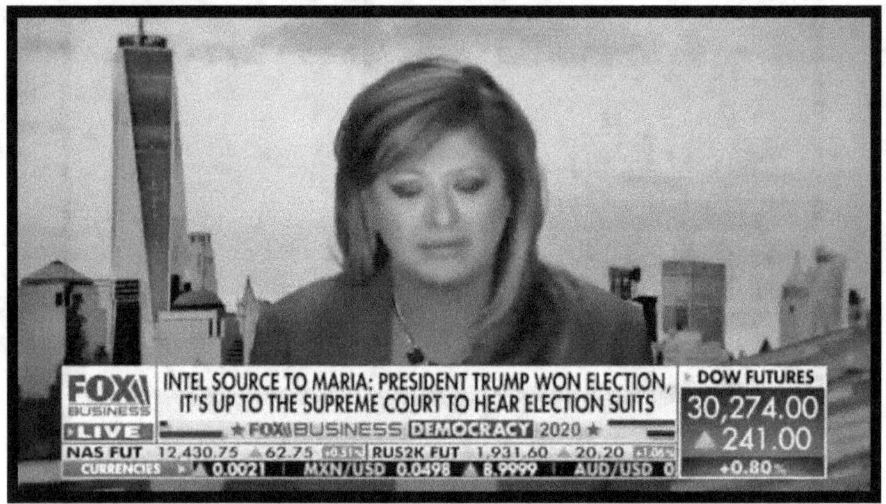

During the "ten days of darkness," it is being theorized that the Internet, radio, television and cell phone networks will be shut down – This will be a last desperate attempt for the "deep state" to prevent the public from learning the truth as they try to escape somehow.

However, the President has already performed a test run of the "Presidential Alert System":

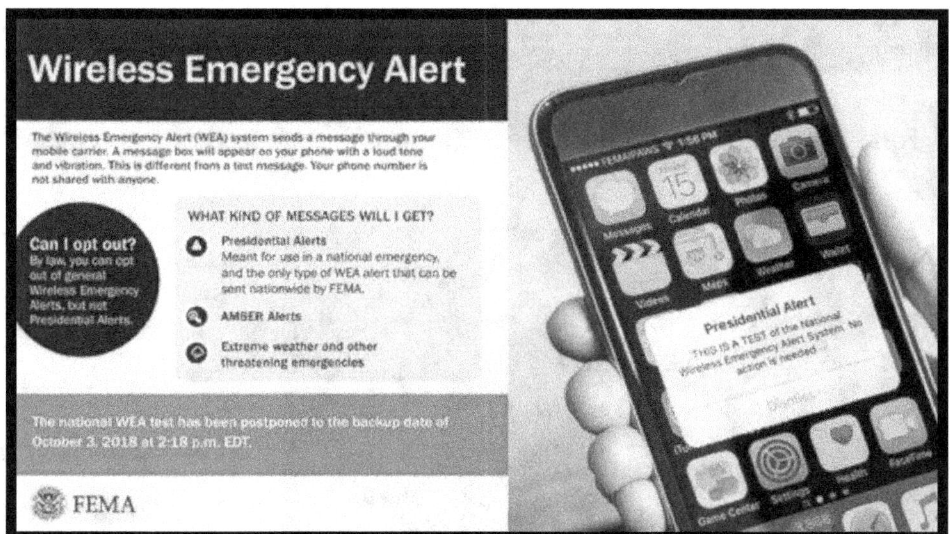

This will broadcast an emergency message to let the public know what is happening and to remain calm – This is likely going to be a "Martial Law" scenario triggered by the "Insurrection Act" that has already been publicly called for by two retired US generals:

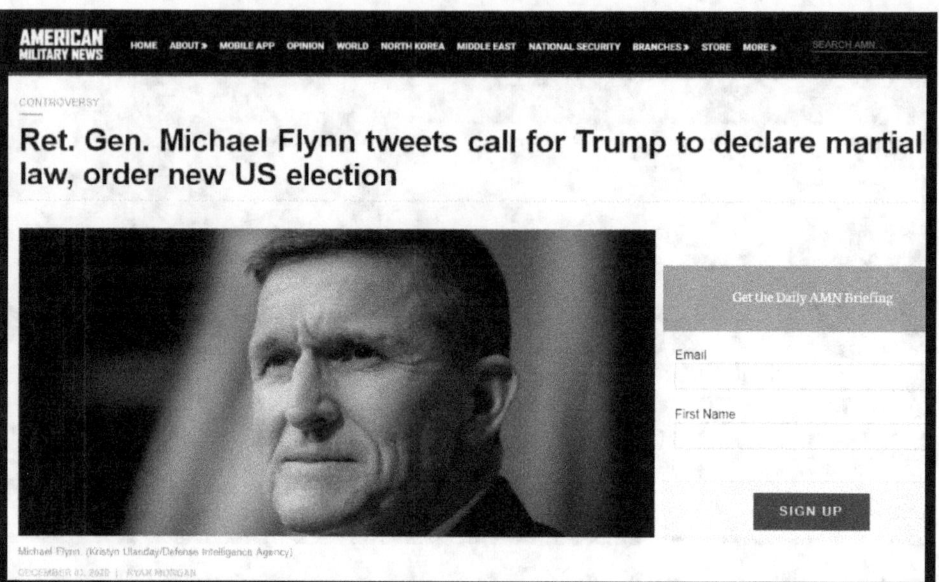

AMERICAN MILITARY NEWS
HOME   ABOUT »   MOBILE APP   OPINION   WORLD   NORTH KOREA   MIDDLE EAST   NATIONAL SECURITY   BRANCHES »   STORE   MORE »   SEARCH AMN

CONTROVERSY

Ret. Gen. Michael Flynn tweets call for Trump to declare martial law, order new US election

Get the Daily AMN Briefing

Email

First Name

SIGN UP

Michael Flynn (Kristyn Ulanday/Defense Intelligence Agency)
DECEMBER 03, 2020 | RYAN MORGAN

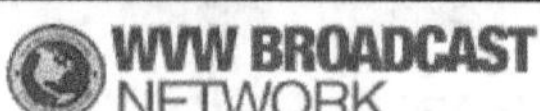
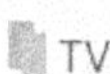
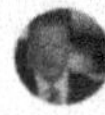

WWW BROADCAST NETWORK   HOME   RADIO ▾   TV ▾   NEWS   SITUATION ROOM ▾

TV

Exclusive: 3-Star General McInerney Calls For Martial Law, Tribunals & Investigation of Treason

By Brannon Howse, 30 November, 2020

(Of course I do not expect these developments to be covered fairly in the "mainstream news")

So the declaration of "Martial Law" will likely last no more than 10 days while the National Guard coordinate with Marines to conduct thousands of arrests and prevent an internal violent insurrection.

When it is conclusively decided that President Trump won reelection, these groups have been armed and instructed to begin using AK-47's instead of urine-filled water bottles that they have been throwing at police – In other words, we are sitting on a powder keg and it is about to explode with the conclusive declaration of President Trump as the next President of the United States for a second term, however he may be the "19th" and not the "45th" President, after all.

Regardless, the revelation of the "Solarwinds" hack is evidence of foreign interference in the election which will trigger the Executive Order to invoke a "National Emergency" and therefore, very likely, 10 days of martial law and no media or Internet – We will be receiving communication from the Presidential Alert System.

On the other side of this we will be able to begin rebuilding our country no longer beholden to the "deep state" and foreign enemies namely China, the Vatican, the United Kingdom, and Washington D.C. itself that had infiltrated our country and had almost completely taken us over before we even knew what was happening.

However, we have been saved by a world-class prizefighter by the name of President Donald J. Trump, and so many ungrateful and unaware individuals allow

their brains to be washed by the "mainstream media" that is controlled and funded by foreign enemies to the United States.

Vladimir Lenin legendarily called such individuals "useful idiots":

COMMENTARY

America's Useful Idiots

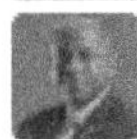

By Allen West | July 13, 2020 | 5:04am EDT

T! ▯ ▯ 🖨 🗎 ✉ f 𝕏

"Useful idiots" is a phrase attributed to Vladimir Lenin, who supposedly used it to describe communist sympathizers in Western Civilization.

It is a very appropriate descriptor when it comes to the so-called "woke" mob of the so-called "resistance" that has overtaken the streets of America. Well, let me rephrase that: They have overtaken the streets of major population centers in America. The infestation of wokeness and idiocy

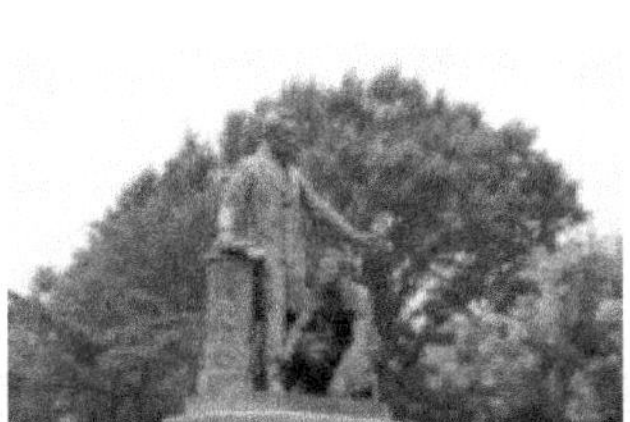

Bronze statue entitled 'Emancipation' depicts US President Abraham Lincoln and a newly liberated slave rising at his feet. The statue in Washington, D.C., was built almost entirely with funds donated by former slaves and dedicated in 1876. (Photo by Carol M. Highsmith/Buyenlarge/Getty Images)

seems concentrated in the very places where progressive socialist policies have failed in America.

Consider the idiocy of a city in Colorado that is incarcerating people who do not wear a mask. Yet these same leftists claimed that criminals had to be released from incarceration due to the threat of COVID-19. Or consider the idiocy of going into the home of private citizens and confiscating their weapon, their right to keep and bear arms, for no apparent reason, other than they defended their property, safety, and security against the invasion of the "woke" mob -- the useful idiots

It may appear that President Trump has been "losing," however that has always been his strategy throughout his lifetime as he has always appeared just prior to striking another victory - This time, it is to save the world from an otherwise all-consuming global communist tyranny.

Kind of like how President Trump's friend Muhammad Ali knocked out George Foreman in the eighth round just as it appeared that he had been losing – The "Rope-A-Dope" – "The Art of War" – "The Art of the Deal" – No coincidence.

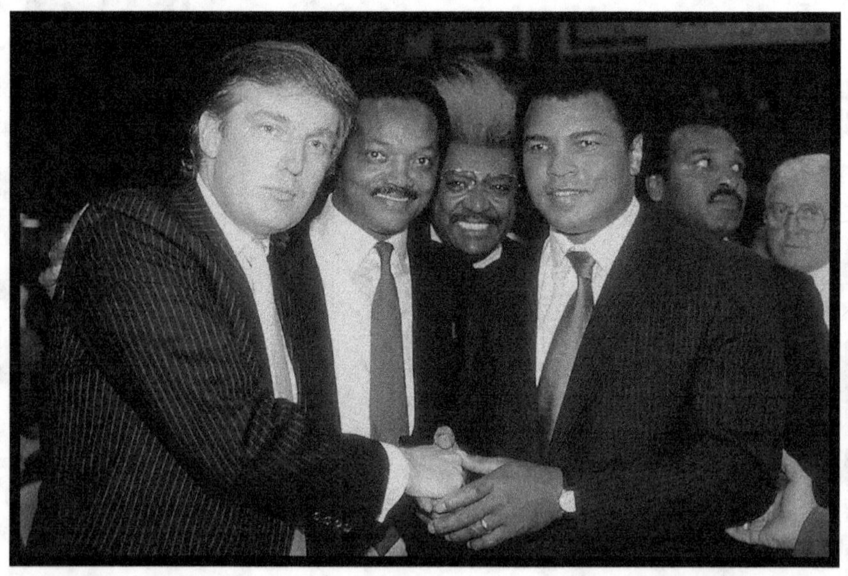

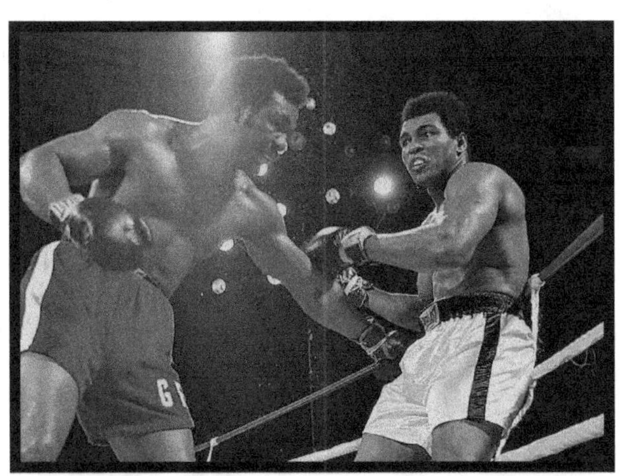

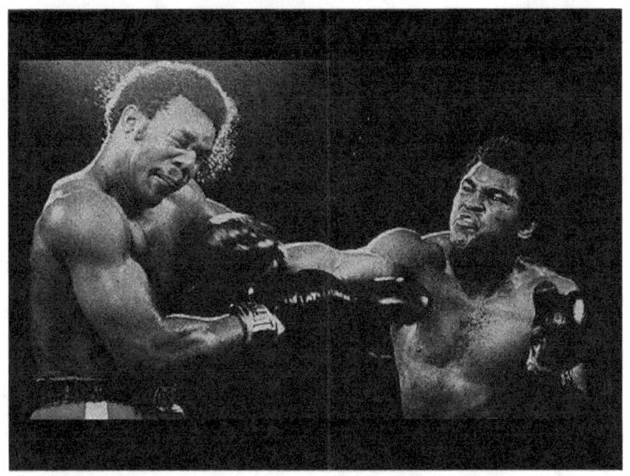

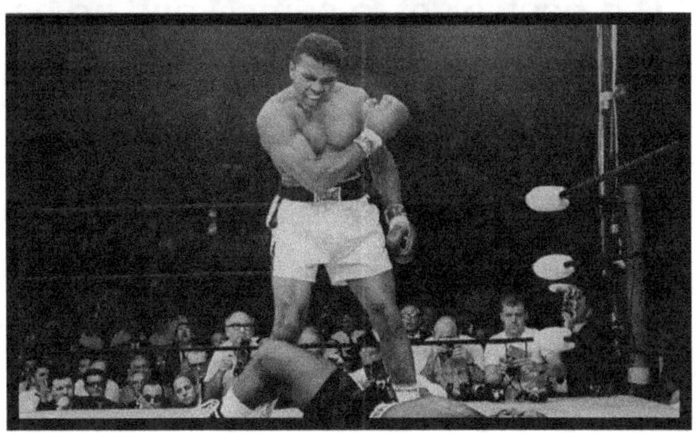

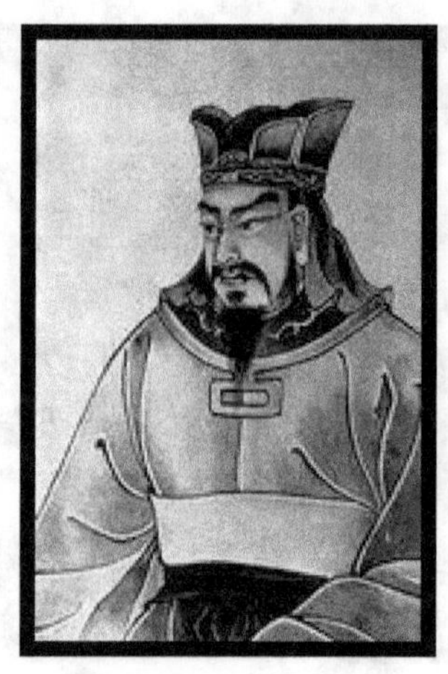

"Appear weak when you are strong, and strong when you are weak." — **Sun Tzu,** The Art of War

Stock up on everything for at least 10 days if we have to hunker down for a little bit – I can only offer you my words, but for whatever they may be worth, do not worry – It is going to get much better just as President Trump often says "The best is yet to come," and he hasn't been wrong yet.

Across the United States, over 200,000 sealed cases – You may know that this is the strategy for arresting the mafia – Sealing cases while turning witnesses to prosecute the head of the organization – With over 200,000 sealed cases, and any of those cases could each include numerous individuals, that is one large criminal organization that is getting arrested.

It is not a "conspiracy theory," the original constitutional United States was taken over by the CORPORATION of the United States of America in 1871:

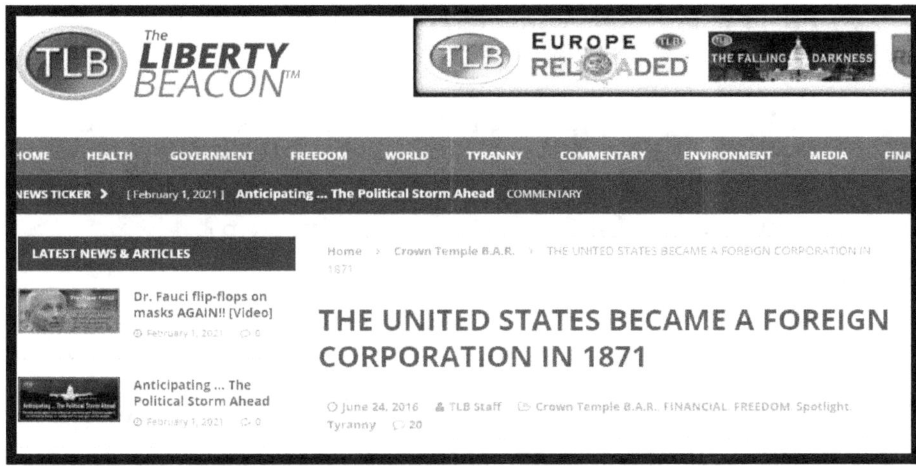

Therefore, we have since 1871 been operating as a corporation, just like General Motors, owned by The United Kingdom at The City of London this entire time, and our tax dollars have been going to "The Rothschilds" who have owned 99% of all the central banks around the entire world.

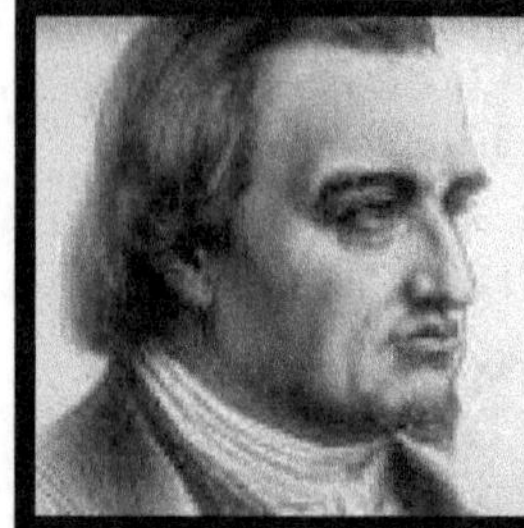

The US Military has recognized this threat since the beginning, however has been prevented from stopping the progressive loss of our liberty due to the civilian control of political power in the country.

Therefore, now reflect upon all of the "booms" and "busts" ever since 1871 – The Great Depression? The World Wars? "The Military Industrial Complex?" – Halliburton?

The reason for the assassination of JFK – The reason for the attempted assassination of President Reagan – The reason for the hundreds of assassination attempts against President Trump, that he had thankfully been protected by his own security force, which happens to be the "Blackwater" military contractor that had originally been hired to invade Iraq – Incidentally, the founder of "Blackwater," Erik Prince, is the brother of the Secretary of Education Betsy DeVos – See how this fits together?

Here is an actual photo from a weather camera in "Skunk Bay" off the coast of Seattle, Washington – This is a missile that was fired from a rogue "deep state" (literally "deep") submarine directed at Air Force One as President Trump was flying overhead on his way to establish peace with North Korea by meeting with Kim Jung Un:

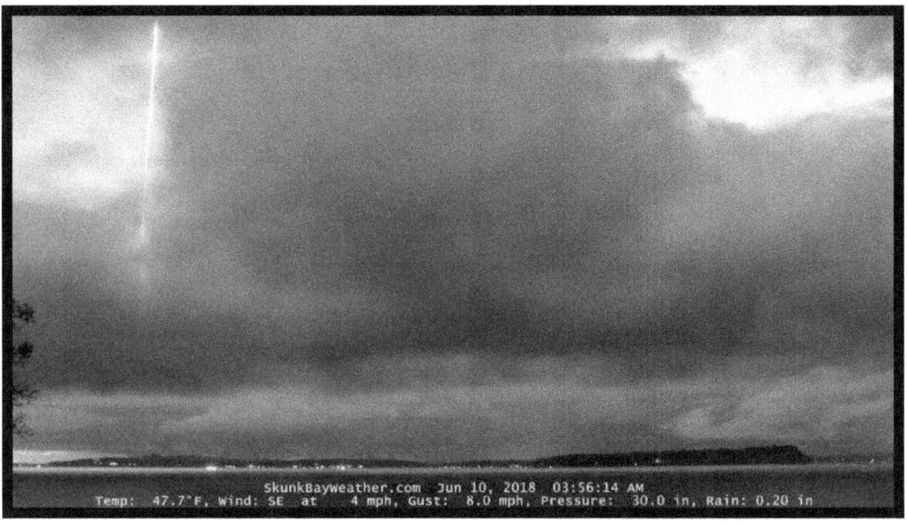

Notice the date? June 10, 2018 – When did President Trump meet with Kim Jung Un?

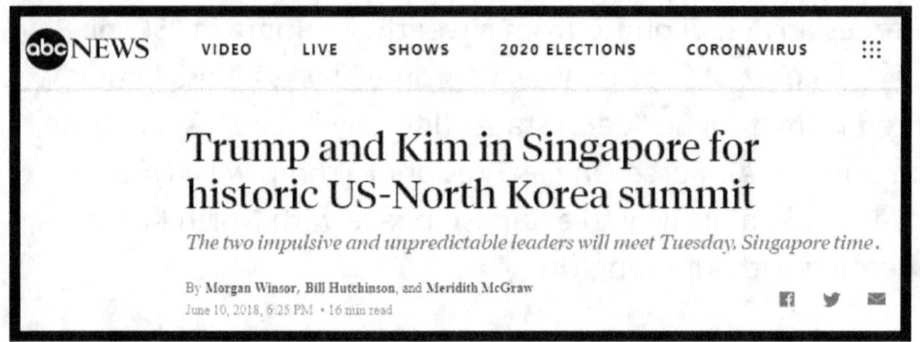

June 10, 2018 – "Trump and Kim in Singapore…"

This information was shared by the "Q" operation, which is an NSA intelligence operation that has been sharing open-source information with the general public in order to inform us of operations "behind the scenes" to defeat the worldwide organizations, globalists, that have been for decades working to destroy the United States so that it will submit with the other nations of the world to become a one world government, a "New World Order" – This is not a "conspiracy theory," this is the truth.

1476

Q !CbboFOtcZs 06/12/2018 17:37:55

ID: 824a6d

Archive Bread/Post Links: 1718008 / 1718290

Direct Link: 1718290

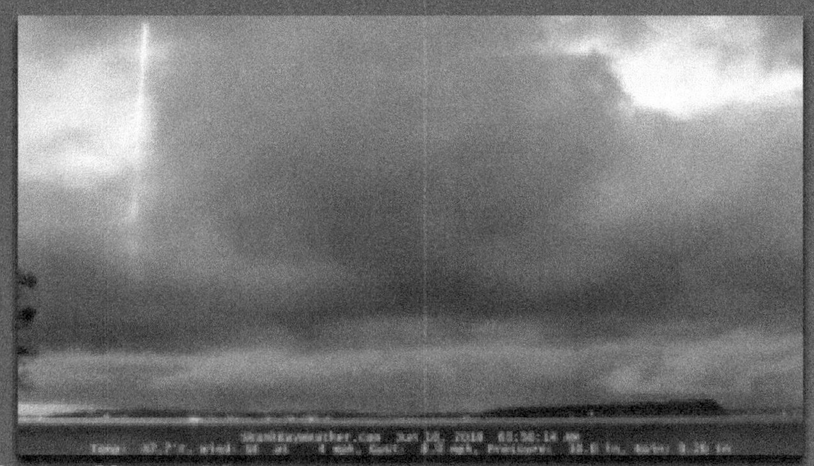

Image Name: *.jpg

Filename:
64b4356d5c829e27078c281d0bcb4edcf61da2814232694ea1b7b716
2d5a9072.jpg

This is not a game.

Certain events were not suppose to take place.

Q

The term "conspiracy theory" itself was invented by the CIA after the JFK assassination to make anyone who questions the original narrative look like a crazy person... Like the Vietnam War... Like "Waco"... Like the "Oklahoma City Bombing"... Like "9/11"

DISPATCH

<table>
<tr><td rowspan="2">TO
Chiefs, Certain Stations and Bases</td><td>CLASSIFICATION
S E C R E T</td><td colspan="2">PROCESSING ACTION
MARKED FOR INDEXING</td></tr>
<tr><td rowspan="3">Document Number 1035-960</td><td>X</td><td>NO INDEXING REQUIRED</td></tr>
<tr><td>INFO.</td><td></td><td>ONLY QUALIFIED DESK
CAN JUDGE INDEXING</td></tr>
<tr><td>FROM
Chief, WOVIEW</td><td colspan="2">for FOIA Review on SEP 1976
CIA HISTORICAL REVIEW PROGRAM
Release In Full 1996</td></tr>
</table>

SUBJECT

O Countering Criticism of the Warren Report

ACTION REQUIRED · REFERENCES

PAUL H.   FOR OSWALD
PSYCH   FILE! 2 COPIES

THIS WAS PULLED TOGETHER BY NED BENNETT OF CA STAFF IN CLOSE CONJUNCTION WITH CI/RYA. WE FURNISHED MOST OF THE SOURCE MATERIAL, PROPOSED MANY OF THE THEMES, AND PROVIDED GENERAL "EXPERTISE" ON THE CASE. THE SPECTATOR ARTICLE WAS WRITTEN BY BENNETT.

G. E. Dou...
23 JAN 196...

1. <u>Our Concern.</u> From the day of President Kennedy's assassination on, there has been speculation about the responsibility for his murder. Although this was stemmed for a time by the Warren Commission report (which appeared at the end of September 1964), various writers have now had time to scan the Commission's published report and documents for new pretexts for questioning, and there has been a new wave of books and articles criticizing the Commission's findings. In most cases the critics have speculated as to the existence of some kind of conspiracy, and often they have implied that the Commission itself was involved. Presumably as a result of the increasing challenge to the Warren Commission's Report, a public opinion poll recently indicated that 46% of the American public did not think that Oswald acted alone, while more than half of those polled thought that the Commission had left some questions unresolved. Doubtless polls abroad would show similar, or possibly more adverse, results.

2. This trend of opinion is a matter of concern to the U.S. government, including our organization. The members of the Warren Commission were naturally chosen for their integrity, experience, and prominence. They represented both major parties, and they and their staff were deliberately drawn from all sections of the country. Just because of the standing of the Commissioners, efforts to impugn their rectitude and wisdom tend to cast doubt on the whole leadership of American society. Moreover, there seems to be an increasing tendency to hint that President Johnson himself, as the one person who might be said to have benefited, was in some way responsible for the assassination. Innuendo of such seriousness affects not only the individual concerned, but also the whole reputation of the American government. Our organization itself is directly involved: among other facts, we contributed information to the investigation. Conspiracy theories have frequently thrown suspicion on our organization, for example by falsely alleging that Lee Harvey Oswald worked for us. The aim of this dispatch is to provide material for countering and discrediting the claims of the conspiracy theorists, so as to inhibit the circulation of such claims in other countries. Background information is supplied in a classified section and in a number of unclassified attachments.

3. <u>Action.</u> We do <u>not</u> recommend that discussion of the assassination question be initiated where it is not already taking place. <u>Where discussion is active, however, addressees are requested:</u>

<table>
<tr><td>AN...FI...</td><td colspan="2"></td><td>CS COPY.</td><td>281-289248</td></tr>
<tr><td>CROSS REFERENCE TO
ABSTRACT X INDEX
9 attachments h/w</td><td></td><td>DISPATCH SYMBOL AND NUMBER
BD 5847</td><td></td><td>DATE
4/1/67</td></tr>
<tr><td>1 - SECRET 8 atts.
8 - Unclassified</td><td></td><td>CLASSIFICATION
S E C R E T</td><td></td><td>HQS FILE NUMBER
DESTROY WHEN NO LONGER
NEEDED</td></tr>
</table>

a. To discuss the publicity problem with liaison and friendly elite contacts (especially politicians and editors), pointing out that the Warren Commission made as thorough an investigation as humanly possible, that the charges of the critics are without serious foundation, and that further speculative discussion only plays into the hands of the opposition. Point out also that parts of the conspiracy talk appear to be deliberately generated by Communist propagandists. Urge them to use their influence to discourage unfounded and irresponsible speculation.

b. To employ propaganda assets to answer and refute the attacks of the critics. Book reviews and feature articles are particularly appropriate for this purpose. The unclassified attachments to this guidance should provide useful background material for passage to assets. Our play should point out, as applicable, that the critics are (i) wedded to theories adopted before the evidence was in, (ii) politically interested, (iii) financially interested, (iv) hasty and inaccurate in their research, or (v) infatuated with their own theories. In the course of discussions of the whole phenomenon of criticism, a useful strategy may be to single out Epstein's theory for attack, using the attached Fletcher Knebel article and Spectator piece for background. (Although Mark Lane's book is much less convincing than Epstein's and comes off badly where contested by knowledgeable critics, it is also much more difficult to answer as a whole, as one becomes lost in a morass of unrelated details.)

4. In private or media discussion not directed at any particular writer, or in attacking publications which may be yet forthcoming, the following arguments should be useful:

a. <u>No significant new evidence</u> has emerged which the Commission did not consider. The assassination is sometimes compared (e.g., by Joachim Joesten and Bertrand Russell) with the Dreyfus case; however, unlike that case, the attacks on the Warren Commission have produced no new evidence, no new culprits have been convincingly identified, and there is no agreement among the critics. (A better parallel, though an imperfect one, might be with the Reichstag fire of 1933, which some competent historians (Fritz Tobias, A.J.P. Taylor, D.C. Watt) now believe was set by Van der Lubbe on his own initiative, without acting for either Nazis or Communists; the Nazis tried to pin the blame on the Communists, but the latter have been much more successful in convincing the world that the Nazis were to blame.)

b. Critics usually overvalue particular items and ignore others. They tend to place more emphasis on the recollections of individual eyewitnesses (which are less reliable and more divergent -- and hence offer more hand-holds for criticism) and less on ballistic, autopsy, and photographic evidence. A close examination of the Commission's records will usually show that the conflicting eyewitness accounts are quoted out of context, or were discarded by the Commission for good and sufficient reason.

c. Conspiracy on the large scale often suggested would be impossible to conceal in the United States, esp. since informants could expect to receive large royalties, etc. Note that Robert Kennedy, Attorney General at the time and John F. Kennedy's brother, would be the last man to overlook or conceal any conspiracy. And as one reviewer pointed out, Congressman Gerald R. Ford would hardly have held his tongue for the sake of the Democratic administration, and Senator Russell would have had every political interest in exposing any misdeeds on the part of Chief Justice Warren. A conspirator moreover would hardly choose a location for a shooting where so much depended on conditions beyond his control: the route, the speed of the cars, the moving target, the risk that the assassin would be discovered. A group of wealthy conspirators could have arranged much more secure conditions.

d. Critics have often been enticed by a form of intellectual pride: they light on some theory and fall in love with it; they also scoff at the Commission because it did not always answer every question with a flat decision one way or the other. Actually, the make-up of the Commission and its staff was an excellent safeguard against over-commitment to any one theory, or against the illicit transformation of probabilities into certainties.

Of course, the head of the CIA at the time of the JFK assassination was George Bush Sr. – Of course he was recorded on national television telling us to look forward to a "New World Order":

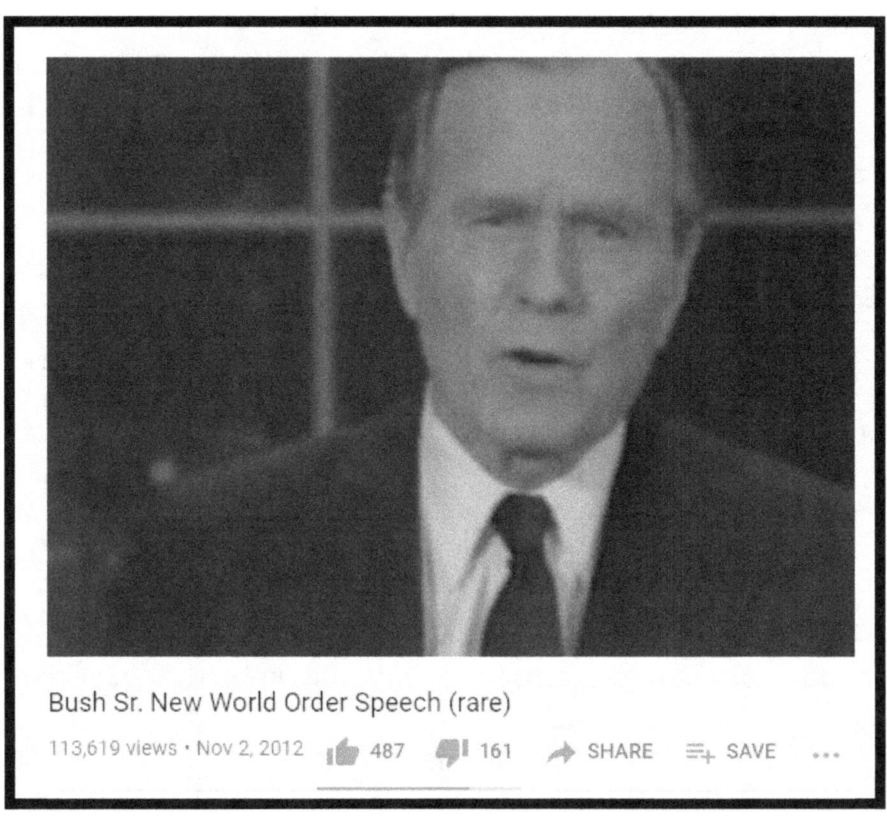

Bush Sr. New World Order Speech (rare)

113,619 views · Nov 2, 2012   487   161   SHARE   SAVE   ...

You may already know much of this, if not much more, however I share this with you to let you know that this story is much bigger than it appears – This obviously has nothing to do with a "virus" that is so scary that we have to completely surrender our constitutional liberties – This is a final attack by the "New World Order," the "Globalists," the "Deep State," the "Shadow Government"… Basically, the banks – The Rothschilds, who have owned The US Federal Reserve Bank and have been collecting our tax dollars for the entire duration of our lifetimes since the establishment of the "Fed" in 1913 – Just a few years after 1871.

What we are now witnessing is the final defeat of this "Globalist Banker Cabal" – Power of the United States was seized by the US Military on January 20, 2021 when "Joe Biden" was supposedly inaugurated to the now bankrupt and non-existent "United States Corporation," and also why President Trump was recently the only man in history ever to walk in front of "The Queen":

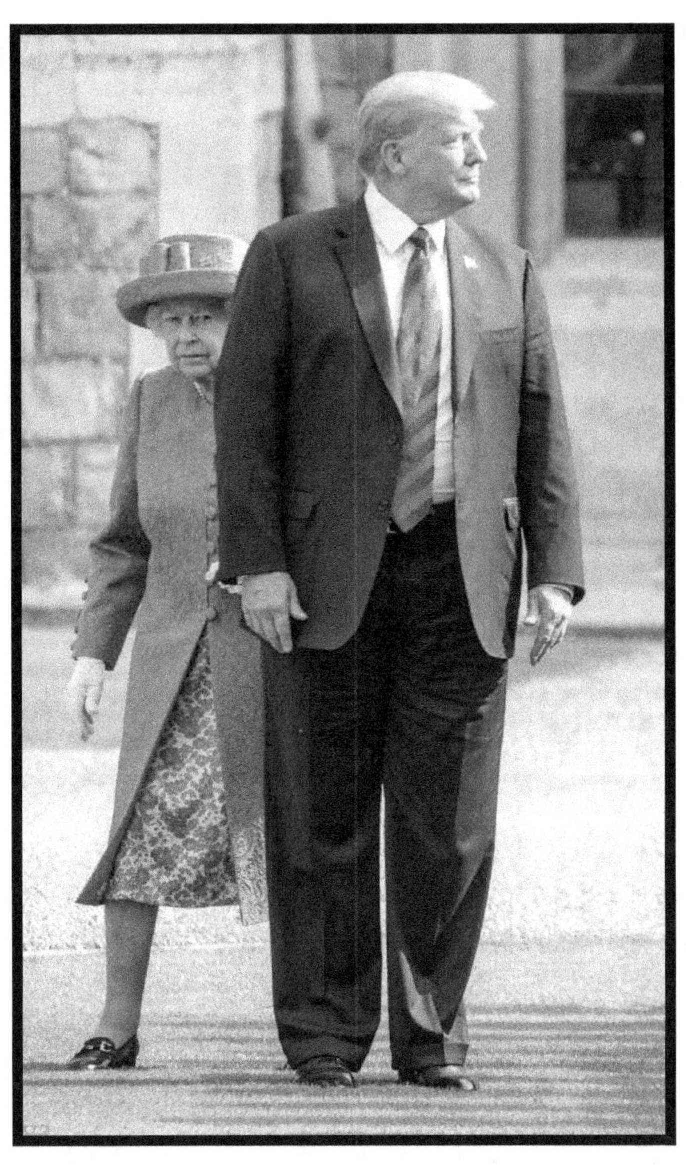

Because she is not "The Queen" anymore

THE SUN, A NEWS UK COMPANY

THE Sun

< WS | MONEY | DEAR DEIDRE | TECH | TRAVEL | MOTORS | PUZZLES

All News | UK News | World News | Brexit | Politics | Opinion

QUEEN'S CASTLE LOCKOUT Queen gets shut out of Windsor Castle in awkward security gaffe

Matt Wilkinson
7 Mar 2020, 2:50 | Updated: 7 Mar 2020, 3:23

56 Comments

THE Queen was locked out of her home at Windsor Castle in an embarrassing security blunder.

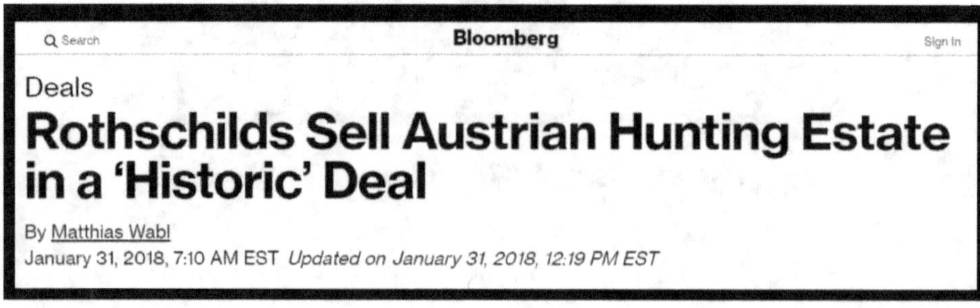

Why do you suppose that the "Rothschilds" sold their Austrian hunting estate for a fraction of what it is worth? A fire sale:

Search | Bloomberg | Sign In

Deals

Rothschilds Sell Austrian Hunting Estate in a 'Historic' Deal

By Matthias Wabl
January 31, 2018, 7:10 AM EST *Updated on January 31, 2018, 12:19 PM EST*

"The Rothschild family sold an Austrian forestry- and hunting estate including a stately lodge and power plants in what the broker called a 'historic transaction' in continental Europe.

"At 5,400 hectares (13,000 acres), the grounds about two hours west of Vienna are 16 times as big as New York's Central Park…"

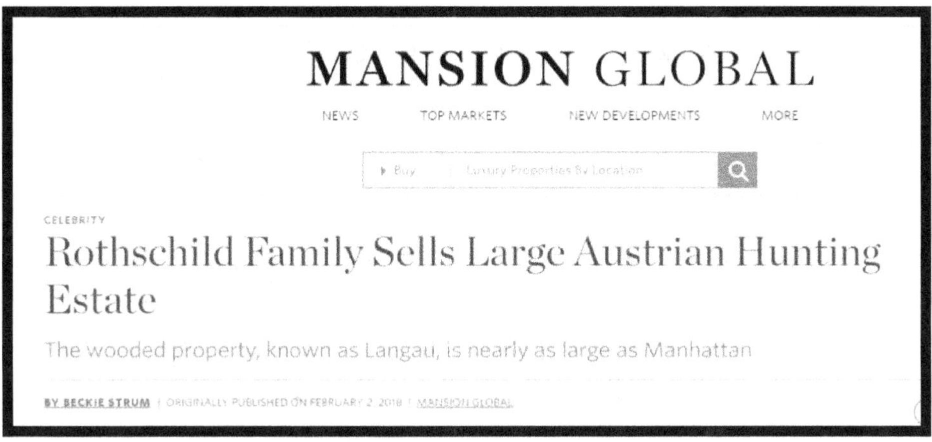

"Austrian media reported the Rothschild heirs sold the property for $112.35 million…"

13,000 acres of a private hunting estate in Austria sold for $112.35 million?

By comparison, have a look at the 82-acre Aspen property owned by the Koch family, worth $100 million.

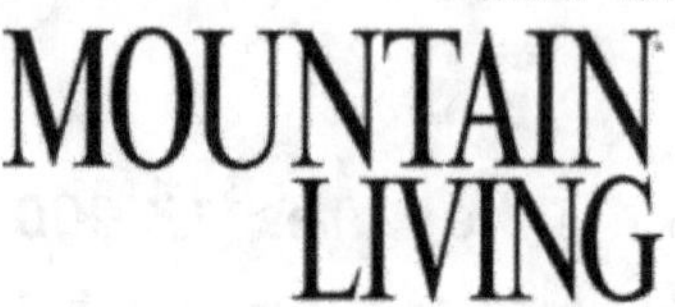

Take a Look at Bill Koch's $100 Million Aspen Compound

April 20, 2015 by Vanessa Richetti

Interested in seeing one of the priciest mountain listings in the country? Well then look no further!

Billionaire businessman William "Bill" Koch (of Koch Industries) recently listed his mountain compound, Elk Mountain Lodge Properties, near Aspen, Colorado, for $100 million.

According to Zillow, the property spans 82.6 acres and includes a log-and-stone main lodge, as well as many single-family homes and historic cabins. The total 43,229 square feet include:

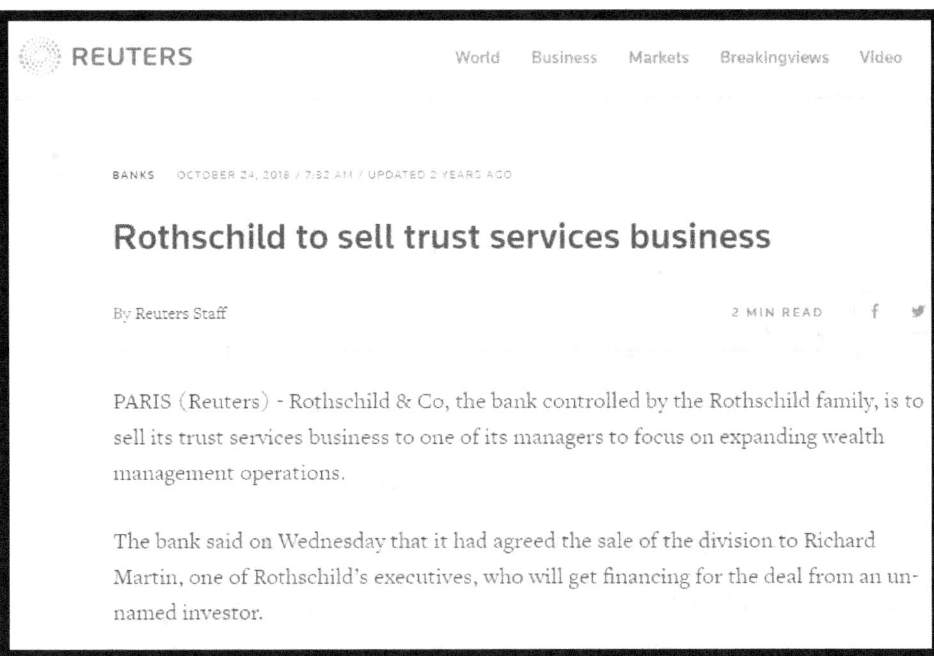

Are we to believe that an 82-acre private ranch in Aspen is worth about the same as a 13,000-acre estate in Austria?

The "Rothschilds" sold this property in a hurry – Here is the reason why – Notice the date of the Rothschild estate sale, February, 2018.

Here is the Executive Order that President Trump had signed just a couple of months beforehand:

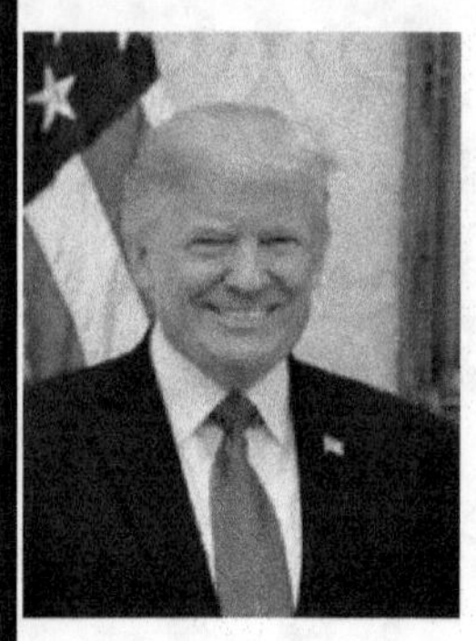

Executive Order 13818— Blocking the Property of Persons Involved in Serious Human Rights Abuse or Corruption

December 20, 2017

"I therefore determine that *serious human rights abuse and corruption around the world constitute an unusual and extraordinary threat* to the national security, foreign policy, and economy of the United States, and *I hereby declare a national* emergency to deal with that threat."

Do you suppose the "Rothschilds" might have been guilty of "human rights abuse?" I do not know, do they look like the kind of people that would be involved in evil and twisted behaviors?

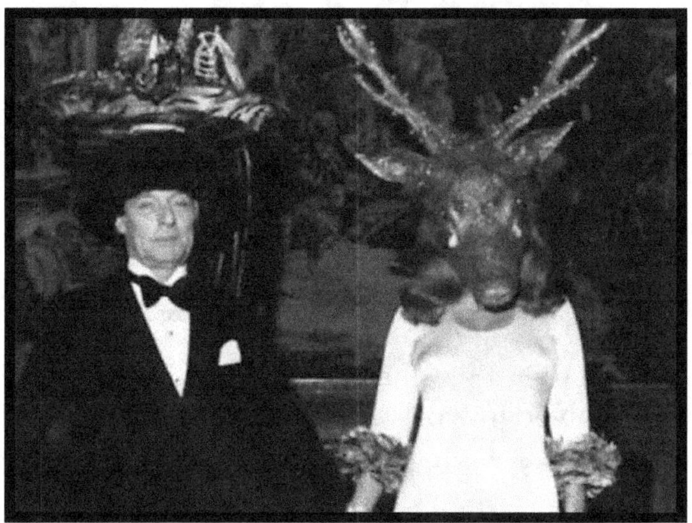

You better believe it – And also why they hate President Trump:

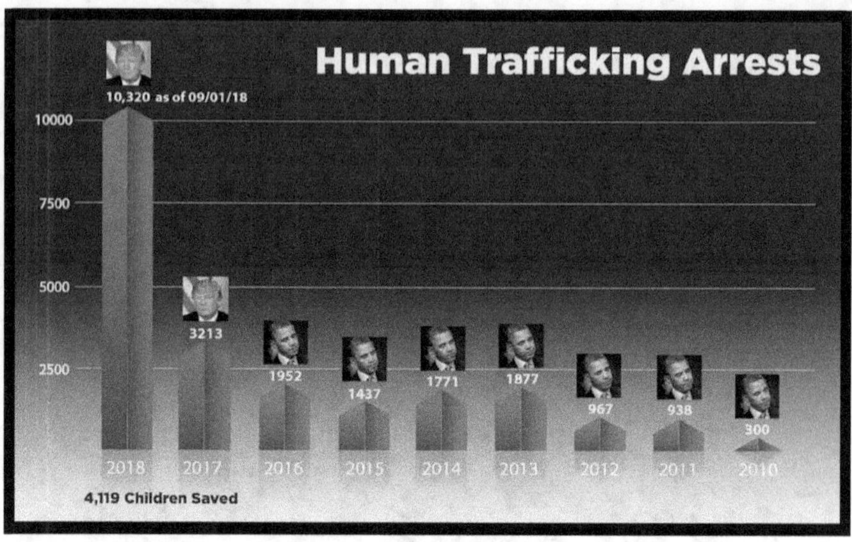

They have been manipulating the banks of the world and not to mention involved in worldwide smuggling of all kinds, particularly humans, for generations causing suffering and widespread death as they have progressively been accumulating personal power with their intention to completely enslave and dominate the entire world... Until President Trump:

(The headline for this article is misleading)

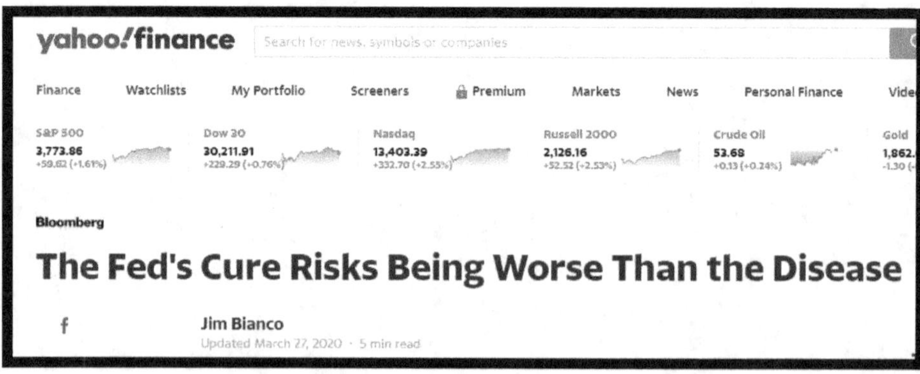

"In other words, the federal government is nationalizing large swaths of the financial markets. The Fed is providing the money to do it. BlackRock will be doing the trades.

"This scheme essentially merges the Fed and Treasury into one organization. So, meet your new Fed chairman, Donald J. Trump."

Notice the timing? March 27, 2020 – Around the same time that the "Queen" had been locked out of the castle – The City of London being the financial hub of the world – The corrupt financial hub of the world – Defeated by President Trump and the United States Military – And most of us do not even know about it - Perhaps you know about the role of The Vatican in all of this - Somehow, like the former "Queen," "The Pope" did not seem to be very happy about the visit, but President Trump appears quite pleased:

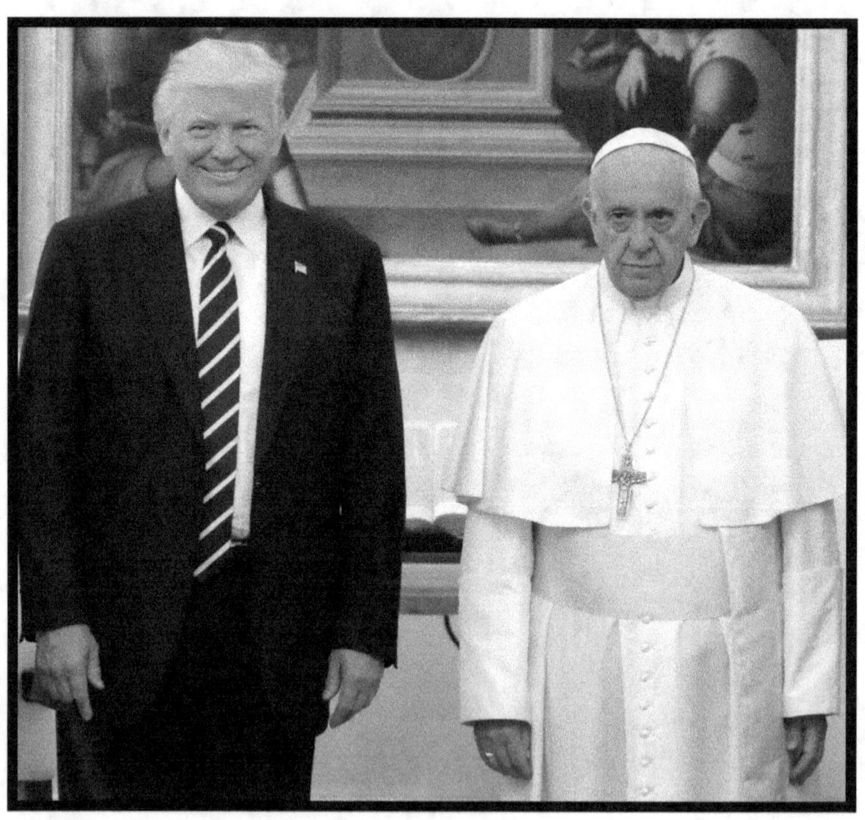

Therefore, the previously foreign-owned "Federal Reserve Bank" is now under the control of the US Government and the Department of the Treasury – See why the "Rothschilds" are so afraid?

There is much, much more to add to this story, and this is all going to break into the public soon, but will happen as "drops" so that the entire public does not get traumatized by realizing that everything that they had believed their entire lives has been a lie, and particularly the Democrat party, but really all US politics has been totally corrupted.

So as the good property developer that he is, President Trump is tearing down the old structure that cannot be rehabilitated and with the US Military beginning a new government of the original constitutional United States of America.

Of course, everybody can have "two sides to every story" – Isn't that true of everyone arrested for a DUI?

There are two sides to this story – The truth, and lies – We have been cowed into submission by the abusive browbeating and incessant push for dominance over our lives that we just surrender that there are "both sides" to everything and all serious debate about anything stops while they continue shamelessly dominating us to death.

Many of them have been infiltrated by the Chinese Communist Party (CCP), that has been working with globalists to become the supreme communist government for the world – But... we will soon learn that is not to be.

However, during their death throes, they are throwing everything and the kitchen sink, and this "COVID" hoax is a desperate attempt to demoralize, bankrupt and cause us to kill ourselves to make their final domination easier – You better believe that they want to confiscate the guns, and the 2nd Amendment is the only reason we are not already ruled by the Chinese.

The CCP infiltration is insidious and has infected US local government to the levels of School Board and County Commissioners – Just look at what they are teaching children in school, about "transgenderism" and the destruction of the traditional family – This is all the same tactics the Nazis used to indoctrinate children – Children are being taught in school to feel guilty for being "white"

our latest
most popular
contributors
subscribe

the
FEDERALIST
A DIVISION OF FDRLST MEDIA

Search ...

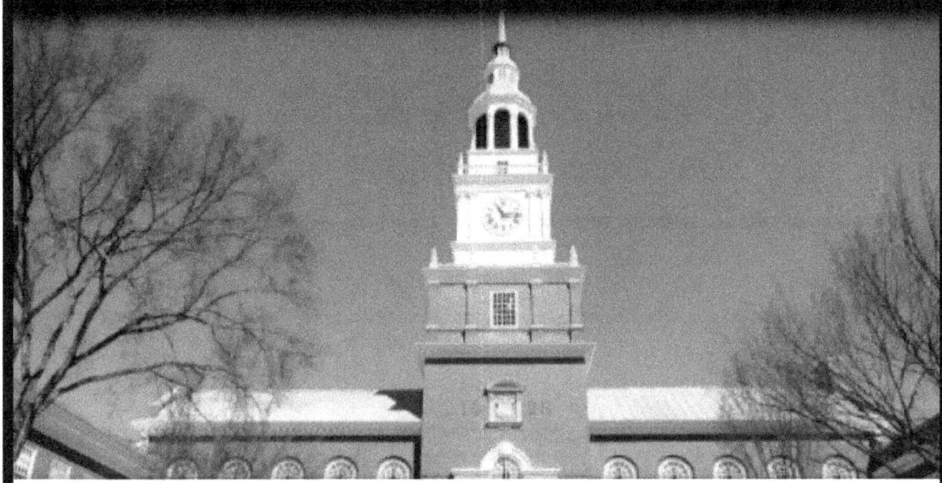

HIGHER EDUCATION

Why Are U.S. Universities Hiding Communist China's Infiltration Of Their Campuses?

Now is the time to demand accountability in America's higher education institutions. Our national security depends on it.

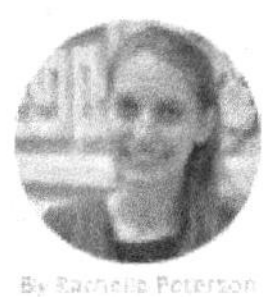

By Rachelle Peterson

FEBRUARY 1, 2021

As President Biden takes office, America faces a new chapter in the China challenge, a major part of which involves protecting American higher education.

China's Thousand Talents Plan has ensnared thousands of American scholars and researchers, including former Harvard University professor and Chemistry Chair Charles Lieber, indicted in June by the Justice Department for lying about China's $50,000 monthly payments to him in exchange for research expertise.

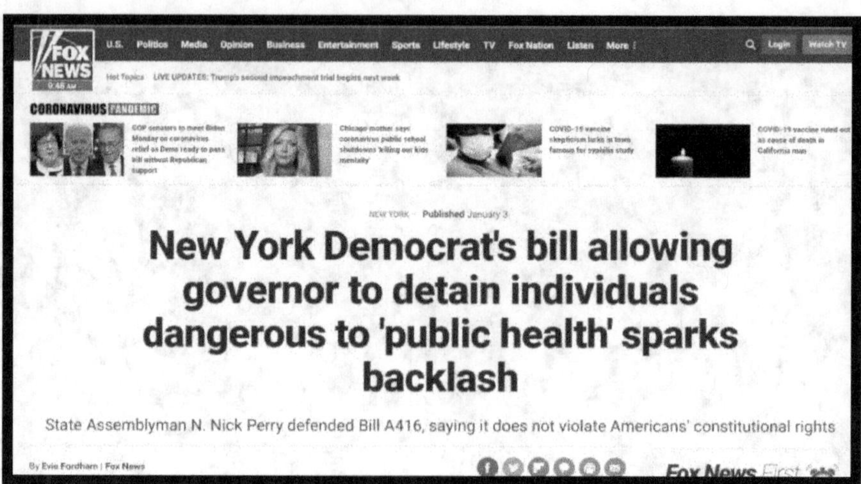

New York Democrat's bill allowing governor to detain individuals dangerous to 'public health' sparks backlash

State Assemblyman N. Nick Perry defended Bill A416, saying it does not violate Americans' constitutional rights

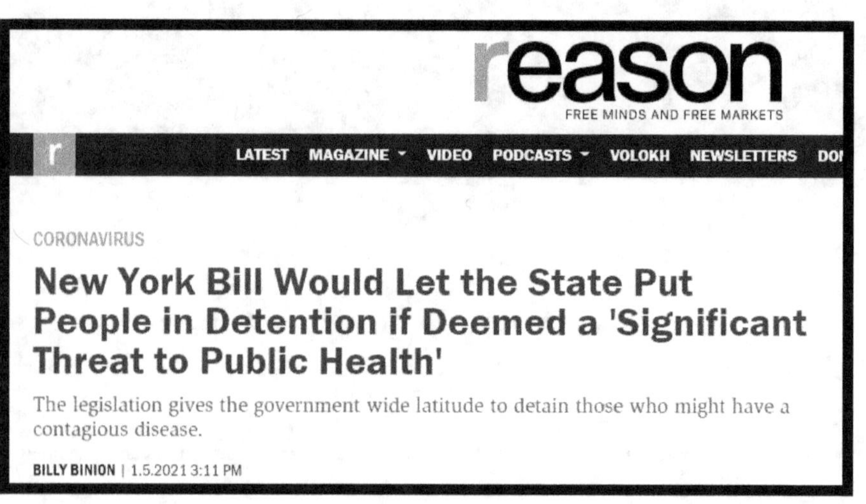

New York Bill Would Let the State Put People in Detention if Deemed a 'Significant Threat to Public Health'

The legislation gives the government wide latitude to detain those who might have a contagious disease.

January 24, 2021:

"CDC" reports <u>*416,010*</u> supposed deaths from "COVID"

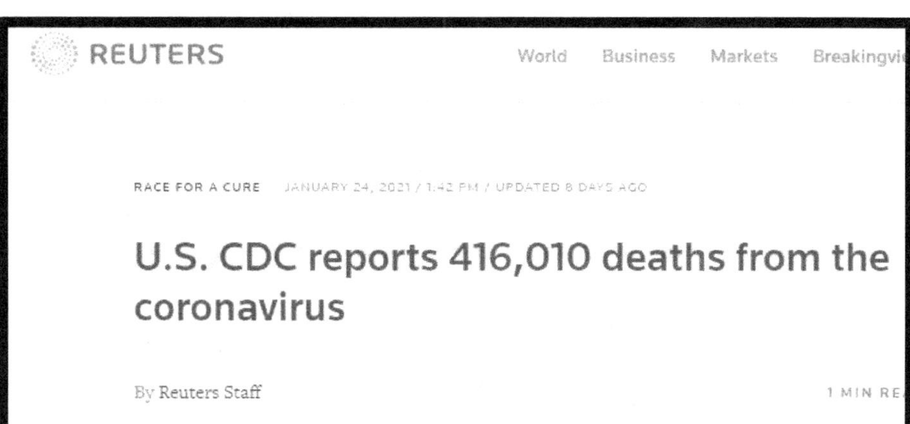

HOW MANY DEATHS HAVE BEEN FALSELY ATTRIBUTED?

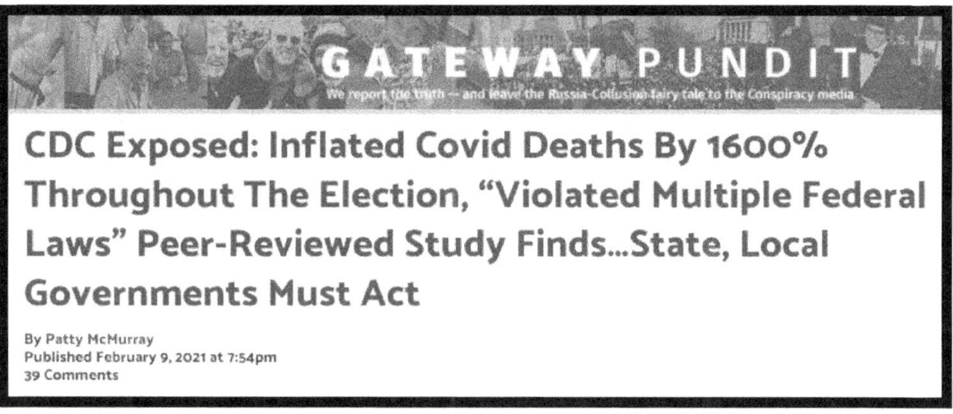

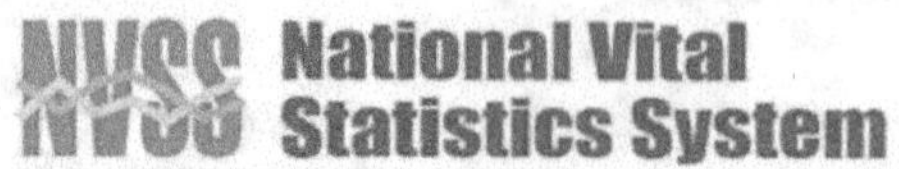 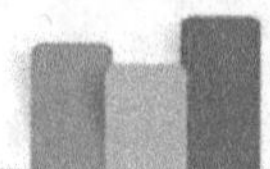

COVID-19 Alert No. 2
March 24, 2020

New ICD code introduced for COVID-19 deaths
This email is to alert you that a newly-introduced ICD code has been implemented to accurately capture mortality data for Coronavirus Disease 2019 (COVID-19) on death certificates.

Please read carefully and forward this email to the state statistical staff in your office who are involved in the preparation of mortality data, as well as others who may receive questions when the data are released.

Should "COVID-19" be reported on the death certificate only with a confirmed test?
COVID-19 should be reported on the death certificate for all decedents where the disease caused **or is assumed to have caused or contributed to death**. Certifiers should include as much detail as possible based on their knowledge of the case, medical records, laboratory testing, etc. If the decedent had other chronic conditions such as COPD or asthma that may have also contributed, these conditions can be reported in Part II. (See attached Guidance for Certifying COVID-19 Deaths)

Steven Schwartz, PhD
Director – Division of Vital Statistics
National Center for Health Statistics
3311 Toledo Rd | Hyattsville, MD 20782

https://www.cdc.gov/nchs/data/nvss/coronavirus/Alert-2-New-ICD-code-introduced-for-COVID-19-deaths.pdf

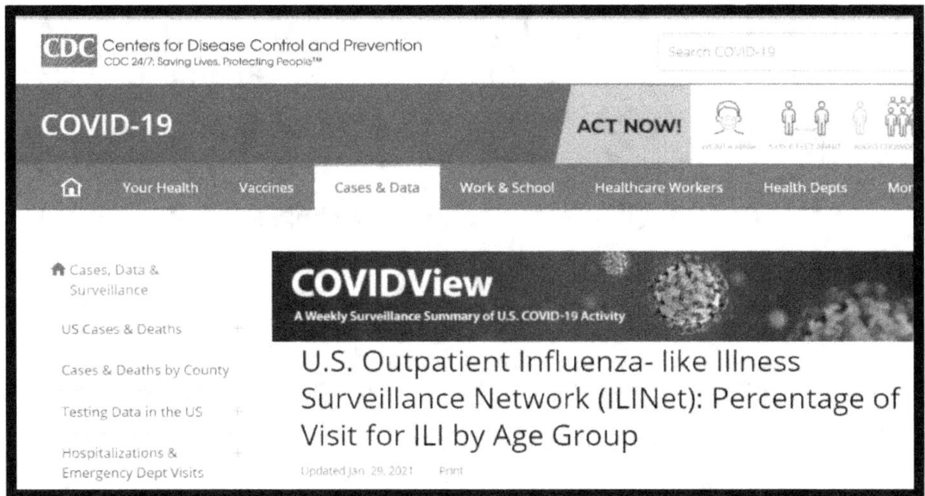

"Percentage of Visits for Influenza-Like Illness (ILI)"

September 29, 2019 – January 23, 2021

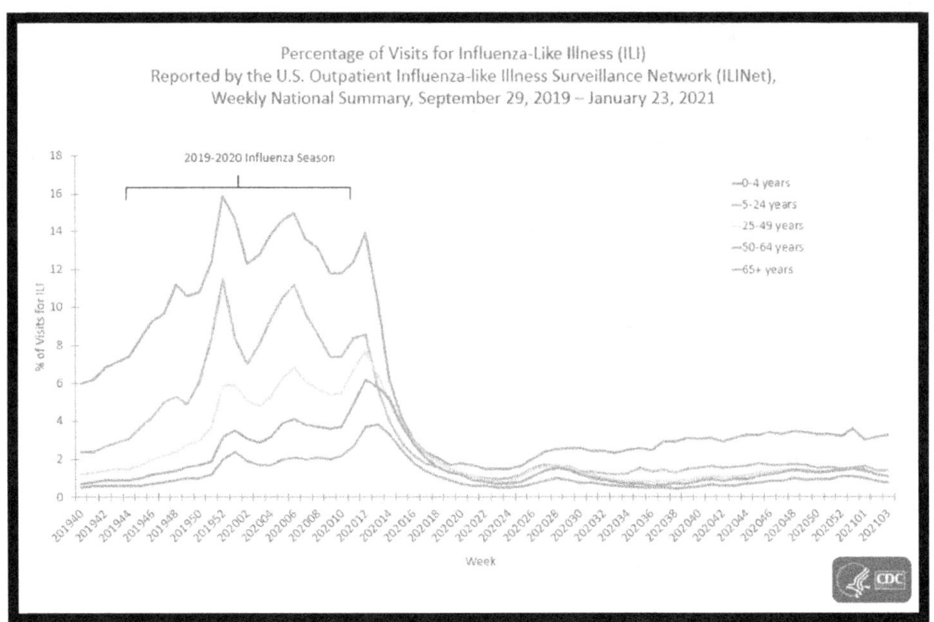

AS YOU CAN PLAINLY SEE, FROM THE OFFICIAL "CDC" DATA ITSELF, THAT AVERAGE YEARLY FLU RATES ARE BEING FRAUDULENTLY REPORTED AS "COVID" FOR POLITICAL REASONS, AND PARTICULARLY TO ADVANCE CONTROL OVER THE AMERICAN PEOPLE BY THE COMMUNIST CHINESE PARTY (CCP)

"COVID DEATHS" ARE ACTUALLY THE AVERAGE NUMBER OF PEOPLE THAT DIE ANNUALLY FROM "THE FLU" IN ADDITION TO THOSE FALSELY-ATTRIBUTED AS "COVID" DEATHS, AND WE HAVE NEVER SURRENDERED OUR PERSONAL FREEDOM FOR THE FLU BEFORE — WHY NOW?

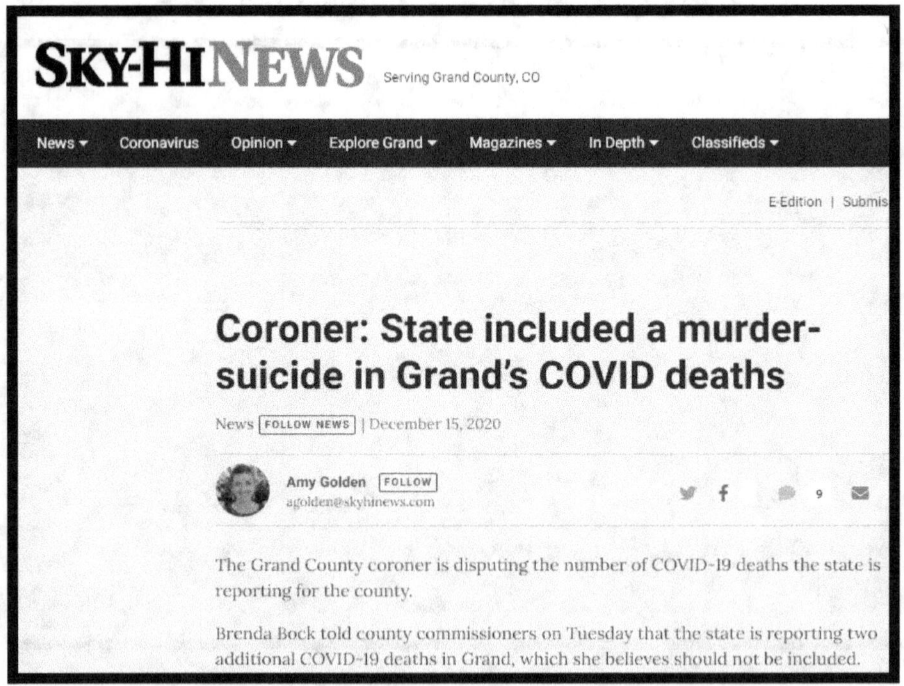

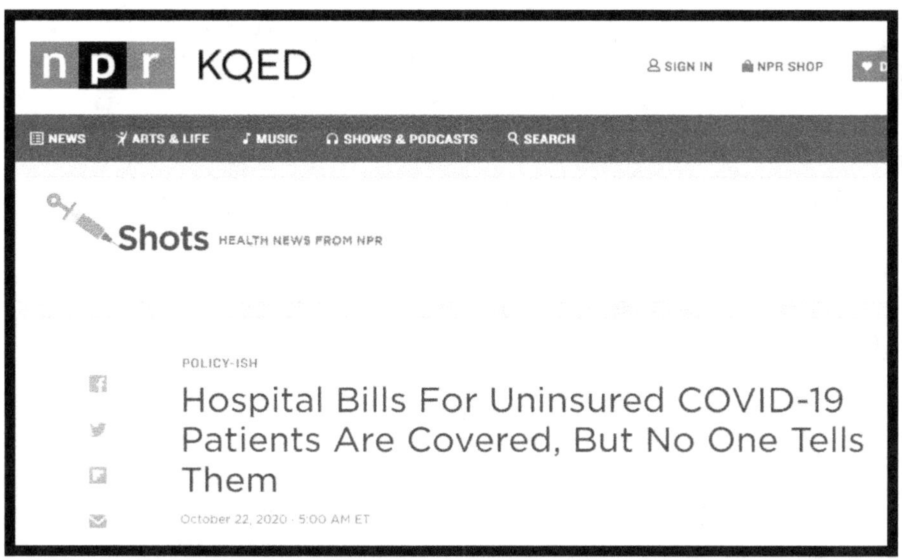

NPR KQED
SIGN IN
NPR SHOP
NEWS
ARTS & LIFE
MUSIC
SHOWS & PODCASTS
SEARCH
Shots HEALTH NEWS FROM NPR
POLICY-ISH
Hospital Bills For Uninsured COVID-19 Patients Are Covered, But No One Tells Them
October 22, 2020 · 5:00 AM ET

Washington Examiner

Politics ▾ Policy ▾ News Opinion ▾ Business MAGAZINE ▾ Multimedia ▾ Beltway C

CDC director acknowledges hospitals have a monetary incentive to overcount coronavirus deaths

by Andrew Mark Miller, Social Media Producer | | August 01, 2020 10:13 AM

U.S. Centers for Disease Control and Prevention Director Robert Redfield agreed that some hospitals have a monetary incentive to overcount coronavirus deaths as they do deaths for other diseases.

"I think you're correct in that we've seen this in other disease processes, too. Really, in the HIV epidemic, somebody may have a heart attack but also have HIV — the hospital would prefer the [classification] for HIV because there's greater reimbursement," Redfield said during a House panel hearing Friday when asked by Rep. Blaine Luetkemeyer about potential "perverse incentives."

Redfield continued: "So, I do think there's some reality to that. When it comes to death reporting, though, ultimately, it's how the physician defines it in the death certificate, and ... we review all of those death certificates. So I think, probably it is less operable in the cause of death, although I won't say there are not some cases. I do think though [that]

THE *"COMMITMENTS TO CONTAINMENT"* HAVE OBVIOUSLY NOT RESULTED IN ANY POSITIVE OUTCOME, AND CERTAINLY NOT REDUCING *"THE NUMBERS"*

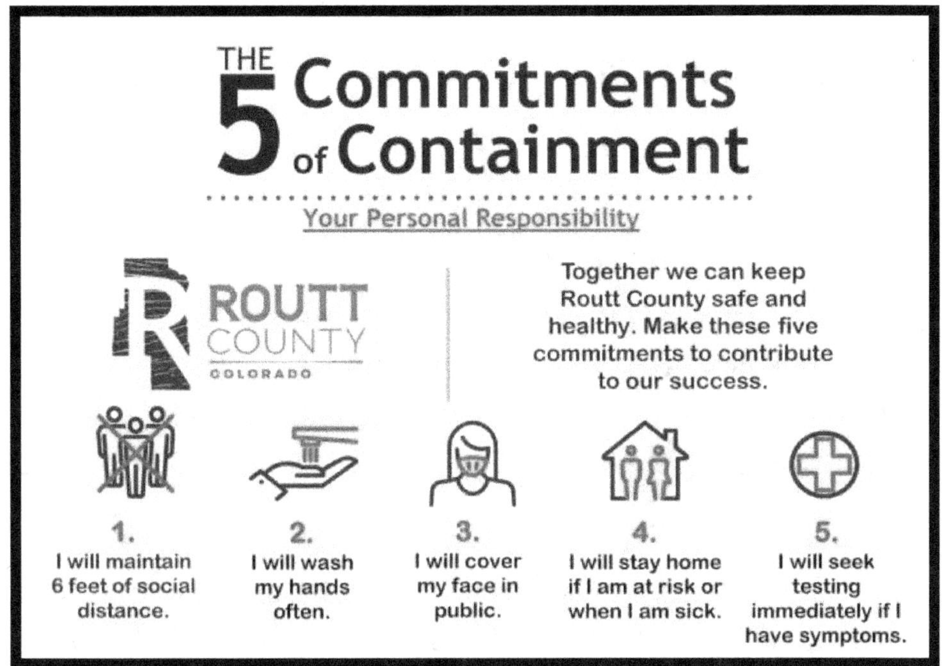

THESE APPEAR TO ME AS COMMITMENTS TO TYRANNY AND SURRENDER OF GOD-GIVEN CONSTITUTIONALLY-PROTECTED PERSONAL LIBERTIES

THE "NUMBERS" WILL NEVER BE REDUCED UNTIL ALL OF THE FRAUDULENT "PCR TESTING" CEASES COMPLETELY

WE ARE SUFFERING THROUGH THIS TYRANNY BY LOCAL GOVERNMENT FOR A "VIRUS" THAT HAS A DEATH RATE LESS THAN ONE-HALF OF ONE PERCENT, AND A "TEST" IS REQUIRED TO LET PEOPLE KNOW THEY EVEN HAVE IT

AND THE AVERAGE AGE OF "COVID" DEATH IS 75 YEARS OLD

 AND THE AVERAGE AGE OF DEATH OVERALL FOR US CITIZENS IS 78 YEARS OLD

ALL OF THIS INFORMATION PORTRAYS THE TRUTH, AND THAT IS WHY THE INFORMATION AS WELL AS THE REST OF THE TRUTH IS CONCEALED FROM THE PUBLIC, BECAUSE PEOPLE WHO ARE FEARFUL AND IGNORANT ARE EASIER TO CONTROL

WHEN DO WE FOLLOW GERMANY, NEW ZEALAND AND CHINA AND BEGIN IMPRISONING FALSELY-DIAGNOSED "COVID-POSITIVE" AMERICANS INTO "QUARANTINE CAMPS?"

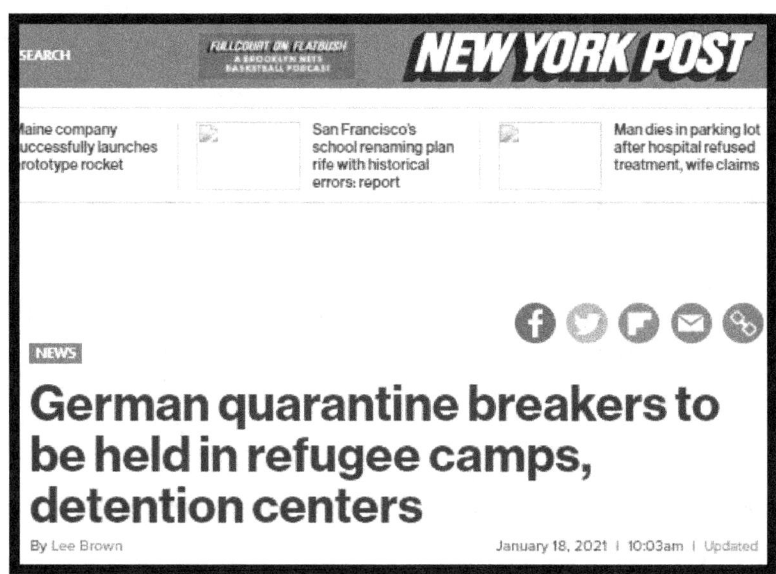

SEARCH
FULLCOURT ON FLATBUSH
A BROOKLYN NETS
BASKETBALL PODCAST
NEW YORK POST
Maine company successfully launches prototype rocket
San Francisco's school renaming plan rife with historical errors: report
Man dies in parking lot after hospital refused treatment, wife claims
NEWS
German quarantine breakers to be held in refugee camps, detention centers
By Lee Brown
January 18, 2021 | 10:03am | Updated

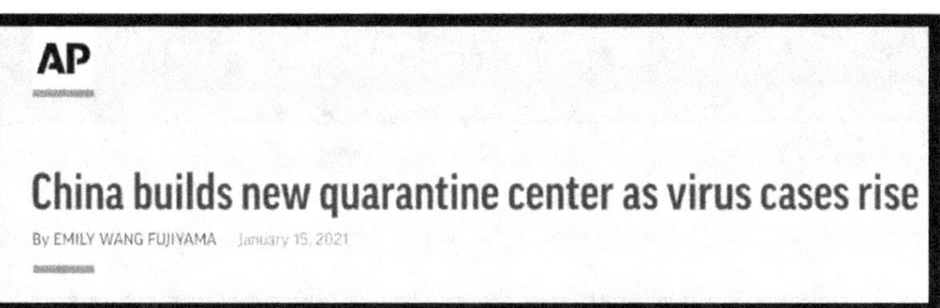

AP
China builds new quarantine center as virus cases rise
By EMILY WANG FUJIYAMA   January 15, 2021

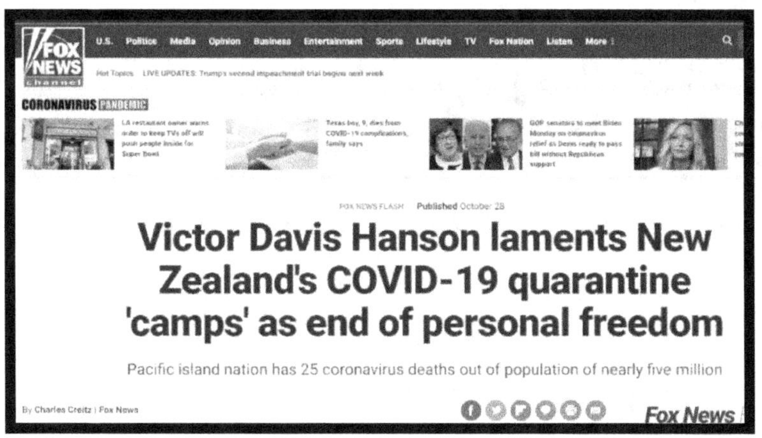

FOX NEWS channel
U.S. Politics Media Opinion Business Entertainment Sports Lifestyle TV Fox Nation Listen More
Hot Topics   LIVE UPDATES: Trump's second impeachment trial begins next week
CORONAVIRUS PANDEMIC
LA restaurant owner warns order to keep TVs off will push people inside for Super Bowl
Texas boy, 9, dies from COVID-19 complications, family says
GOP senators to meet Biden Monday on coronavirus relief as Dems ready to pass bill without Republican support
FOX NEWS FLASH   Published October 28
Victor Davis Hanson laments New Zealand's COVID-19 quarantine 'camps' as end of personal freedom
Pacific island nation has 25 coronavirus deaths out of population of nearly five million
By Charles Creitz | Fox News
Fox News

A GLASS OF COLA, A GOAT, AND AN AFRICAN FRUIT ALL TESTED POSITIVE FOR "COVID"

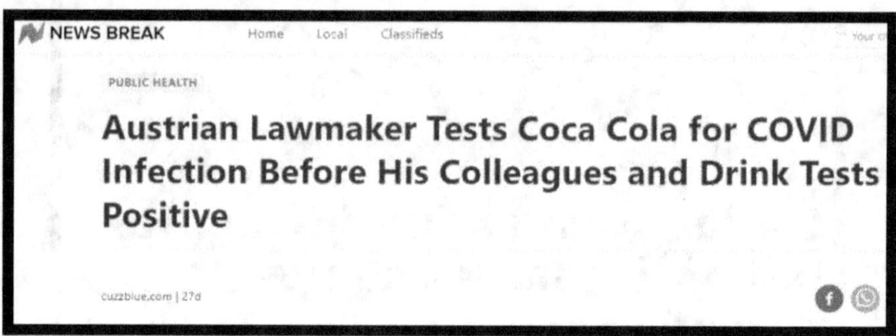

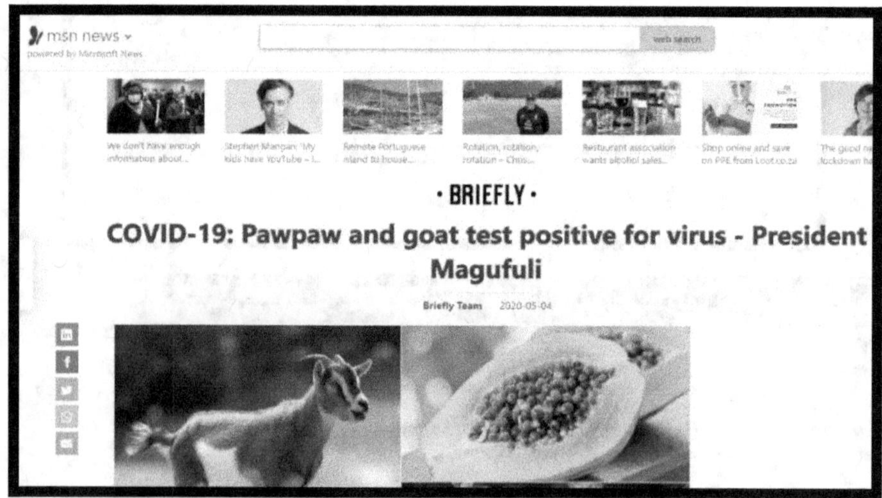

THE "FDA" ITSELF WARNED ABOUT FALSE-POSITIVE "COVID" TESTING

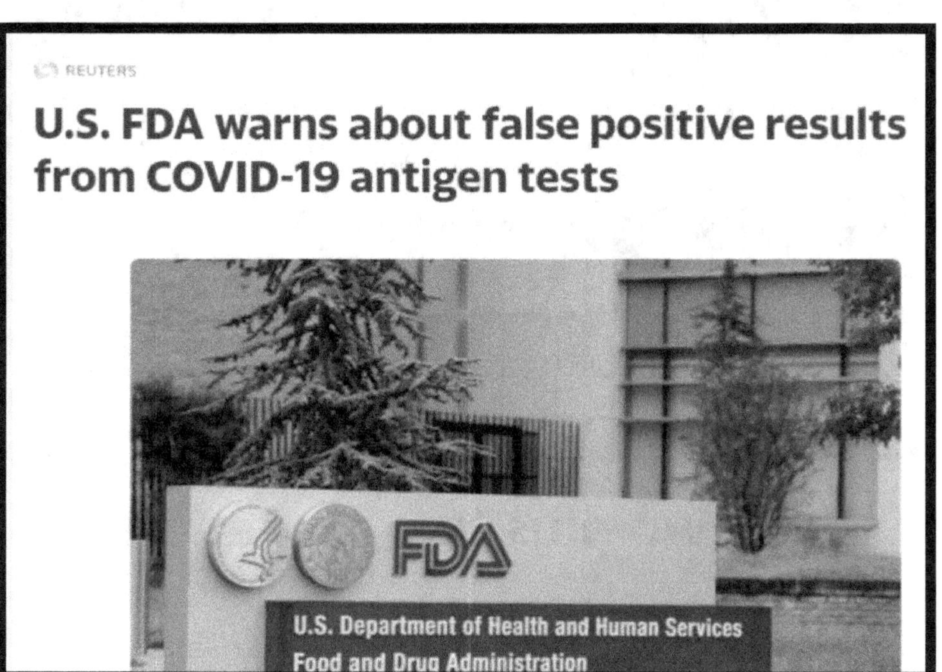

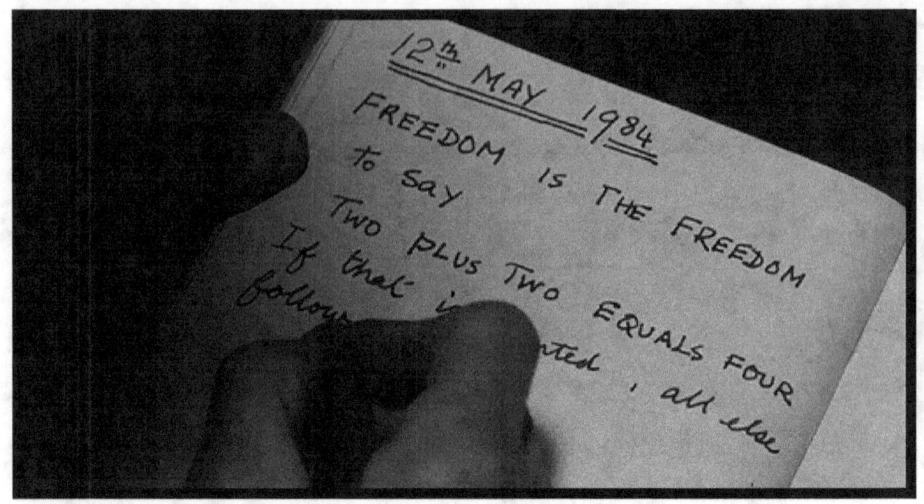

"Freedom is the freedom to say that two plus two make four."

– "1984," George Orwell

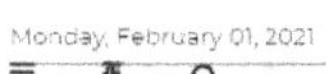

GATEWAY PUNDIT

We report the truth — and leave the Russia-Collusion fairy tale to the Conspiracy media

BREAKING: Evidence of Biden Payments from China Support Tony Bobulinski and Show the Bidens Made Millions Swindling America

By Joe Hoft
Published November 2, 2020 at 12:00pm
504 Comments

Monday, February 01, 2021

Washington Examiner

Politics ▾   Policy ▾   News   Opinion ▾   Business   MAGAZINE ▾   Multimedia ▾   Beltway Confid

Senate investigators: New records 'confirm' troubling Biden family links to China and Russia

by | November 18, 2020 06:31 PM

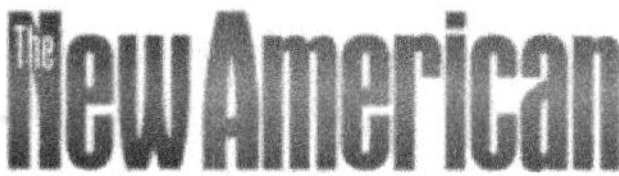

📧 Get E-Mail Updates

HOME   SECTIONS ⌄   MAGAZINE ⌄   FREEDOM INDEX

The New American » Science & Technology » Biden Terminates Trump Order that Kept China Out of America's Po

Biden Terminates Trump Order that Kept China Out of America's Power Grid

👤 by Luis Miguel   ✏ January 25, 2021

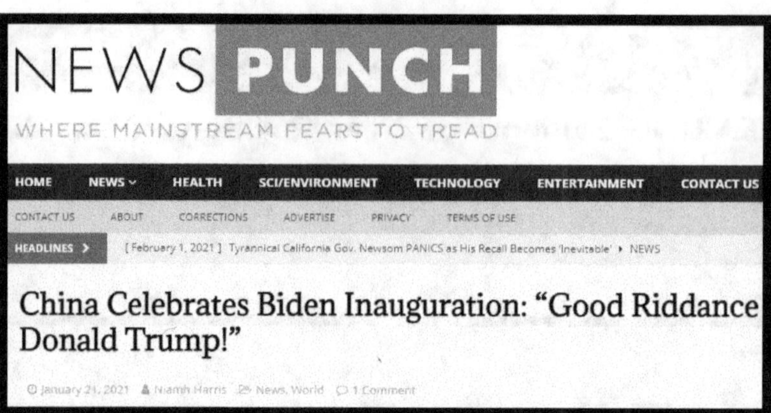

NEWS PUNCH

WHERE MAINSTREAM FEARS TO TREAD

HOME   NEWS ⌄   HEALTH   SCI/ENVIRONMENT   TECHNOLOGY   ENTERTAINMENT   CONTACT US

CONTACT US   ABOUT   CORRECTIONS   ADVERTISE   PRIVACY   TERMS OF USE

HEADLINES ❯   [February 1, 2021] Tyrannical California Gov. Newsom PANICS as His Recall Becomes 'Inevitable' ▸ NEWS

China Celebrates Biden Inauguration: "Good Riddance Donald Trump!"

January 21, 2021   Niamh Harris   News, World   1 Comment

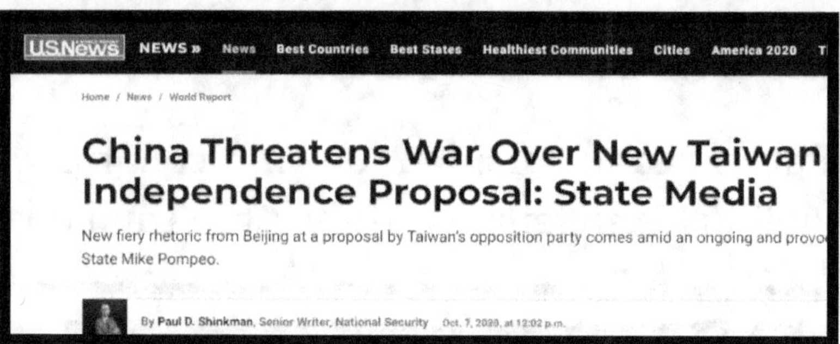

U.S.News   NEWS »   News   Best Countries   Best States   Healthiest Communities   Cities   America 2020   T

Home / News / World Report

China Threatens War Over New Taiwan Independence Proposal: State Media

New fiery rhetoric from Beijing at a proposal by Taiwan's opposition party comes amid an ongoing and provoc State Mike Pompeo.

By **Paul D. Shinkman**, Senior Writer, National Security   Oct. 7, 2020, at 12:02 p.m.

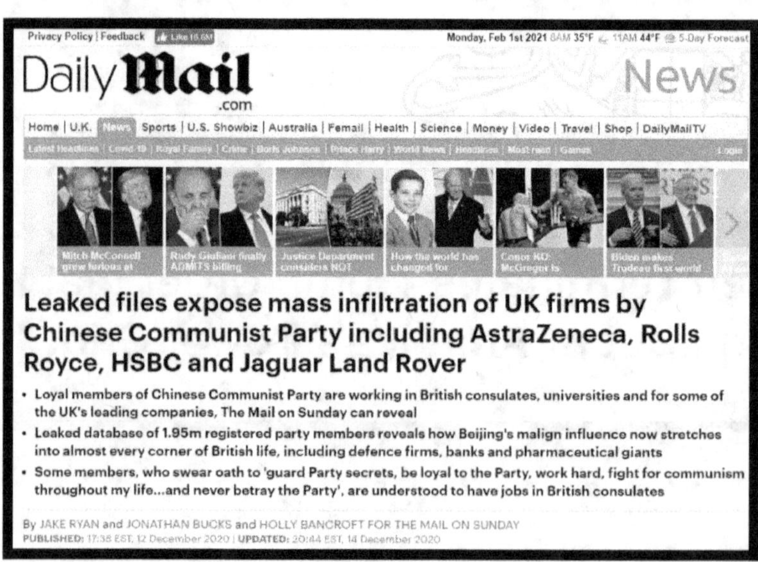

Privacy Policy | Feedback   Like 16.6M   Monday, Feb 1st 2021 8AM 35°F   11AM 44°F   5-Day Forecast

Daily Mail .com

News

Home | U.K. | News | Sports | U.S. Showbiz | Australia | Femail | Health | Science | Money | Video | Travel | Shop | DailyMailTV

Latest Headlines | Covid-19 | Royal Family | Crime | Boris Johnson | Prince Harry | World News | Headlines | Most read | Games | Login

Leaked files expose mass infiltration of UK firms by Chinese Communist Party including AstraZeneca, Rolls Royce, HSBC and Jaguar Land Rover

- Loyal members of Chinese Communist Party are working in British consulates, universities and for some of the UK's leading companies, The Mail on Sunday can reveal
- Leaked database of 1.95m registered party members reveals how Beijing's malign influence now stretches into almost every corner of British life, including defence firms, banks and pharmaceutical giants
- Some members, who swear oath to 'guard Party secrets, be loyal to the Party, work hard, fight for communism throughout my life...and never betray the Party', are understood to have jobs in British consulates

By JAKE RYAN and JONATHAN BUCKS and HOLLY BANCROFT FOR THE MAIL ON SUNDAY
PUBLISHED: 17:38 EST, 12 December 2020 | UPDATED: 20:44 EST, 14 December 2020

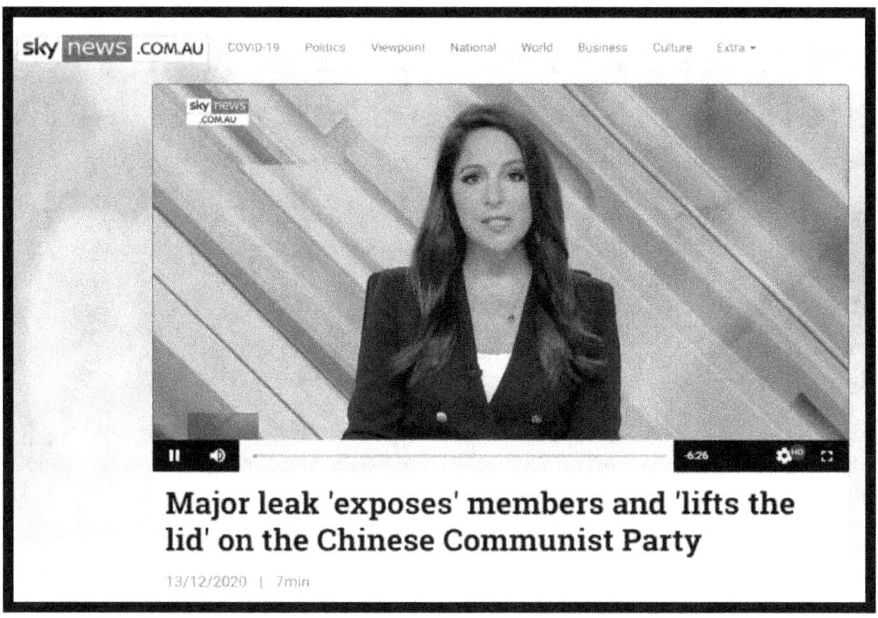

Major leak 'exposes' members and 'lifts the lid' on the Chinese Communist Party

13/12/2020 | 7min

Major leak 'exposes' members and 'lifts the lid' on the Chinese Communist Party

13/12/2020 | 7min

A major leak containing a register with the details of nearly two million CCP members has occurred – exposing members who are now working all over the world, while also lifting the lid on how the party operates under Xi Jinping, says Sharri Markson.

Ms Markson said the leak is a register with the details of Communist Party members, including their names, party position, birthday, national ID number and ethnicity.

"It is believed to be the first leak of its kind in the world," the Sky News host said.

"What's amazing about this database is not just that it exposes people who are members of the communist party, and who are now living and working all over the world, from Australia to the US to the UK," Ms Markson said.

"But it's amazing because it lifts the lid on how the party operates under President and Chairman Xi Jinping".

Ms Markson said the leak demonstrates party branches are embedded in some of the world's biggest companies and even inside government agencies.

"Communist party branches have been set up inside western companies, allowing the infiltration of those companies by CCP members - who, if called on, are answerable directly to the communist party, to the Chairman, the president himself," she said.

"Along with the personal identifying details of 1.95 million communist party members, mostly from Shanghai, there are also the details of 79,000 communist party branches, many of them inside companies".

Ms Markson said the leak is a significant security breach likely to embarrass Xi Jinping.

"It is also going to embarrass some global companies who appear to have no plan in place to protect their intellectual property from theft. From economic espionage," she said.

Ms Markson said the data was extracted from a Shanghai server by Chinese dissidents, whistleblowers, in April 2016, who have been using it for counter-intelligence purposes.

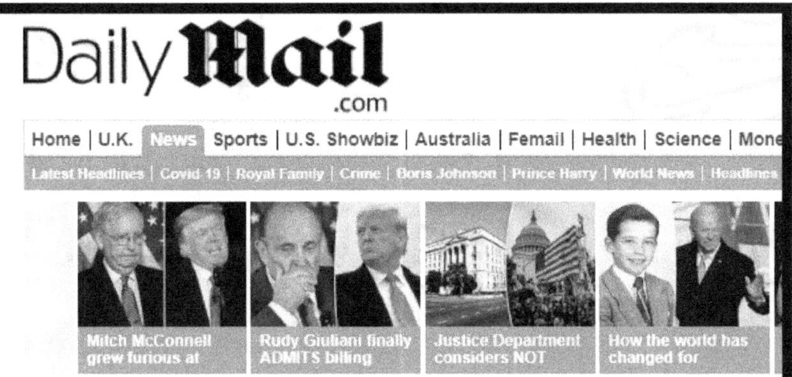

Mike Pompeo reveals intelligence that researchers at Wuhan Institute of Virology fell ill in late 2019 and demands WHO investigate the lab as possible origin point of COVID-19

- Pompeo issued a public call to investigate the notorious Wuhan lab on Friday
- WHO team of international COVID researchers arrived in Wuhan on Thursday
- The visit is shrouded in secrecy but there are no plans to investigate the lab
- Pompeo said new evidence suggests virus accidentally escaped from lab
- Intelligence indicates several workers there fell ill in the fall of 2019
- US says researchers there studied a bat coronavirus that's 96% similar to COVID
- They were also conducting 'gain of function' research to modify viruses
- Pompeo demands a full investigation of whether COVID escaped from lab
- Accuses Beijing of withholding vital information about the pandemic

By KEITH GRIFFITH FOR DAILYMAIL.COM
PUBLISHED: 23:56 EST, 15 January 2021 | UPDATED: 03:04 EST, 16 January 2021

CAN YOU SEE WHAT IS HAPPENING?

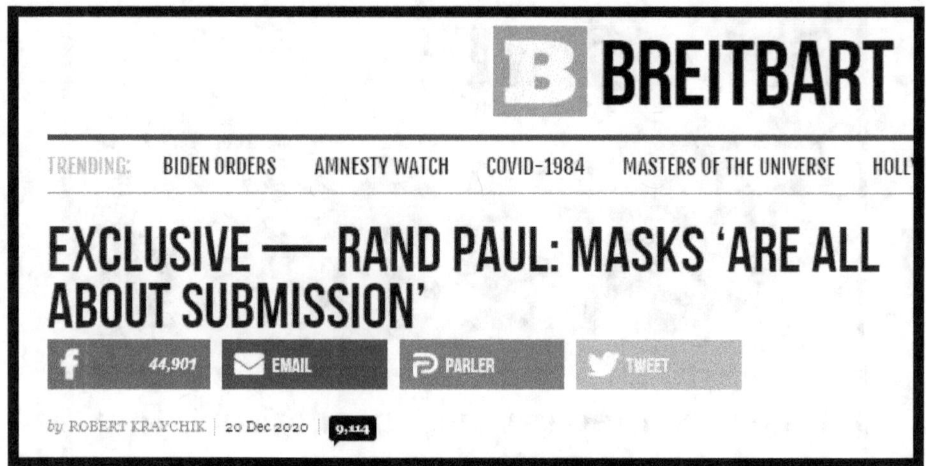

"PAUL: It'd be one thing if we were told you have to give up your liberty, you have to give up your freedom, we're going to save your life. But what if you have to give up all your freedoms and they're wrong on the science? "

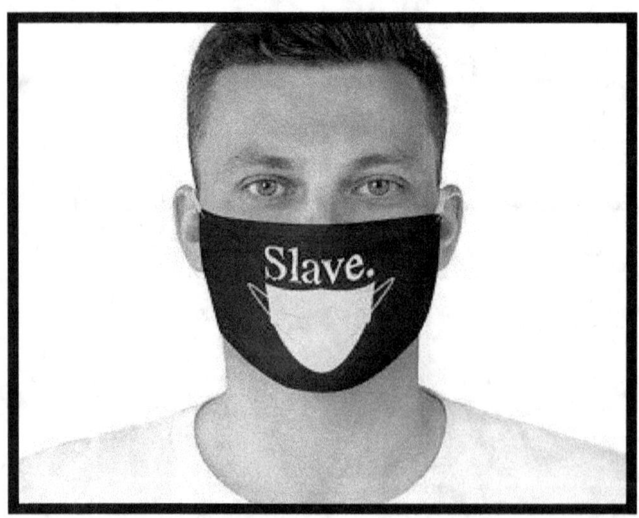

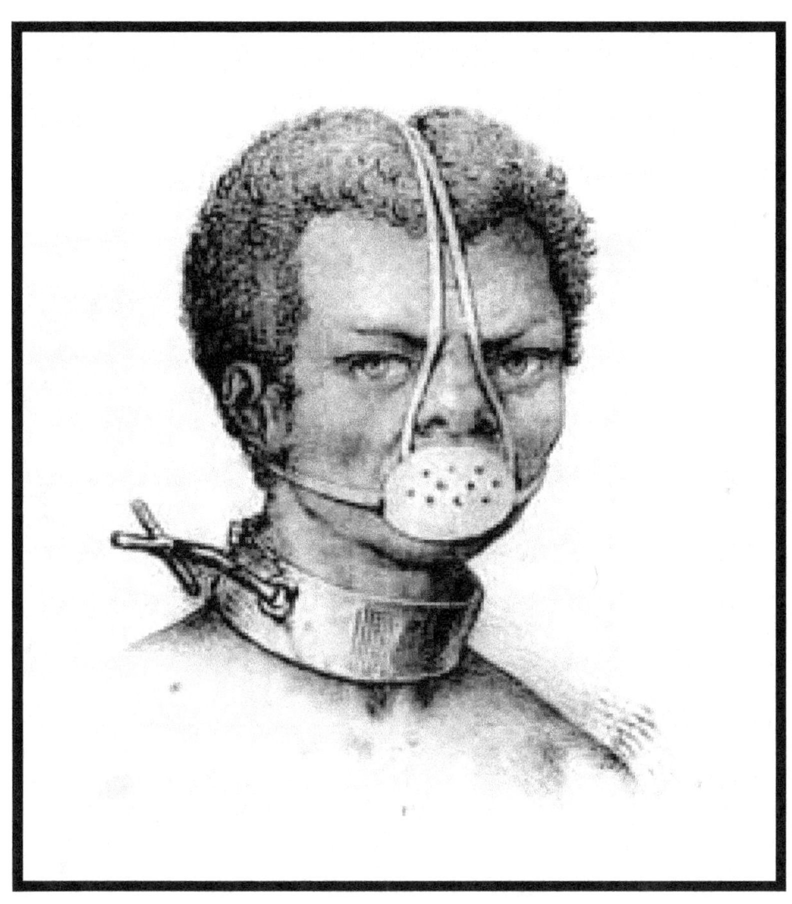

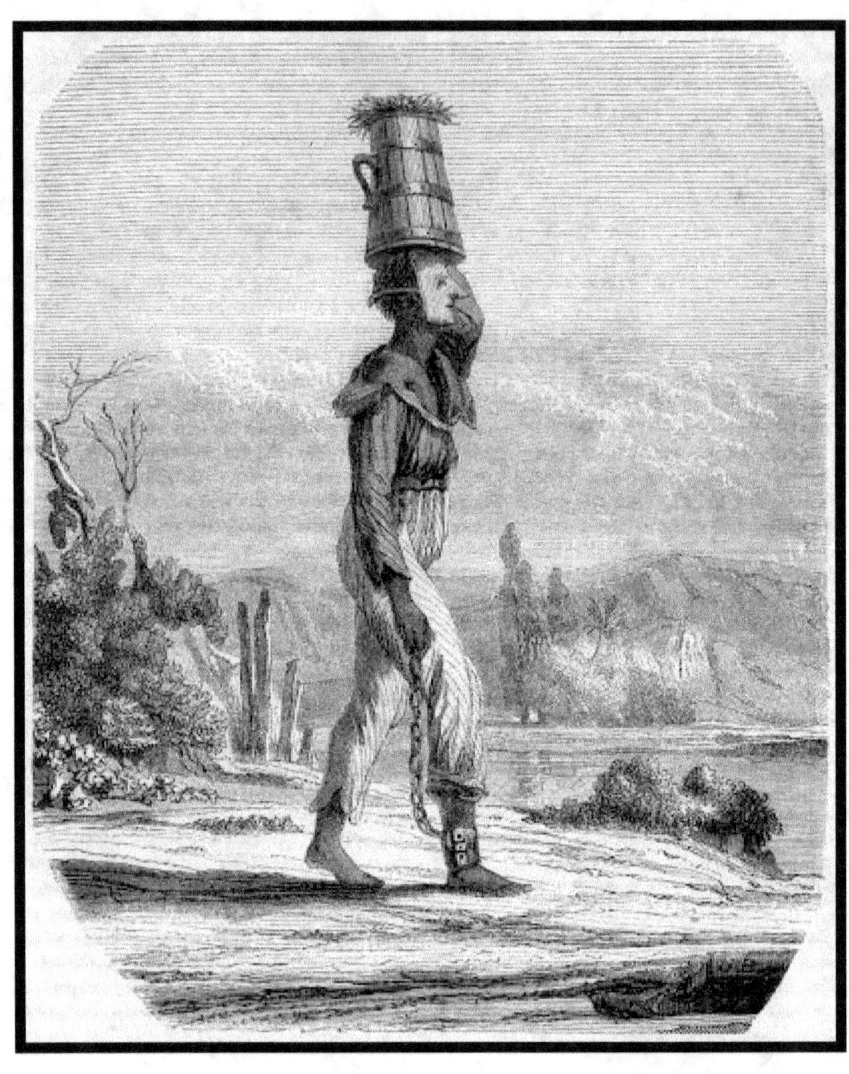

Is it time to say no to masks?

January 6, 2021

To the editor:

Is it time to say no to masks, Indiana?

Mandatory masking isn't slowing Covid in Indiana. Since Governor Holcomb instituted the mandate in July, Covid cases and Covid deaths have not decreased. This was true even two to four weeks after the institution of the mandate, when universal masking should have caused a drop in new Covid cases, but didn't. What we did see was two months of no change, followed by an increase in caseload starting in late September. Today, rates of Covid appear to be at their highest ever — despite widespread masking. Why?

I think, because masks don't work.

This is not an anti-science position. Science supports it. In 2015, a study in the British Medical Journal showed that cloth masks were basically useless, penetrated by nearly 97% of particles; the authors added the "caution" that cloth masks may be more harmful than no masks at all. In 2019, the NIH published a study concluding that cloth masks are "not recommended" because of the high "bioburden" of germs they carry. In 2020 the CDC reviewed evidence from 14 randomized controlled trials and concluded that masking the public was basically useless at slowing the spread of the flu: "Our systematic review found no significant effect of face masks on transmission."

Studies from this year confirm this. In September 2020, the NIH published a review of 15 studies involving nearly 24,000 people showing that "Surgical mask wearing among individuals in non-healthcare settings is not significantly associated with reduction in [respiratory infections]." In June 2020, the WHO said, "There is no direct evidence ... on the effectiveness of universal masking of healthy people in the community to prevent infection with ... COVID-19." A May 2020 study in the New England Journal of Medicine states flatly, "We know that wearing a mask outside health care facilities offers little, if any, protection from infection ... In many cases, the desire for widespread masking is a reflexive reaction to anxiety over the pandemic."

Why was this evidence not considered in forming Indiana's mask policy? It's all publicly available. Decide for yourselves.

—Jessica Warden
Dale

A representation of a slave at work cruelly accoutred, with a Head-frame and Mouth-piece to prevent his eating—with Boots and Spurs round his legs, and half a hundred weight chained to his body to prevent his absconding.

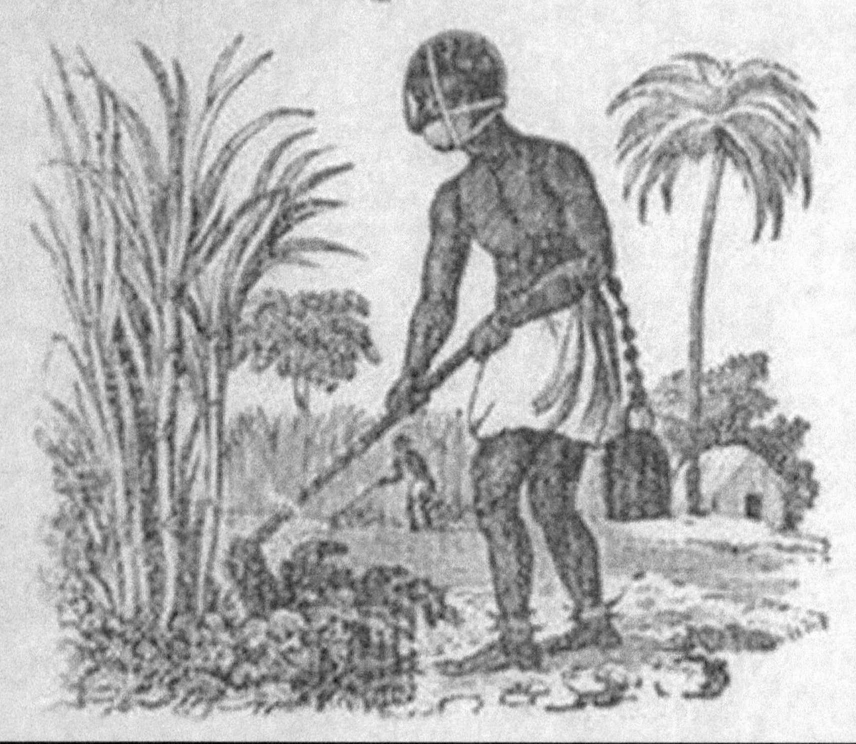

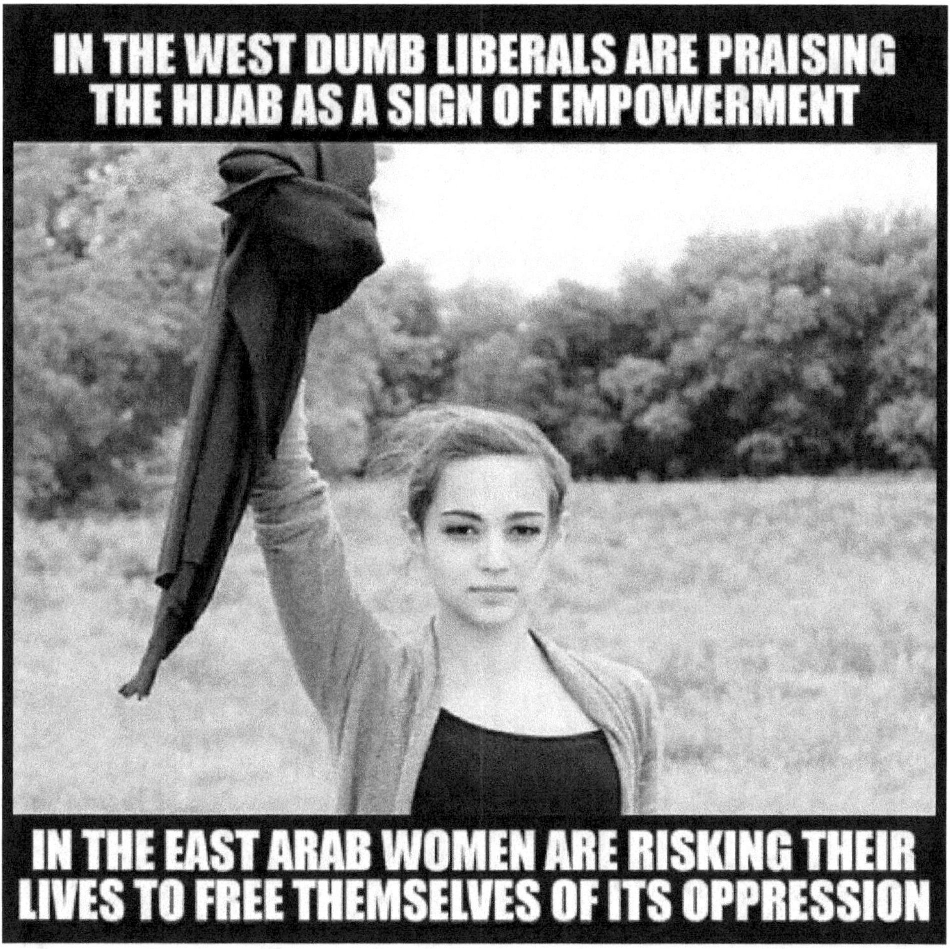

IN THE WEST DUMB LIBERALS ARE PRAISING THE HIJAB AS A SIGN OF EMPOWERMENT
IN THE EAST ARAB WOMEN ARE RISKING THEIR LIVES TO FREE THEMSELVES OF ITS OPPRESSION

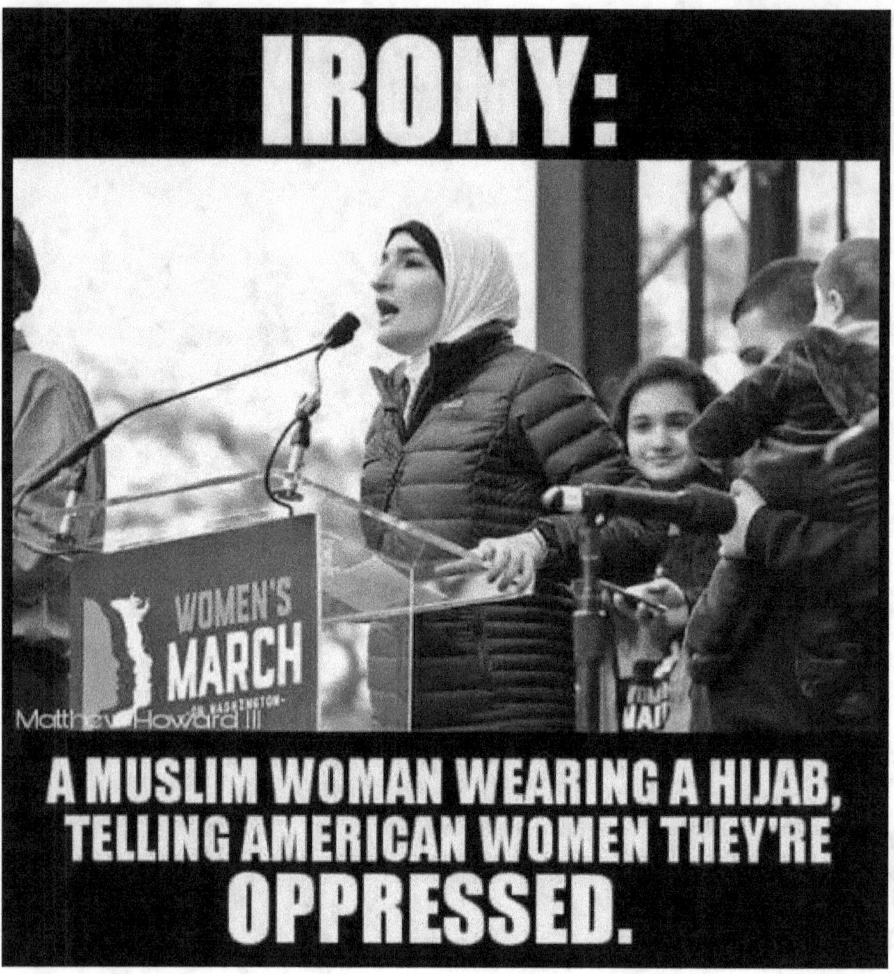

IRONY:
WOMEN'S MARCH
ON WASHINGTON
Matthew Howard III
A MUSLIM WOMAN WEARING A HIJAB,
TELLING AMERICAN WOMEN THEY'RE
OPPRESSED.

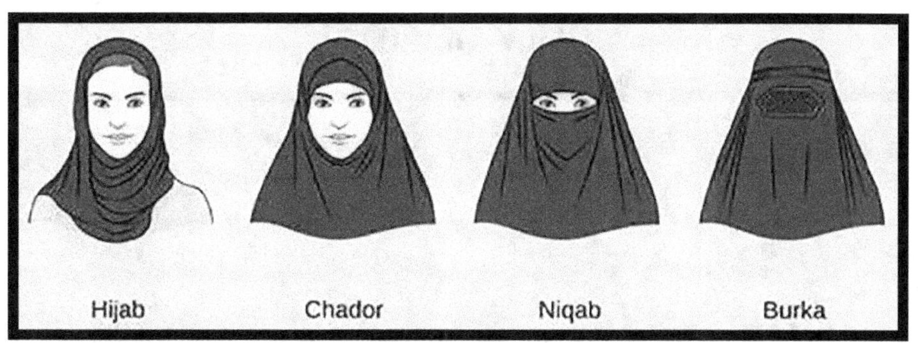

("PROGRESSION" OF OPPRESSION = "PROGRESSIVES")

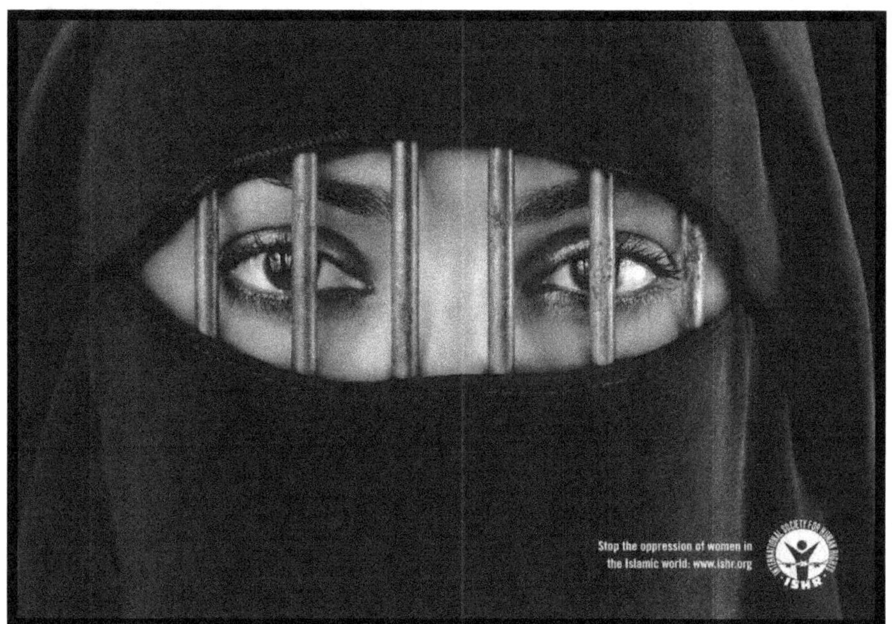

(JULY 14, 2020)

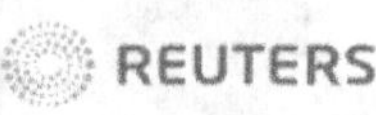

"4-8 WEEKS?"

NOT SO MUCH

HOW MUCH LONGER?

FOREVER?

UNTIL WHEN?

DO NOT ASK QUESTIONS

OBEY AUTHORITY

AS OF THE DATE OF THIS WRITING, THE "MASK REQUIREMENTS" CONTINUE TO BE ENFORCED, DESPITE EVIDENCE THAT "MASKS" ARE MORE LIKELY TO CAUSE INFECTION, AND OFFER NO PROTECTION TO THE WEARER OR TO OTHERS – THE "MASKS" THAT INDIVIDUALS ARE FORCED TO WEAR ARE INSTRUMENTS OF OPPRESSION, JUST AS THEY ALWAYS HAVE BEEN AROUND THE WORLD THROUGHOUT HISTORY

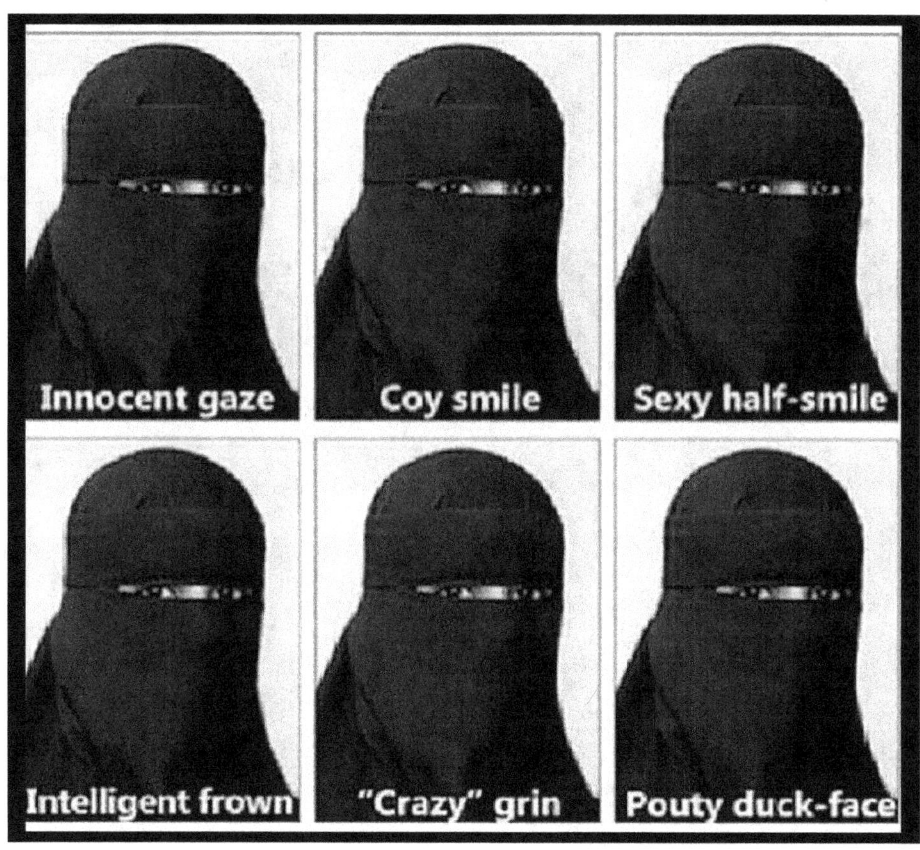

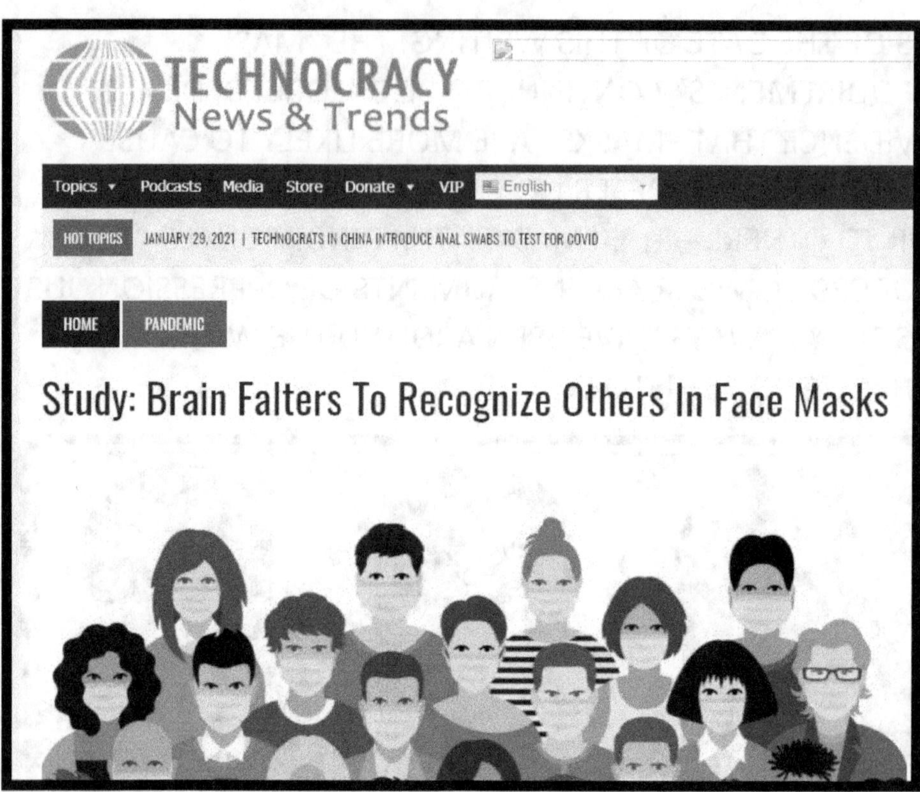

TECHNOCRACY
News & Trends
Topics ▼   Podcasts   Media   Store   Donate ▼   VIP   English
HOT TOPICS   JANUARY 29, 2021 | TECHNOCRATS IN CHINA INTRODUCE ANAL SWABS TO TEST FOR COVID
HOME   PANDEMIC
Study: Brain Falters To Recognize Others In Face Masks

Home > Comment > Columnists > Richard and Judy

Richard and Judy

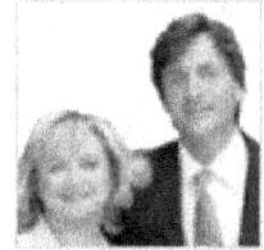

Britain's best-loved TV couple

The burka is a sign of degradation and has no place on our streets

WHENEVER I see a woman wearing a burka or the niqab veil I feel uneasy.

By RICHARD AND JUDY
PUBLISHED: 06:24, Sat, Sep 21, 2013

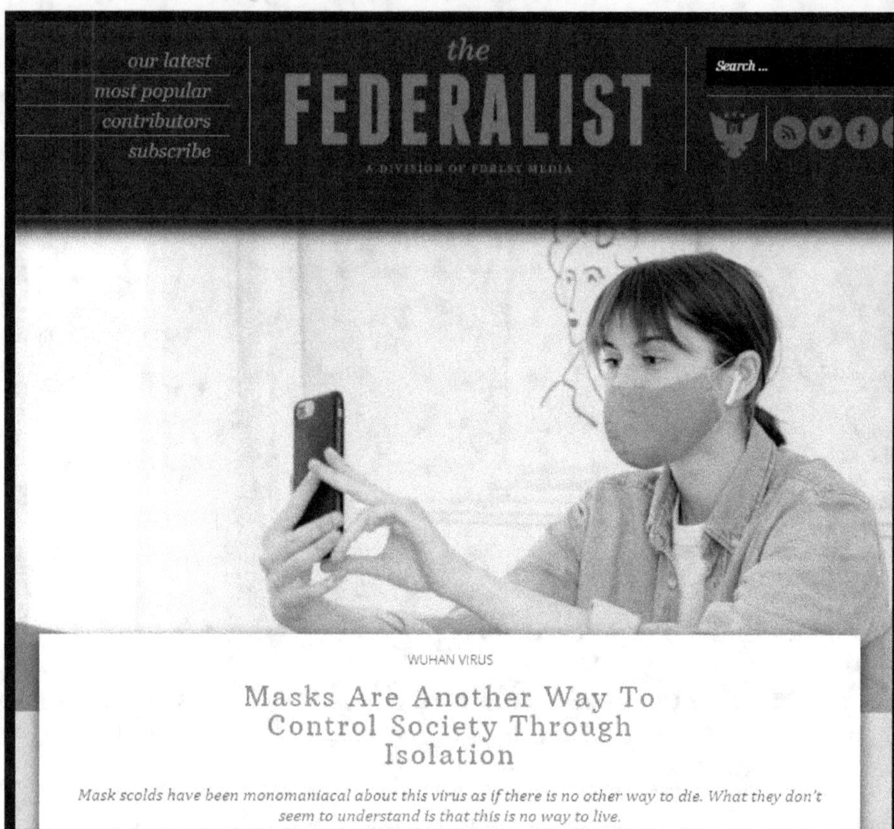

the
FEDERALIST
A DIVISION OF FDRLST MEDIA
our latest
most popular
contributors
subscribe
Search ...
WUHAN VIRUS
Masks Are Another Way To Control Society Through Isolation
Mask scolds have been monomaniacal about this virus as if there is no other way to die. What they don't seem to understand is that this is no way to live.

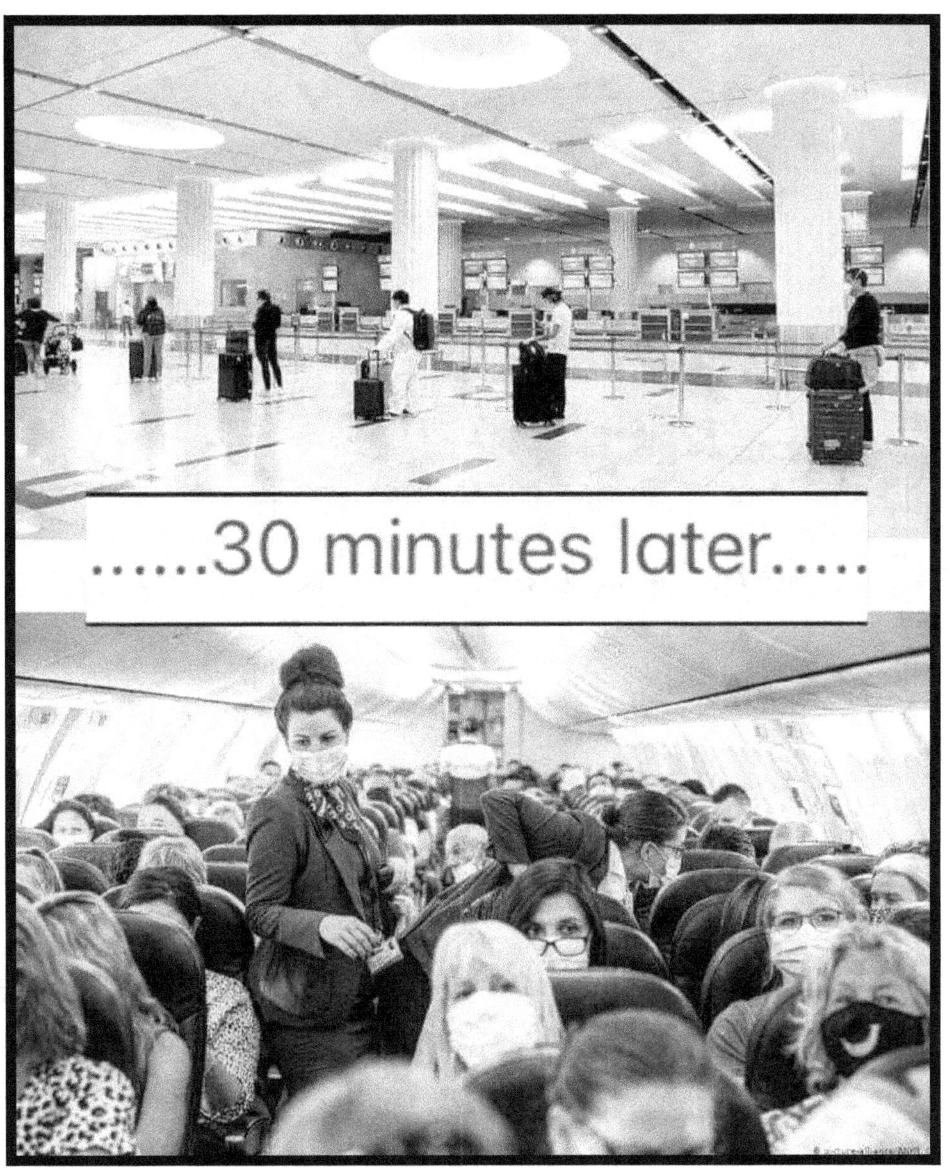
.......30 minutes later......

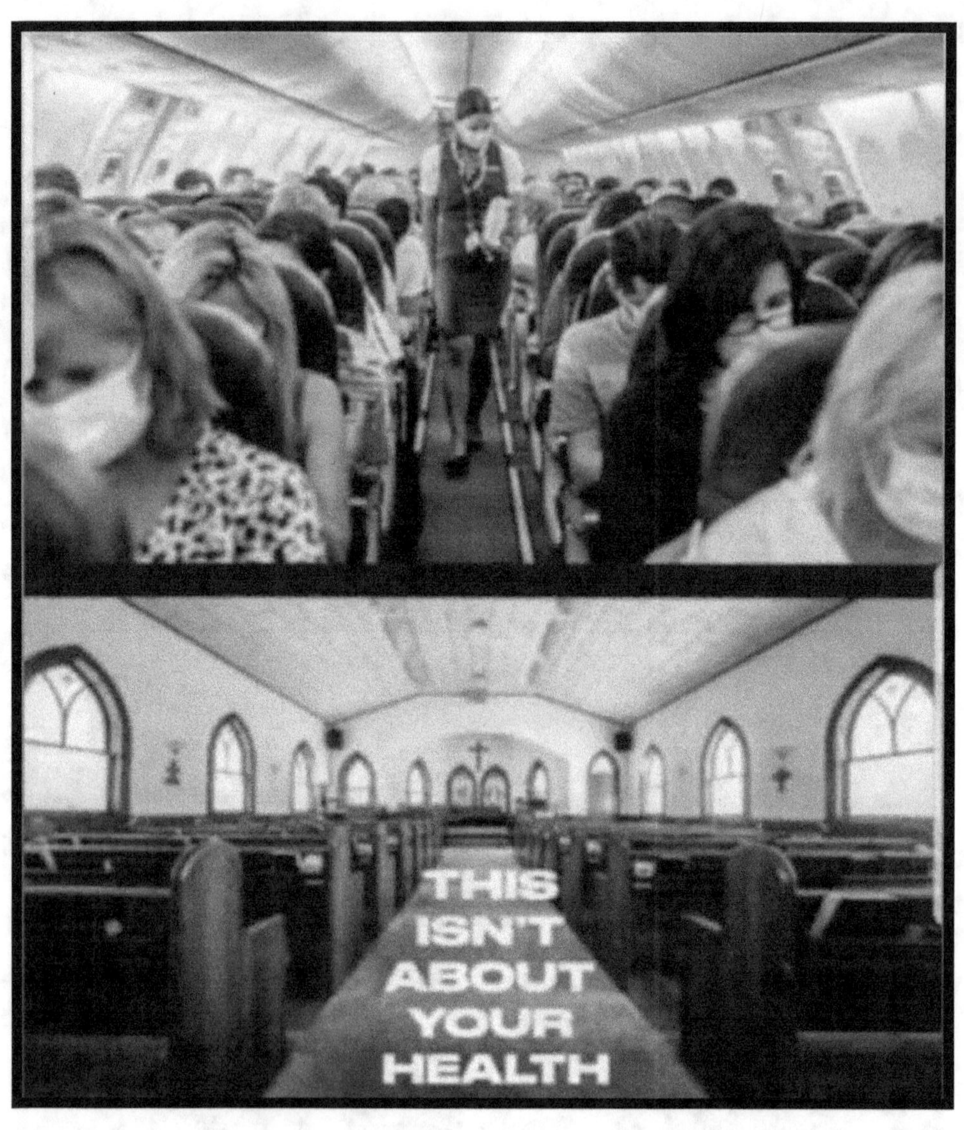
THIS
ISN'T
ABOUT
YOUR
HEALTH

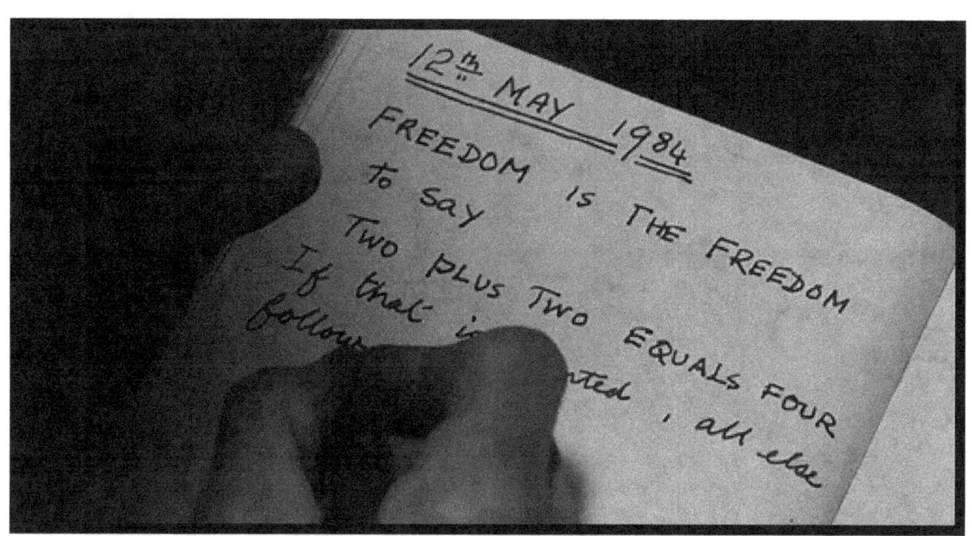

12th MAY 1984
FREEDOM IS THE FREEDOM
to say
TWO PLUS TWO EQUALS FOUR
If that is granted, all else
follows

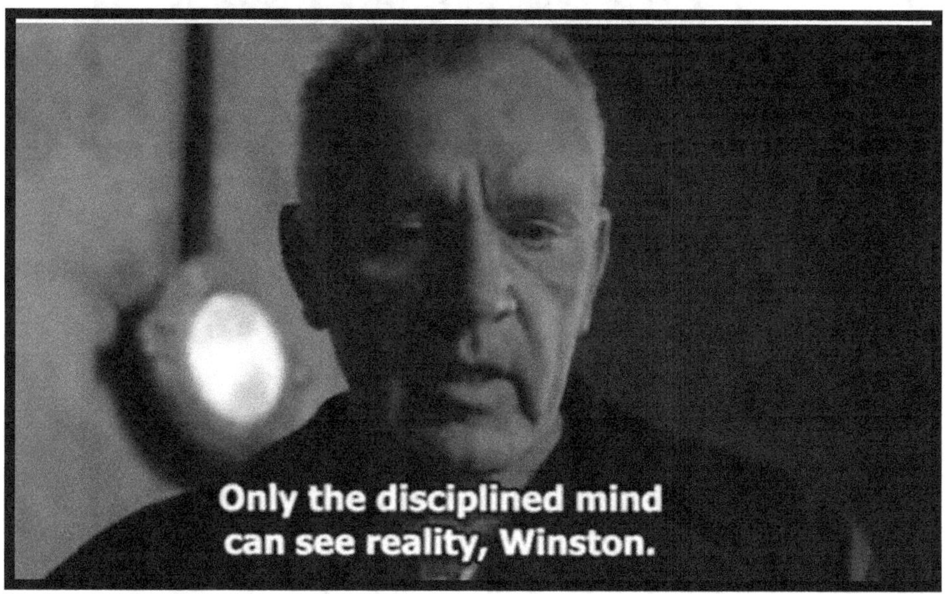

Only the disciplined mind
can see reality, Winston.

"MASKS" PROTECT AGAINST THE SPREAD OF "COVID"

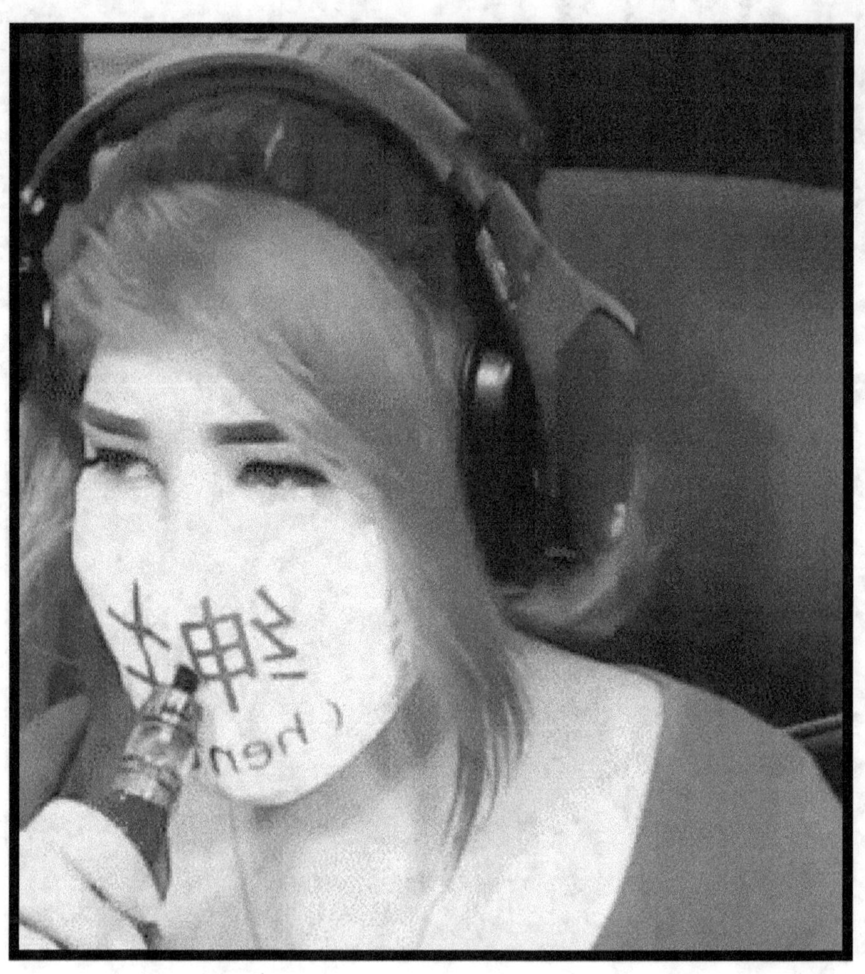

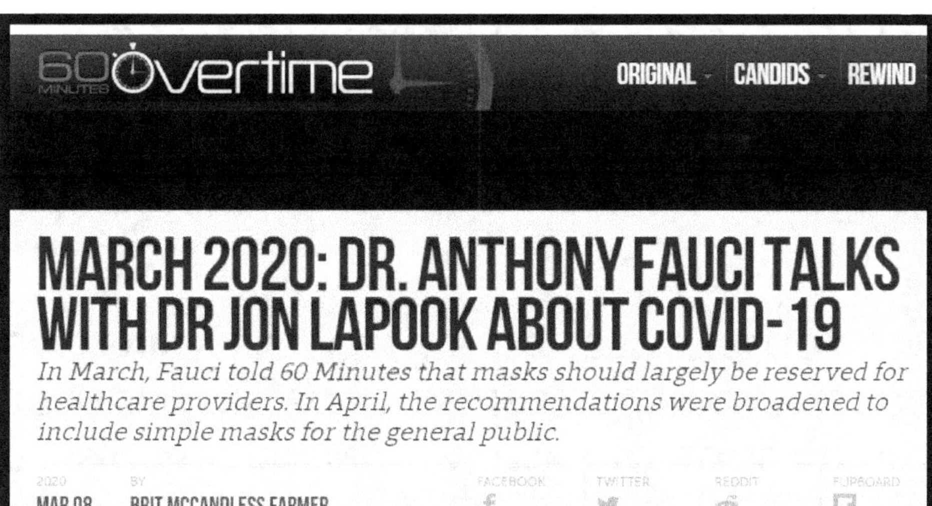

MARCH 2020: DR. ANTHONY FAUCI TALKS WITH DR JON LAPOOK ABOUT COVID-19

In March, Fauci told 60 Minutes that masks should largely be reserved for healthcare providers. In April, the recommendations were broadened to include simple masks for the general public.

2020
MAR 08

BY
BRIT MCCANDLESS FARMER

FACEBOOK   TWITTER   REDDIT   FLIPBOARD

MEDPAGE TODAY

Home   Specialties   CME/CE   Election 2020   Meetings   COVID-19   Videos   Opinion   Condition Centers   Careers   Society Partners

Infectious Disease > COVID-19

Study: Masks Fail to Filter Virus in Coughing COVID-19 Patients

— About that mask recommendation...

by Molly Walker, Associate Editor, MedPage Today   April 6, 2020

MAY I PLEASE SEE THE EVIDENCE THAT MASKS ARE EFFECTIVE AGAINST THE TRANSMISSION OF "COVID?"

NO - YOU WILL OBEY THE STATE, WEAR A MASK, DO NOT QUESTION THE LEGITIMACY OF THIS ORDER BY THE STATE, OR YOU WILL BE CRIMINALLY PUNISHED

"MASKS" THAT CAUSE ASTHMATICS LIKE ME TO SUFFER HYPOXIA?

"MASKS" THAT CAUSE SKIN INFECTIONS AND ORAL HEALTH PROBLEMS?

"MASKS" THAT PREVENT THE NORMAL RECOGNITION OF HUMAN FACES AND ABILITY TO SEE FACIAL EXPRESSIONS?

"MASKS" THAT PREVENT EFFECTIVE COMMUNICATION, NOT ONLY MAKING EVERYDAY LIFE MORE UNBEARABLE, BUT ALSO PREVENT INDIVIDUALS LIKE ME FROM ACTUALLY SPEAKING TO OTHERS ABOUT THE TRUTH OF THE CONSTITUTIONAL CRISIS CURRENTLY TAKING PLACE - IT DEFIES ANY LOGICAL REASONING, AND THAT IS THE POINT - IT DOESN'T NEED TO MAKE SENSE - IT IS BETTER IF IT DOES NOT MAKE SENSE - THAT MAKES THE OBSERVATION OF MASS PUBLIC COMPLIANCE TO FRAUDULENT GOVERNMENTAL AUTHORITY ALL THE MORE OBVIOUS, AS THE PUBLIC EVEN THEMSELVES ARE HUMILIATED TRULY KNOWING THAT THEY ARE SUBMITTING TO AUTHORITARIAN LIES.

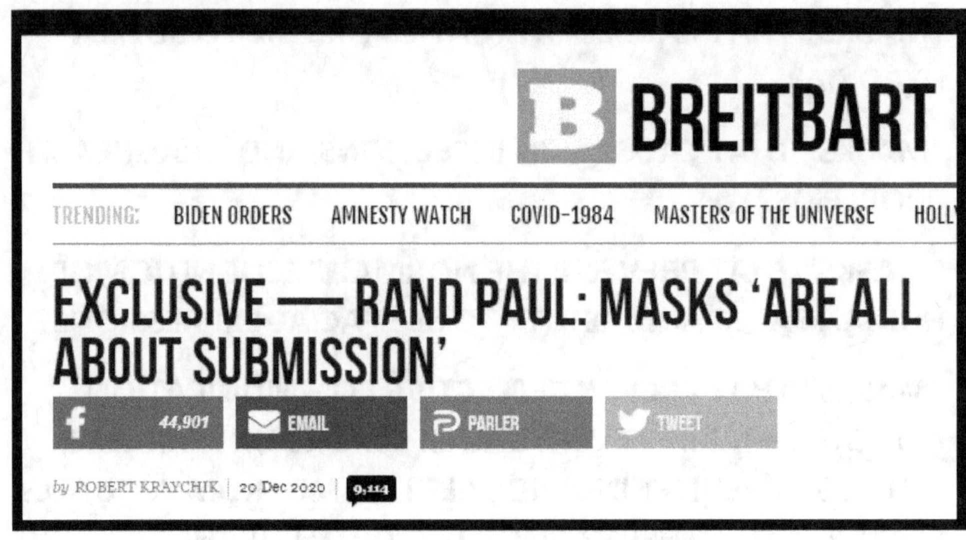

BUT WHAT MUST THEY SAY PUBLICLY, TO THEIR EMPLOYERS, TO THEIR FRIENDS, OR FACE RIDICULE, OR WORSE?

HOW MANY FINGERS AM I HOLDING UP?

HOW MANY FINGERS AM I HOLDING UP?

IS THE "COVID" PANDEMIC REAL?

DO "MASKS" WORK?

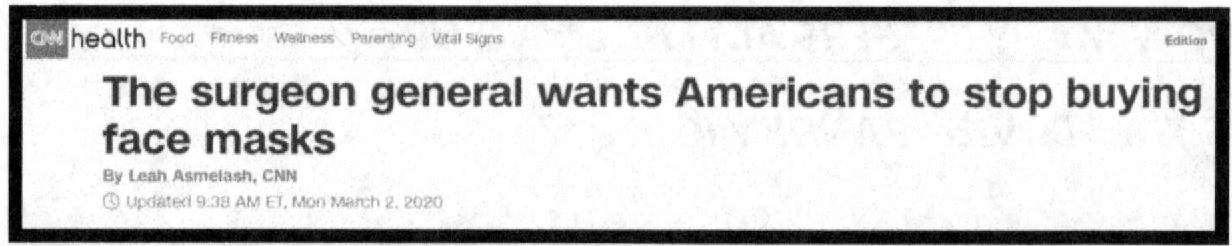

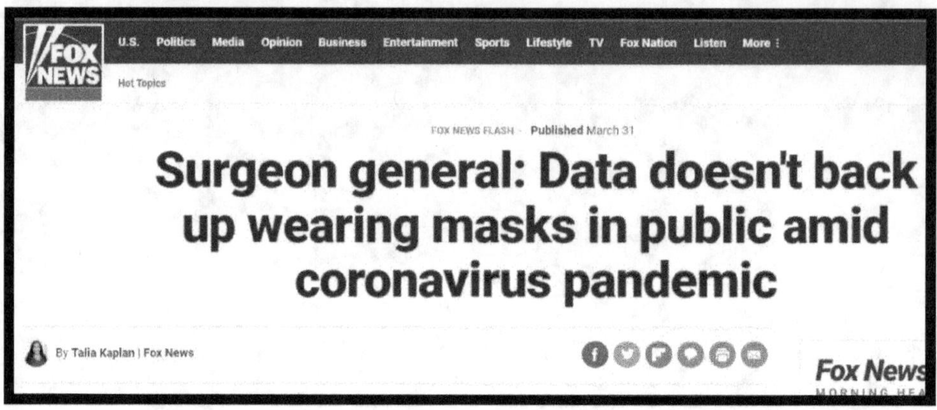

BUT THE SURGEON GENERAL SAID THAT MASKS DO NOT WORK

IT DOES NOT MATTER - THAT WAS "TRUMP'S SURGEON GENERAL," AND HE DOES NOT UNDERSTAND SCIENCE

BUT HE WAS THE <u>SURGEON GENERAL</u>

<u>"TRUMP'S SURGEON GENERAL"</u> - THE ARGUMENT IS OVER - EVERYTHING ASSOCIATED WITH "TRUMP" IS IMMEDIATELY TO BE UNDERSTOOD AS WRONG - HOW MANY FINGERS AM I HOLDING UP?

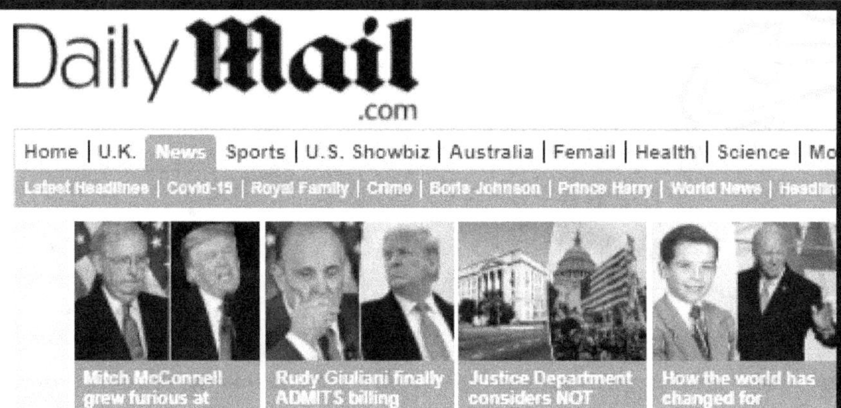

Daily Mail
.com

Surgeon General Jerome Adams says people still need to wear masks and socially distance after they've been vaccinated because it doesn't prevent infection just severe illness

- Surgeon General Jerome Adams appeared on GMA on Monday as the first vaccines were rolled out across the US
- He said that Pfizer vaccine protects people against severe disease but not from getting infected
- It means that after people have been vaccinated, they still need to be careful
- The government says it'll roll out 100million vaccinations by March
- But that's only a third of the country and many are unwilling to take the vaccine
- The first doses are being administered across the country on Monday morning
- Intensive care nurse Sandra Lindsay received the first Pfizer shot in the U.S. at the Long Island Jewish Medical Center in Queens just before 9.30am

By JENNIFER SMITH FOR DAILYMAIL.COM
PUBLISHED: 08:57 EST, 14 December 2020 | UPDATED: 13:38 EST, 14 December 2020

THAT IS BETTER - WE GOT HIM BACK INTO LINE

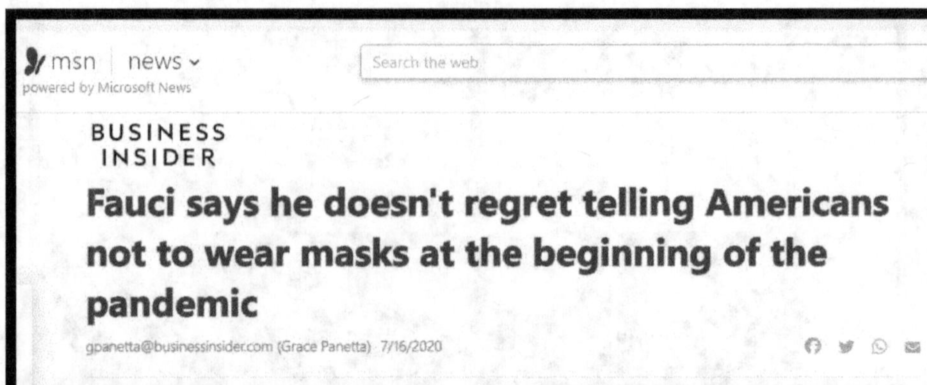

BUSINESS INSIDER

Fauci says he doesn't regret telling Americans not to wear masks at the beginning of the pandemic

gpanetta@businessinsider.com (Grace Panetta) 7/16/2020

IT DOES NOT MATTER WHAT WE TOLD YOU EVEN A FEW MONTHS AGO - YOU WILL ACCEPT AND FOLLOW WHAT WE TELL YOU NOW

YOU ARE NOT ALLOWED TO FOLLOW YOUR OWN REASONING NOR WHAT YOU PREVIOUSLY UNDERSTOOD AS "COMMON SENSE" - OBEY THE STATE

MASKS WORK...

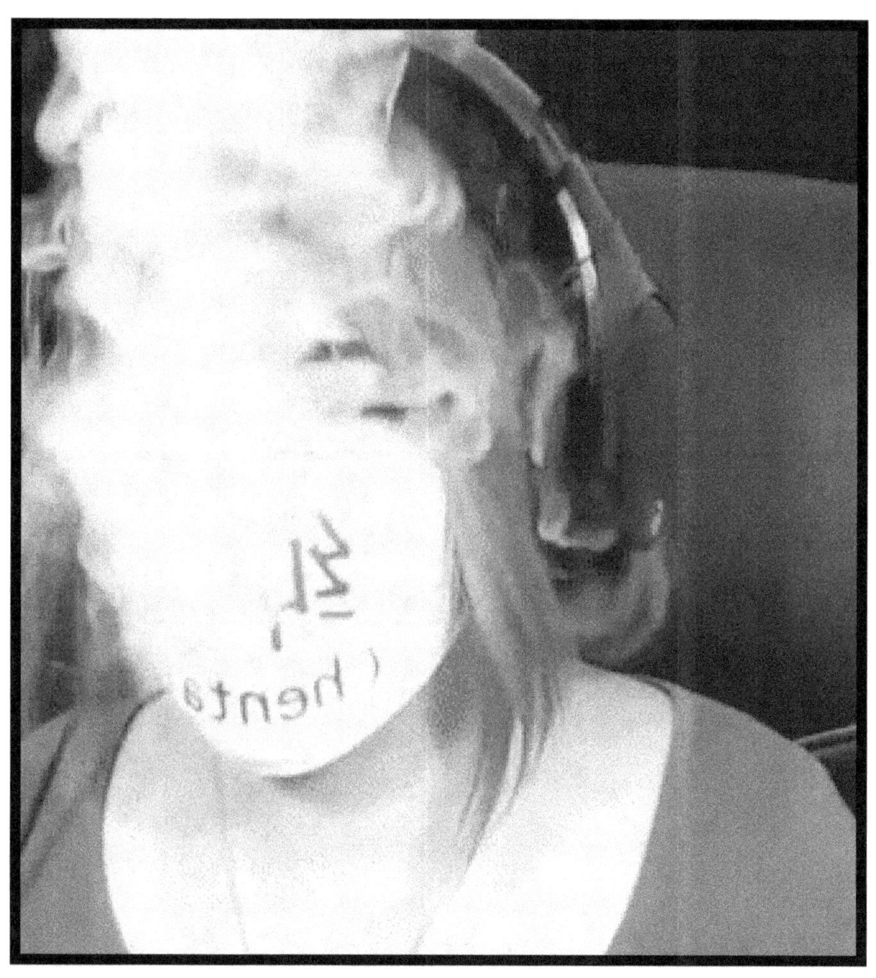

(THEY "WORK" AS ANTI-CONSTITUTIONAL INSTRUMENTS OF GOVERNMENTAL ABUSE AND CONTROL OVER THE LIVES OF AMERICAN CITIZENS)

Parameter	Scenario 1	Scenario 2	Scenario 3	Scenario 4	Scenario 5: Current Best Estimate
R_0*	2.0		4.0		2.5
Infection Fatality Ratio[†]	0-19 years: 0.00002 20-49 years: 0.00007 50-69 years: 0.0025 70+ years: 0.028		0-19 years: 0.0001 20-49 years: 0.0003 50-69 years: 0.010 70+ years: 0.093		0-19 years: 0.00003 20-49 years: 0.0002 50-69 years: 0.005 70+ years: 0.054

(FROM THE "CDC" ITSELF)

70+ years: 0.054

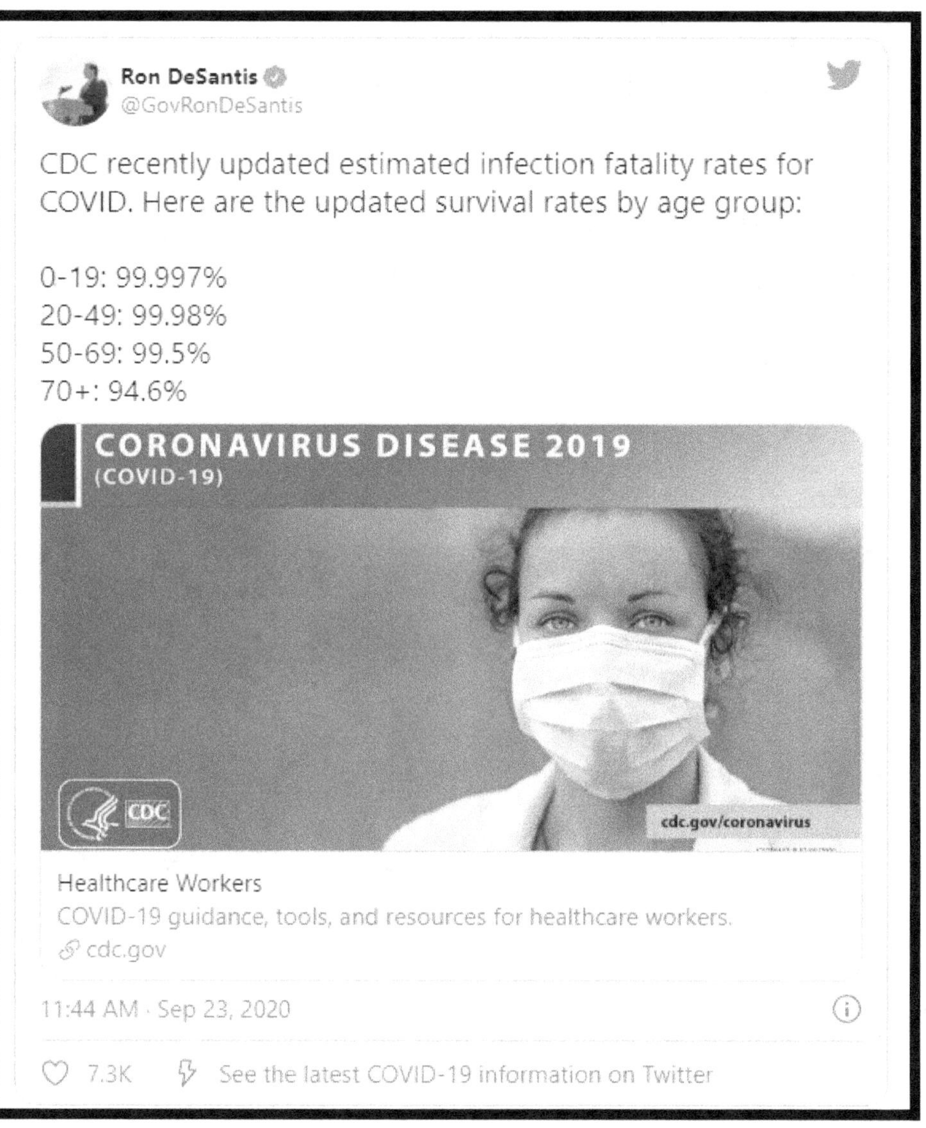
Ron DeSantis
@GovRonDeSantis

CDC recently updated estimated infection fatality rates for COVID. Here are the updated survival rates by age group:

0-19: 99.997%
20-49: 99.98%
50-69: 99.5%
70+: 94.6%

CORONAVIRUS DISEASE 2019
(COVID-19)

CDC

cdc.gov/coronavirus

Healthcare Workers
COVID-19 guidance, tools, and resources for healthcare workers.
cdc.gov

11:44 AM · Sep 23, 2020

7.3K   See the latest COVID-19 information on Twitter

YOU SEE **THE AVERAGE SURVIVABILITY RATE OF "COVID" IS OVER <u>99.5%</u>**, AND IS MUCH HIGHER UPON AVERAGE FOR THE ENTIRE POPULATION

THE AVERAGE OVERALL AGE OF DEATH FOR UNITED STATES CITIZENS IS 78 YEARS OLD, APPROXIMATELY THREE YEARS OLDER THAN THE AVERAGE AGE OF SUPPOSEDLY "COVID"-RELATED DEATHS, WHICH IS 75

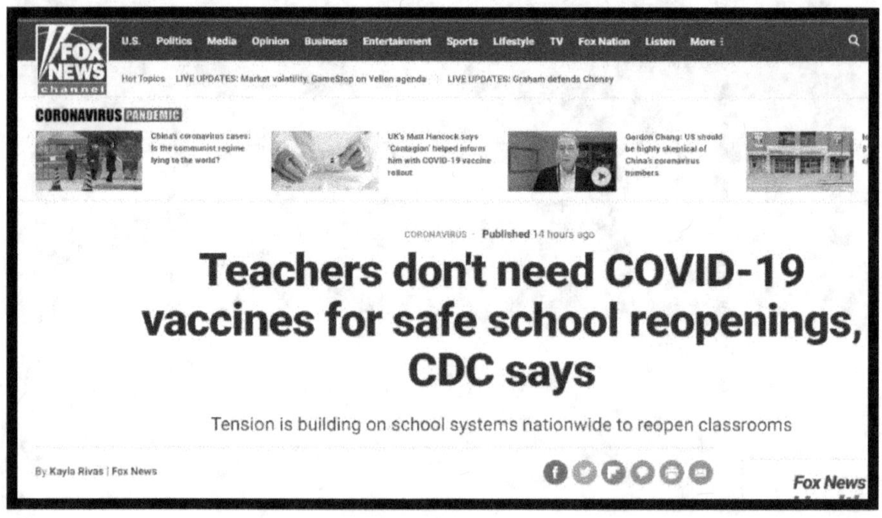

I HAVE SHOWN YOU THE EVIDENCE FROM THE "CDC" ITSELF THAT "COVID" DEATHS ARE DETERMINED IF A HEALTH PROFESSIONAL MAKES AN "*ASSUMPTION*" THAT "COVID" WAS THE CAUSE OF DEATH

WHAT DOES THIS ADD UP TO?

PEOPLE ARE NOT DYING OF "COVID" – PEOPLE ARE DYING FROM GOVERNMENT IMPOSITION OF BOGUS RESTRICTIONS

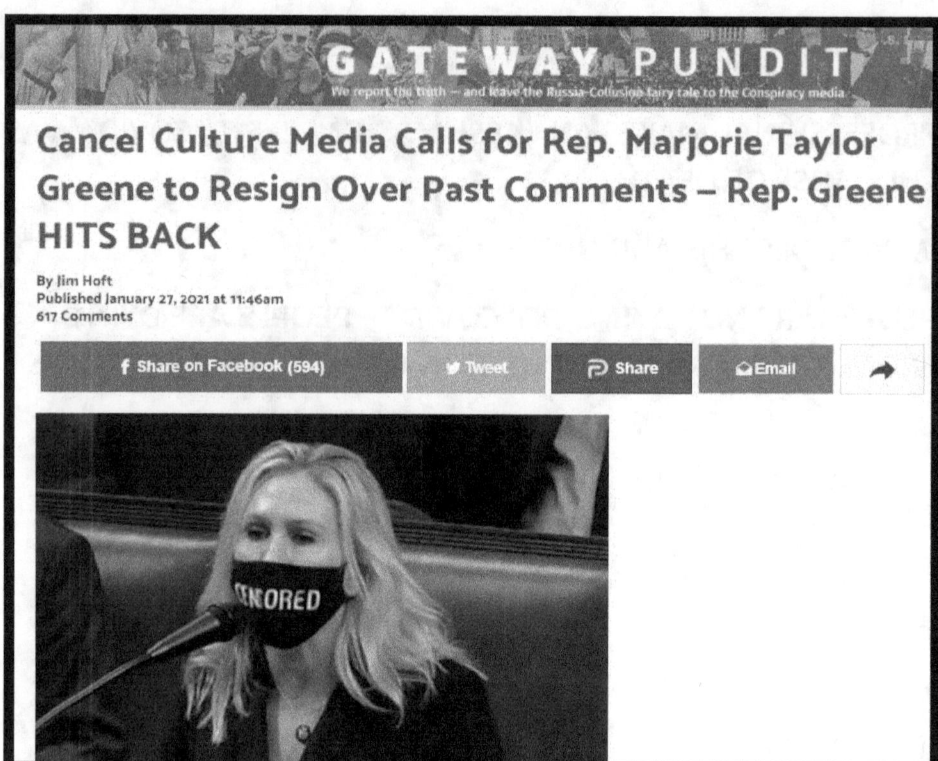

Cancel Culture Media Calls for Rep. Marjorie Taylor Greene to Resign Over Past Comments – Rep. Greene HITS BACK

By Jim Hoft
Published January 27, 2021 at 11:46am
617 Comments

Democrats and their media are very upset with Marjorie Taylor Greene after she introduced articles of impeachment against corrupt pervert Joe Biden last week following his virtual inauguration.

According to **CNN** Rep. Greene "liked" Facebook comments that threatened crooked Democrats and FBI operatives.

> *Greene, who represents Georgia's 14th Congressional District, frequently posted far-right extremist and debunked conspiracy theories on her page, including the baseless QAnon conspiracy which casts former President Donald Trump in an imagined battle against a sinister cabal of Democrats and celebrities who abuse children.*
>
> *TRENDING: EXCLUSIVE: Independent Journalist Tayler Hansen: A Riot that Turned Deadly, What I Witnessed at the US Capitol Riot*
>
> *In one post, from January 2019, Greene liked a comment that said "a bullet to the head would be quicker" to remove House Speaker Nancy Pelosi. In other posts, Greene liked comments about executing FBI agents who, in her eyes, were part of the "deep state" working against Trump.*

AND WHAT HORRIBLE THINGS DID MARJORIE TAYLOR GREENE SAY TO THE PUBLIC?

THE HORRIBLE TRUTH

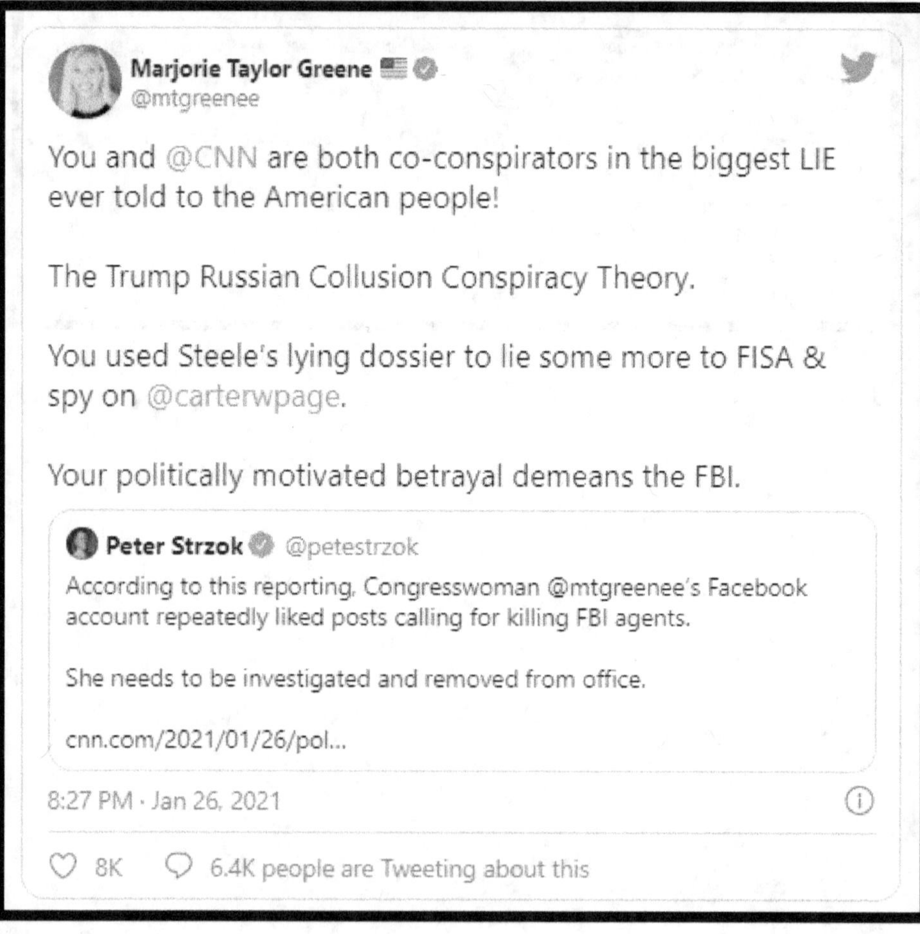

THAT MAKES SENSE - SHE HAS BEEN ATTACKED BY CORRUPT POLITICIANS AND MEDIA TRAITORS TO THE UNITED STATES

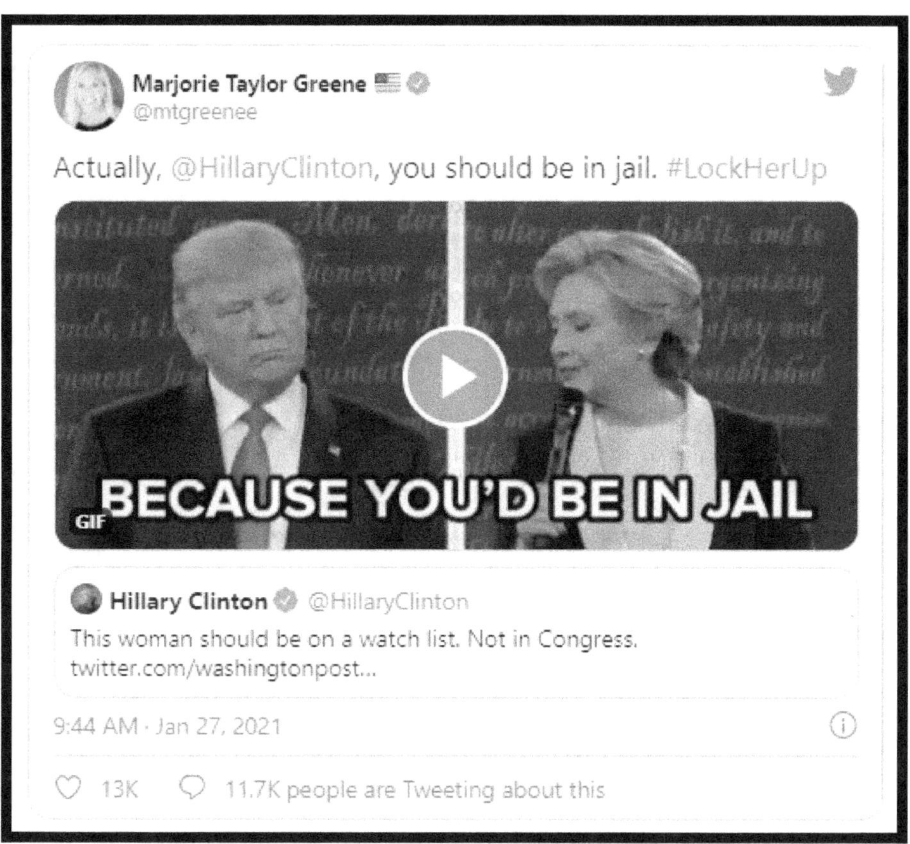

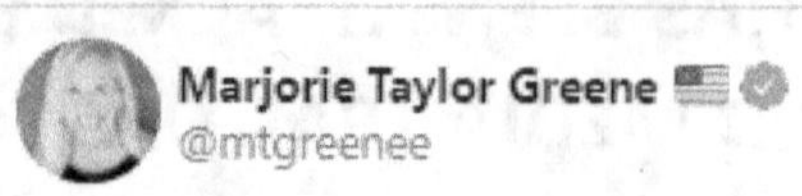

Marjorie Taylor Greene 🇺🇸 ✅
@mtgreenee

You, of all people, that preaches abortion from the pulpit should not judge.

You don't believe the very word of God that created us male and female in His image and declares, "Before I formed you in the womb I knew you."

"Pastor," being a heretic is far worse than fake news.

> 🌐 **Senator Reverend Raphael Warnock** ✅ @ReverendWarnock
> This is dangerous and unacceptable for a member of Congress. We're entrusted to serve and represent all of our constituents. This extreme and violent rhetoric only fans the flames of division, and we've just seen how deadly those flames can be. twitter.com/KFILE/status/1...

7:40 PM · Jan 26, 2021 

♡ 6.2K 💬 4.7K people are Tweeting about this

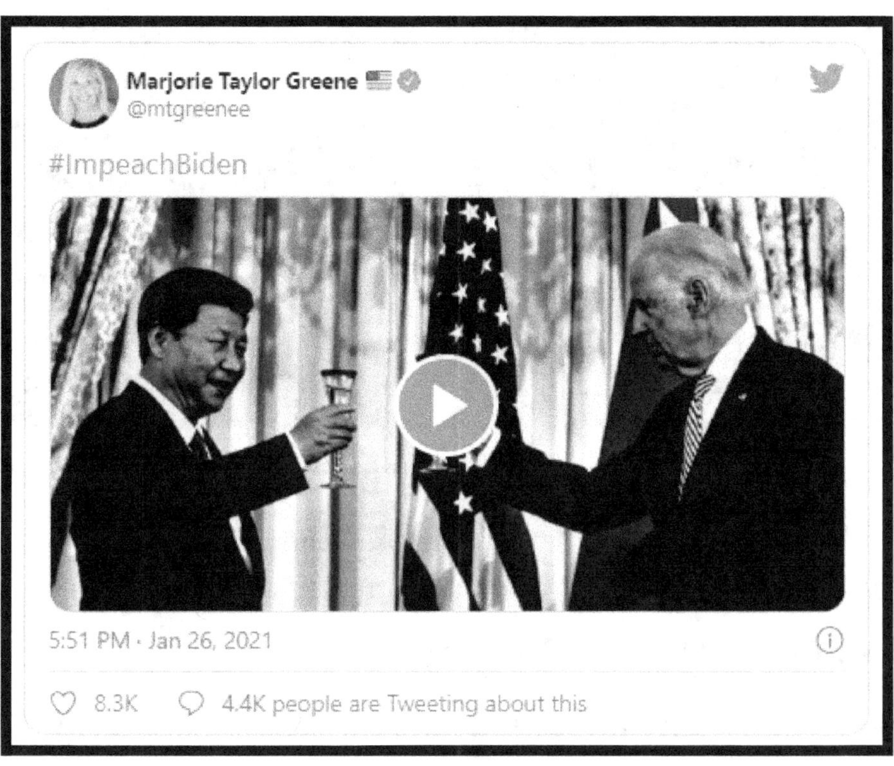

STRIKE ANOTHER VICTORY FOR TYRANNICAL CENSORSHIP:

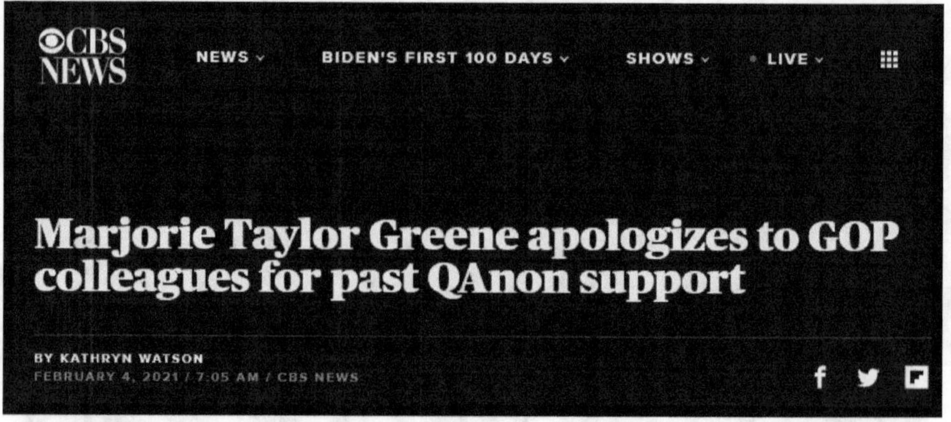

MEANWHILE, SUPPORT FOR "BLACK LIVES MATTER" IS ENCOURAGED – ANOTHER EXAMPLE OF "PROJECTION," CONFLATING POSITIONS - "I KNOW YOU ARE, BUT WHAT AM I?"

BECAUSE "BLACK LIVES MATTER" ARE ACTUALLY SUPPORTED AND CONTROLLED BY FOREIGN ENEMIES TO THE UNITED STATES – THEY BURN CITIES – THEY SHOUT CHANTS CALLING FOR THE MURDER OF POLICE OFFICERS - LOOK AT MINNEAPOLIS AND PORTLAND, BUT ALL ACROSS THE COUNTRY – AND NOW THEY ARE BEGINNING TO CONTROL THE MINDS OF OUR CHILDREN – HAVE THEY ALREADY CAPTURED CONTROL OVER YOURS?

MEANWHILE WE FORCE CHILDREN TO MISS CRITICAL TIME OUT OF SCHOOL – WE FORCE

CHILDREN TO WEAR HARMFUL MASKS – AND THE REASON WHY?

"COVID"

AND IS THE THREAT OF "COVID" A THREAT TO THE CHILDREN?

NO, THEIR IMMUNE SYSTEMS ARE TOO STRONG AND CHILDREN ARE SHOWN NOT TO BE SUSCEPTIBLE TO "COVID"

SO, WE ARE FORCING CHILDREN TO MISS SCHOOL, WEAR HARMFUL MASKS AND EVEN FORCE CHILDREN TO TAKE DANGEROUS "VACCINES," ALL THE WHILE CHILDREN ARE COMMITTING SUICIDE IN RECORD NUMBERS, ALL FOR THE SAKE OF SAVING ADULTS FROM CATCHING "COVID?"

THAT IS CORRECT

WHY IS IT BAD IF ADULTS CATCH COVID?

BECAUSE ADULTS CAN DIE FROM "COVID"

WHAT IS THE AVERAGE AGE OF DEATH FROM "COVID?"

THE AVERAGE AGE OF DEATH FROM "COVID" IS 75 YEARS OLD

WHAT IS THE AVERAGE AGE OF DEATH OVERALL FOR AMERICAN CITIZENS?

THE AVERAGE AGE OF DEATH FOR AMERICANS IS 78 YEARS OLD

SO, THEREFORE THERE MUST BE A LOT OF 75-YEAR-OLDS DYING FROM "COVID"

ACTUALLY, THE RATE OF SURVIVABILITY OF INDIVIDUALS WHO CONTRACT "COVID" IS OVER 99.5%

SO, THAT MEANS THAT EVERYONE YOUNGER THAN 75 YEARS OLD HAS A MUCH BETTER CHANCE OF SURVIVING "COVID"

CORRECT – THE OVERALL SURVIVABILITY RATE OF INDIVIDUALS WHO CONTRACT "COVID" IS 99.7%

SO THEN WHY ARE CHILDREN BEING KEPT HOME FROM SCHOOL AND BEING FORCED TO WEAR HARMFUL MASKS AND BEING FORCED TO RECEIVE DANGEROUS "VACCINES" WHILE THE CHILDREN ARE

COMMITTING SUICIDE IN ALARMINGLY HIGH RATES?

AS IT WAS EXPLAINED BEFORE, THE CHILDREN MUST SUFFER THIS ABUSE IN ORDER TO PREVENT THE TRANSMISSION OF THE "COVID" DISEASE, BECAUSE THE CHILDREN MIGHT BE CONTAGIOUS AND INFECT AN ADULT, WHO MAY HAVE A .05% CHANCE OF DYING, BUT ONLY IF AT AN AVERAGE AGE OF 75 YEARS OLD.

SO, THEREFORE, WE ARE NEEDLESSLY ABUSING OUR CHILDREN

CORRECT

Children in Iowa's Ames Community School District, from preschool through high school, are going to be part of a Black Lives Matter "week of action" beginning February 1st.

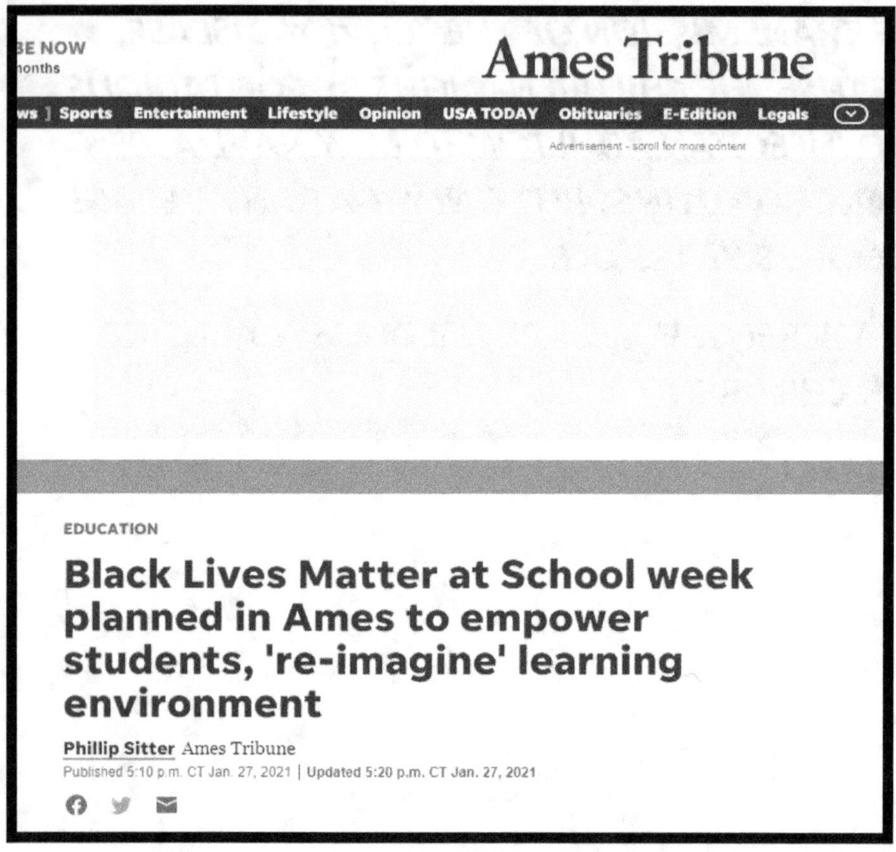

"OH, THAT'S A GOOD IDEA," YOU THINK, SINCE *"BLACK LIVES"* OBVIOUSLY *"MATTER,"* RIGHT?

WHICH IS IDENTICAL TO NAMING "OBAMACARE" AS "THE AFFORDABLE CARE ACT," BECAUSE EVERYBODY IS IN SUPPORT OF "AFFORDABLE CARE," RIGHT?

EXCEPT THAT "OBAMACARE" CAUSED MILLIONS OF AMERICAN CITIZENS TO LOSE THEIR HEALTH INSURANCE AND INCREASE MEDICAL COSTS – GREAT FOR THE PHARMACEUTICAL COMPANIES, AND THEY LOVED OBAMA – BUT THEY HATE PRESIDENT TRUMP – WHY? COULD IT BE BECAUSE PRESIDENT TRUMP LOWERED DRUG PRICES?

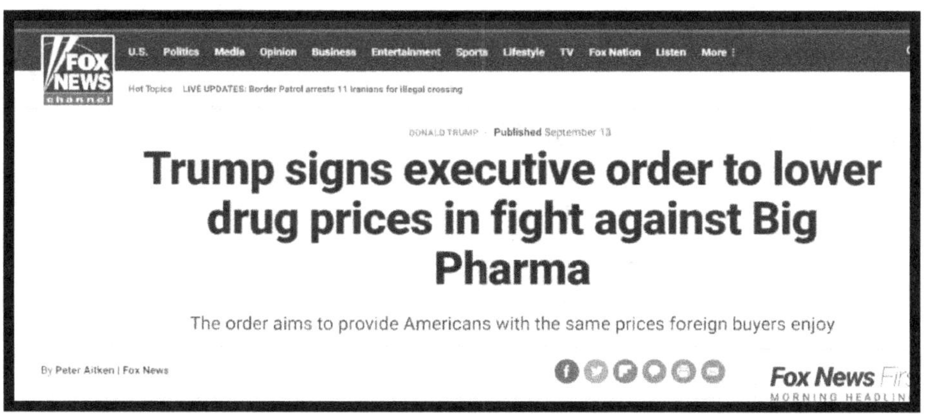

DO PHARMACEUTICAL COMPANIES PAY FOR ADVERTISING ON MAINSTREAM NEWS NETWORKS?

OF COURSE YOU KNOW THAT PHARMACEUTICAL COMPANIES ARE PRACTICALLY THE ONLY ADVERTISERS ON MAINSTREAM NEWS NETWORKS.

WHY DO YOU SUPPOSE THAT MAINSTREAM NEWS NETWORKS HAVE RELENTLESSLY ATTACKED PRESIDENT TRUMP EVER SINCE HE RAN FOR PRESIDENT, BUT THE MAINSTREAM NETWORKS LOVED DONALD TRUMP FOR DECADES BEFOREHAND?

USE LOGICAL REASONING.

THIS IS JUST AN INTRODUCTION – YOU HAVE BEEN DECEIVED.

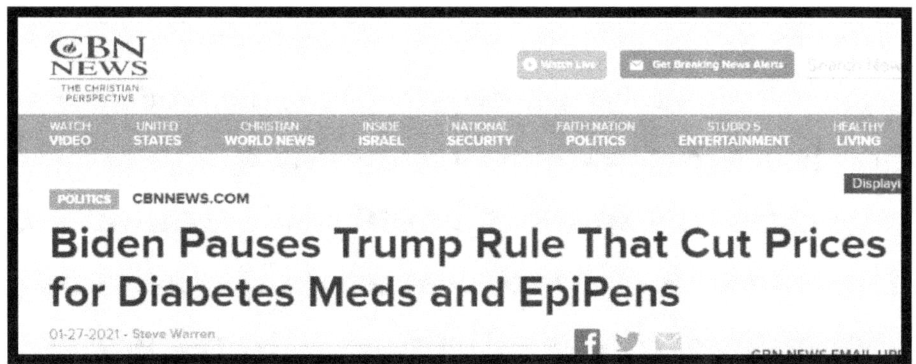

CBN NEWS
THE CHRISTIAN PERSPECTIVE
Watch Live
Get Breaking News Alerts
WATCH VIDEO
UNITED STATES
CHRISTIAN WORLD NEWS
INSIDE ISRAEL
NATIONAL SECURITY
FAITH NATION POLITICS
STUDIO 5 ENTERTAINMENT
HEALTHY LIVING
POLITICS CBNNEWS.COM
Biden Pauses Trump Rule That Cut Prices for Diabetes Meds and EpiPens
01-27-2021 - Steve Warren

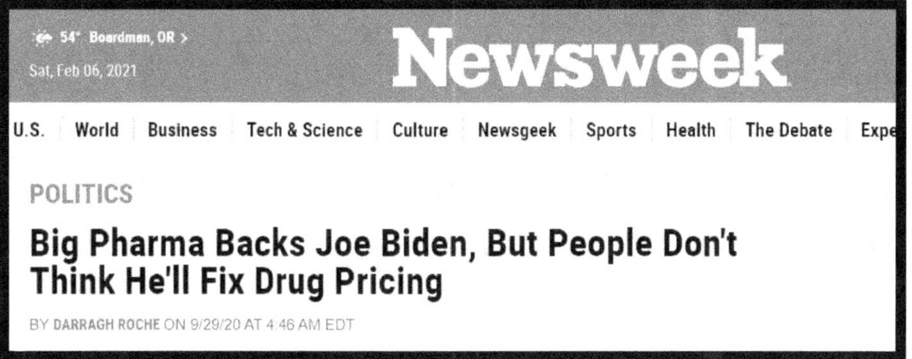

54° Boardman, OR
Sat, Feb 06, 2021
Newsweek
U.S.   World   Business   Tech & Science   Culture   Newsgeek   Sports   Health   The Debate   Expe
POLITICS
Big Pharma Backs Joe Biden, But People Don't Think He'll Fix Drug Pricing
BY DARRAGH ROCHE ON 9/29/20 AT 4:46 AM EDT

According to the public school district's website, students from preschool through high school **"will engage in … a 5-day guide to expand student understanding of the Black Lives Matter at School Principles,"** including **"queer affirming," "transgender affirming," "globalism,"** and ***"disruption of Western nuclear family dynamics."***

DO WE CARE ABOUT PRESERVING "WESTERN NUCLEAR FAMILY DYNAMICS?

DO WE WANT TO TEACH CHILDREN IN SCHOOL HOW TO DISRUPT WESTERN FAMILY DYNAMICS?

DO WE WANT TO DESTROY EVERYTHING ABOUT AMERICA?

"BLACK LIVES MATTER" WANT TO DESTROY EVERYTHING ABOUT AMERICA, INCLUDING THE MINDS OF OUR CHILDREN

AND YOUR MINDS AS WELL – TIME TO WAKE UP

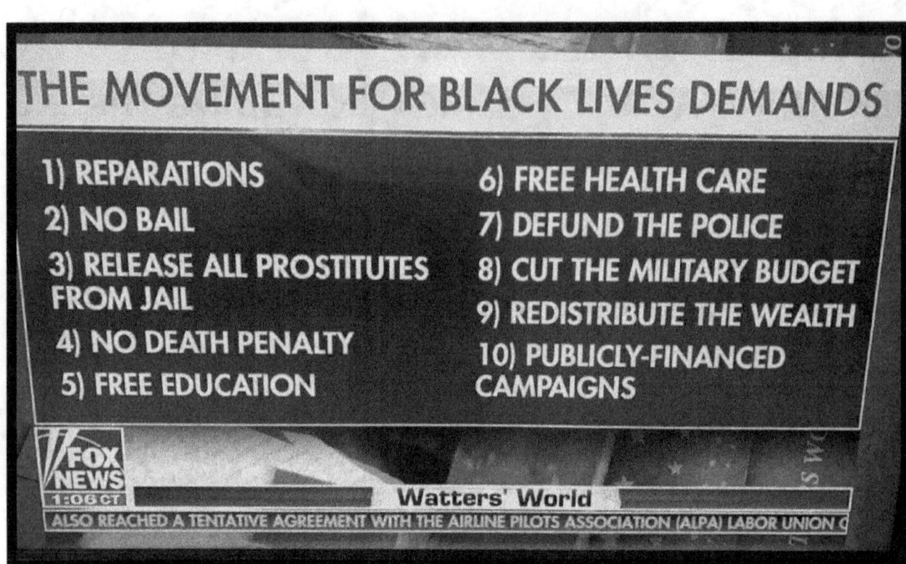

Less Than One Percent of 1,200 Reported Racial Incidents in Last Five Years at Michigan State Were Valid

Posted by Mike LaChance   Monday, February 1, 2021 at 12:00pm

"Only eight instances, however, truly violated the school's bias and discrimination policies."

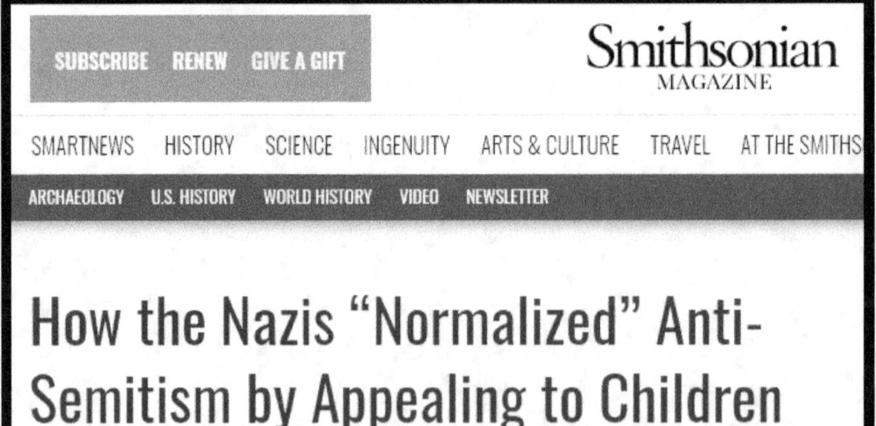

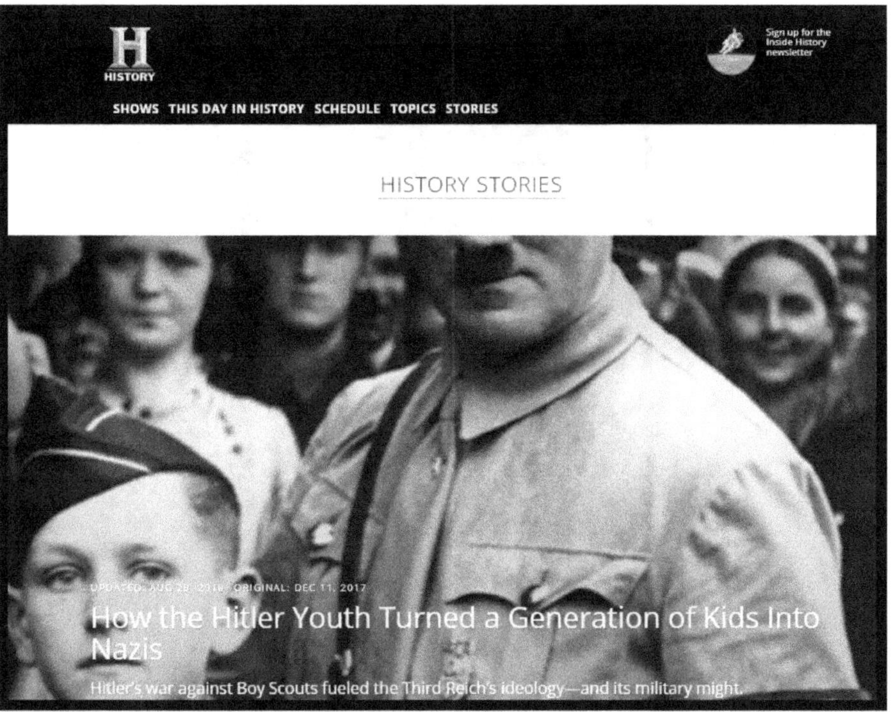

Shaping the Future: Indoctrinating Youth

"These boys and girls enter our organizations [at] ten years of age, and often for the first time get a little fresh air; after four years of the Young Folk they go on to the Hitler Youth, where we have them for another four years . . . And even if they are still not complete National Socialists, they go to Labor Service and are smoothed out there for another six, seven months . . . And whatever class consciousness or social status might still be left . . . the Wehrmacht [German armed forces] will take care of that."
—Adolf Hitler (1938)

STUDENTEN
SEID
PROPA-
GANDISTEN
DES
FÜHRERS
HOCH-u. FACHSCHULEN BEKENNEN SICH AM 29. MÄRZ
ZUR DEUTSCHEN FREIHEITSBEWEGUNG

SAME =

EDUCATED LOVING
TEACHER
DEDICATED
LOVING
PATIENT
SKILLED
POWER TO THE PEOPLE
POWER & EQUALITY
BLACK LIVES MATTER
CHICANAS FOR
BLACK LIVES
ALL LIVES MATTER

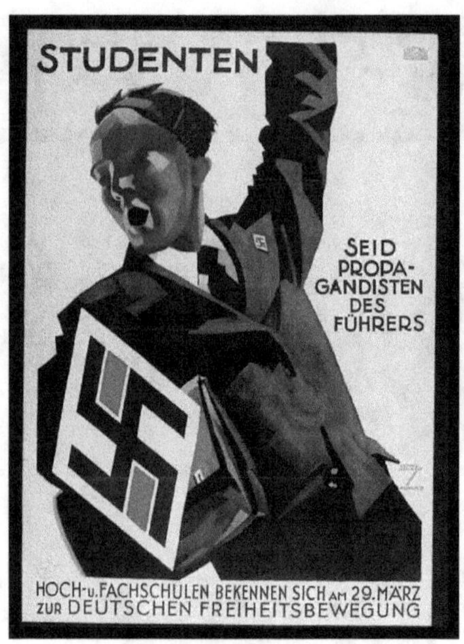

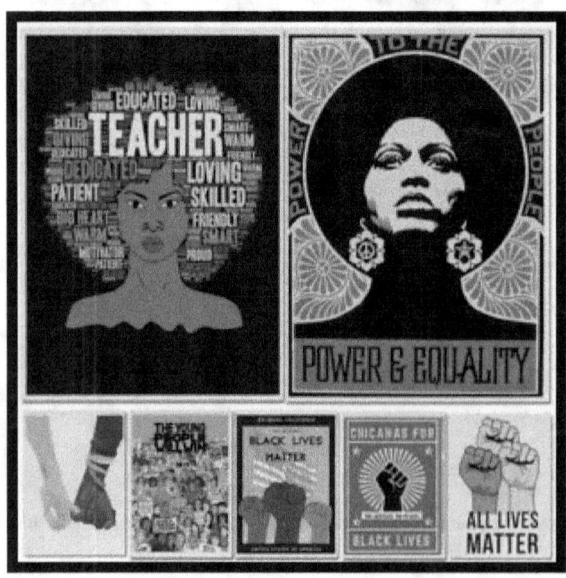

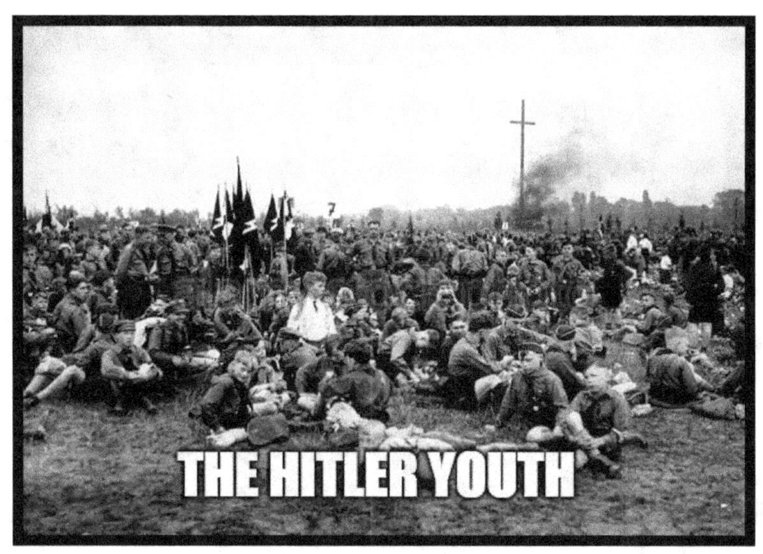

SAME =

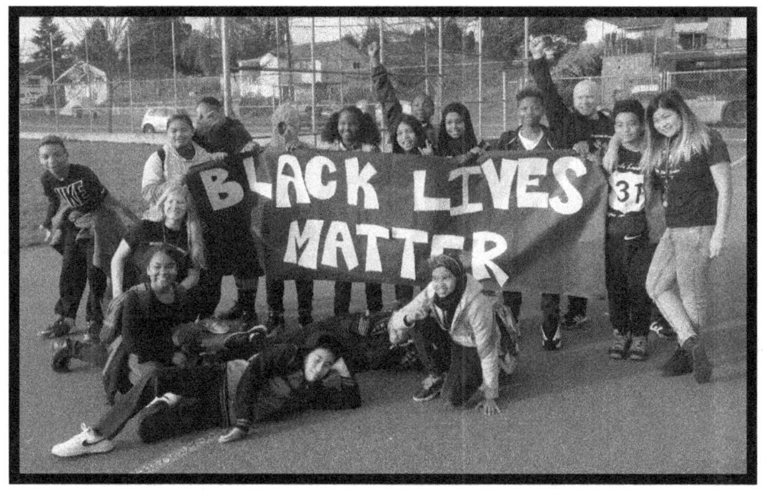

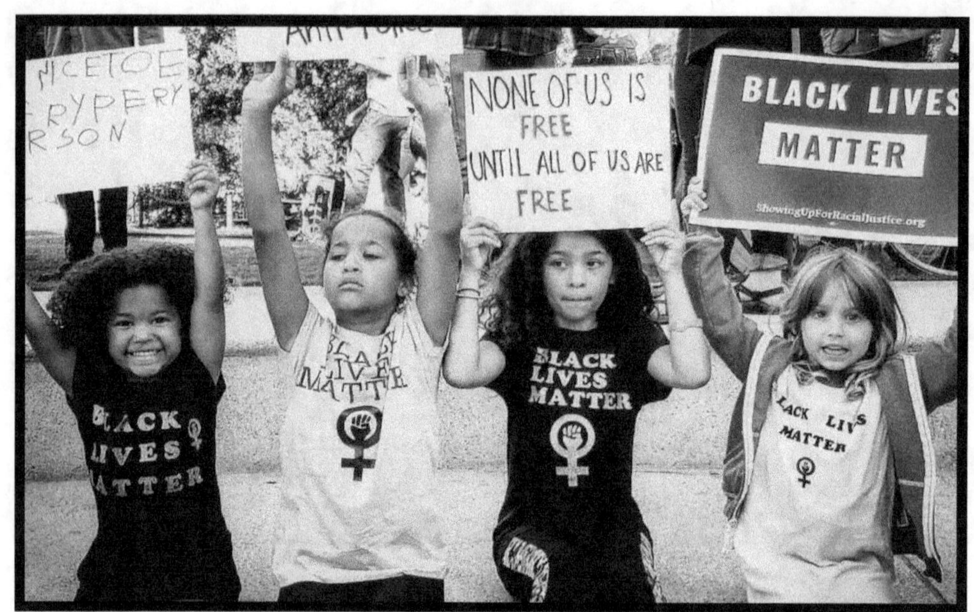
ANTI POLICE
NONE OF US IS
FREE
UNTIL ALL OF US ARE
FREE
BLACK LIVES
MATTER
ShowingUpForRacialJustice.org
BLACK
LIVES
MATTER
BLACK
LIVES
MATTER
BLACK
LIVES
MATTER
LACK LIVS
MATTER

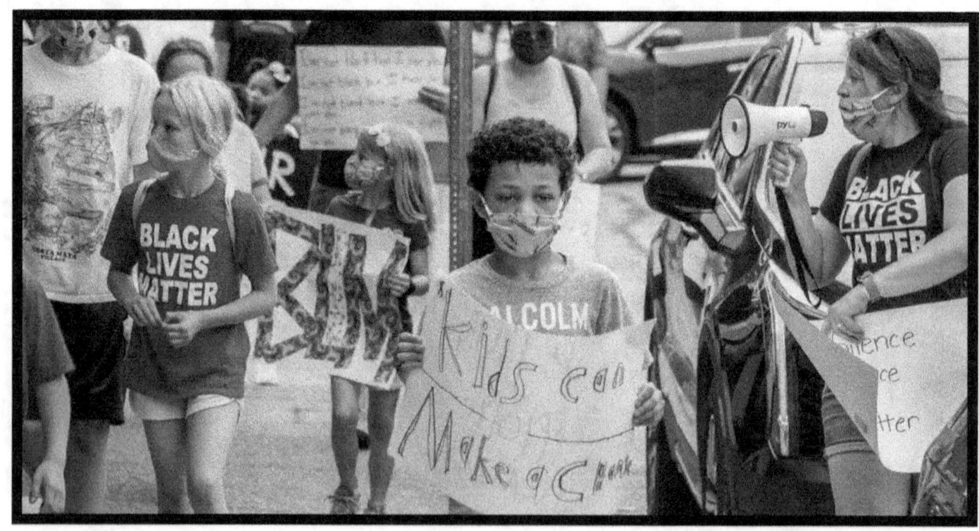
BLACK
LIVES
MATTER
BLACK
LIVES
ATTER
MALCOLM
Kids can
Make a Change

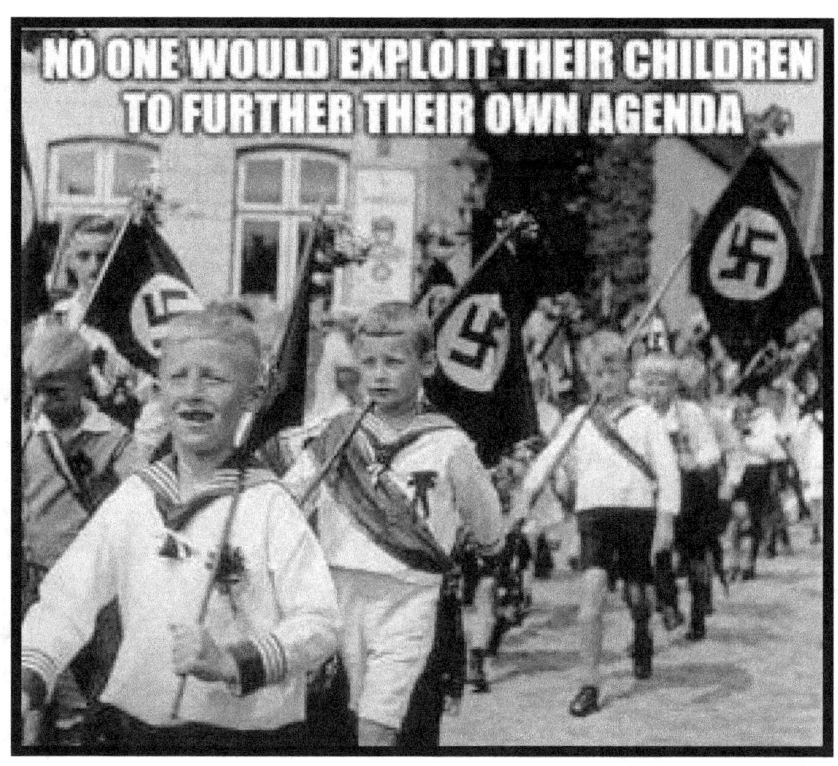

NO ONE WOULD EXPLOIT THEIR CHILDREN
TO FURTHER THEIR OWN AGENDA

Drag queen with demon-like horns reads to children at Michelle Obama Neighborhood Library

DAVE URBANSKI | October 17, 2017

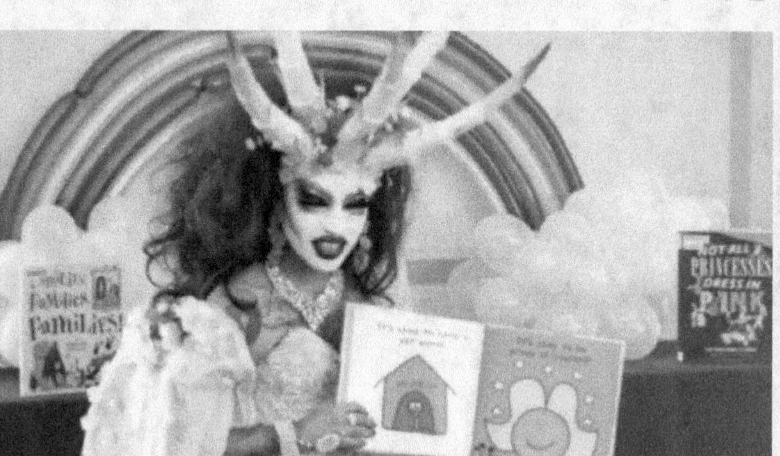

I wear a mask to protect you from the virus
I refuse to wear a mask, in order to protect you from tyranny and stupidity.
THE COVID PANDEMIC IS A HOAX

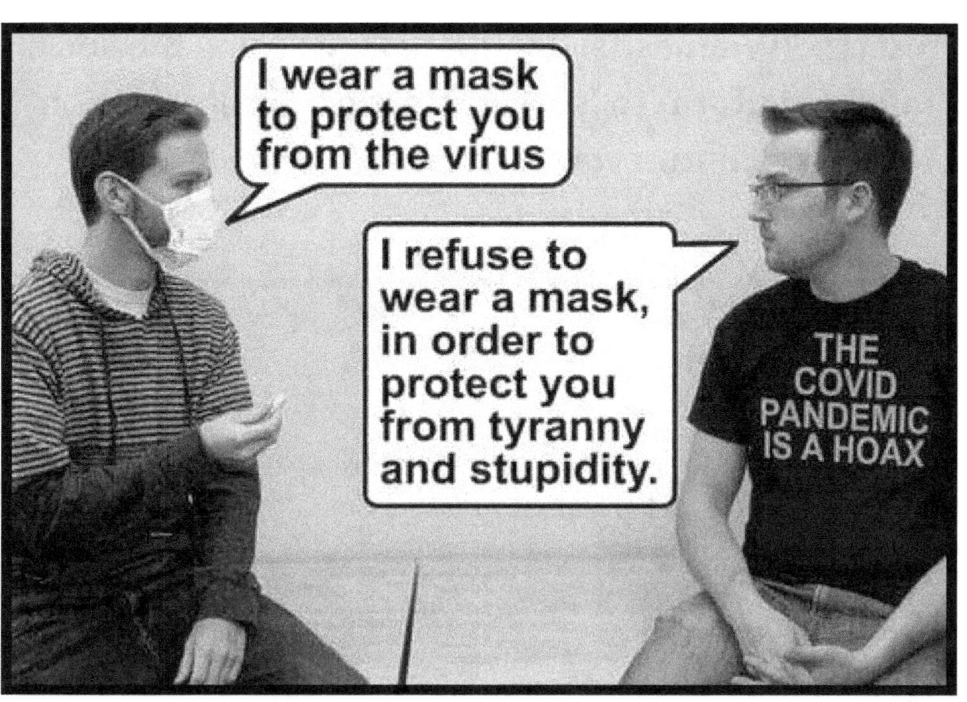

114

"A pro-Trump meme maker and Twitter troll was indicted Wednesday by the feds for using the social media platform to 'spread election disinformation' to Hillary Clinton voters in 2016."

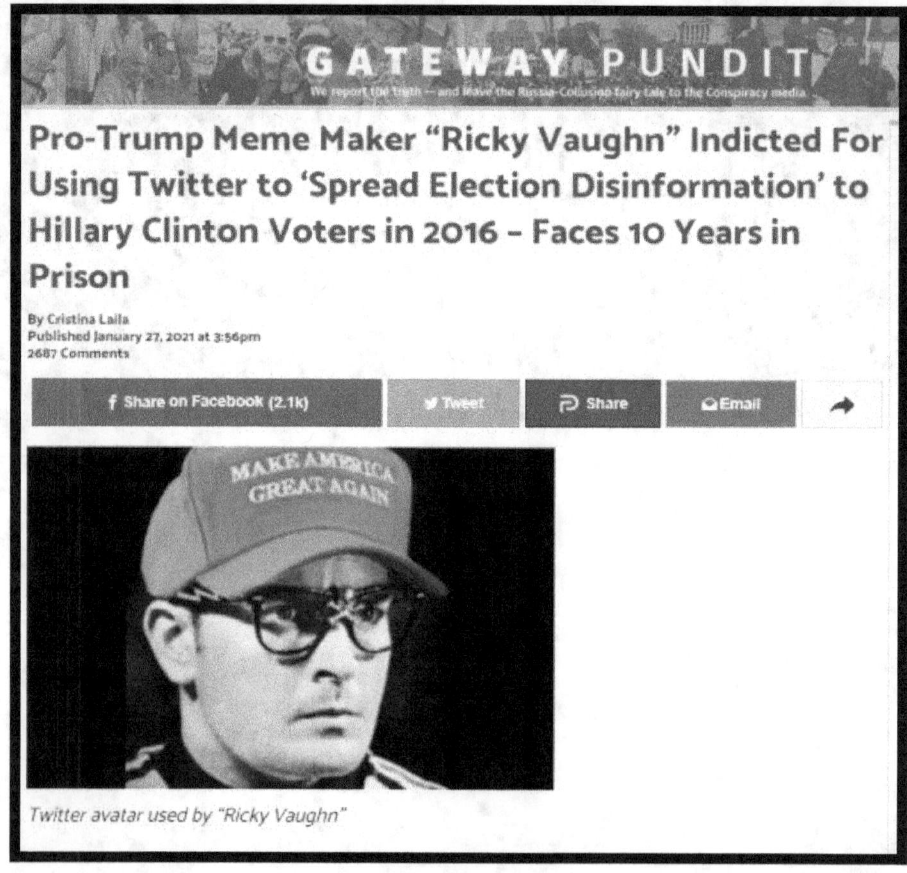

GATEWAY PUNDIT
We report the truth -- and leave the Russia-Collusion fairy tale to the Conspiracy media

Pro-Trump Meme Maker "Ricky Vaughn" Indicted For Using Twitter to 'Spread Election Disinformation' to Hillary Clinton Voters in 2016 – Faces 10 Years in Prison

By Cristina Laila
Published January 27, 2021 at 3:56pm
2687 Comments

f Share on Facebook (2.1k)   🐦 Tweet   ⮂ Share   ✉ Email

Twitter avatar used by "Ricky Vaughn"

"'Ricky Vaughn' AKA, Douglass Mackey, used Twitter to post memes and troll Hillary Clinton during the 2016 presidential election cycle.

"31-year-old Mackey was arrested in West Palm Beach on one charge of conspiracy against rights and **faces up to 10 years in prison.**"

WHO ELSE COMMITTED "ELECTION INTERFERENCE" BY USE OF MEDIA?

THE "MAINSTREAM MEDIA" – "THE RUSSIAN COLLUSION HOAX" – THE 2018 ELECTION

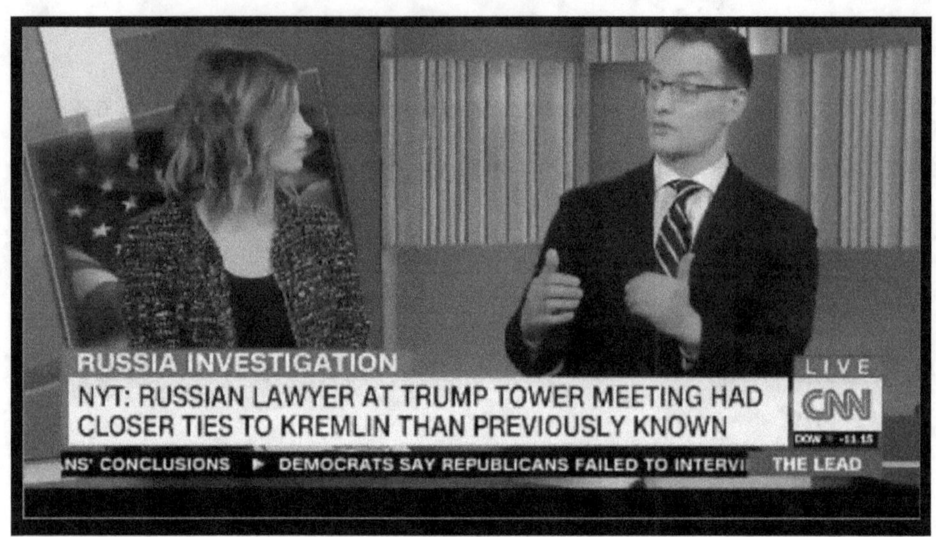

RUSSIA INVESTIGATION
NYT: RUSSIAN LAWYER AT TRUMP TOWER MEETING HAD
CLOSER TIES TO KREMLIN THAN PREVIOUSLY KNOWN
LIVE
CNN
NS' CONCLUSIONS   DEMOCRATS SAY REPUBLICANS FAILED TO INTERVI   THE LEAD

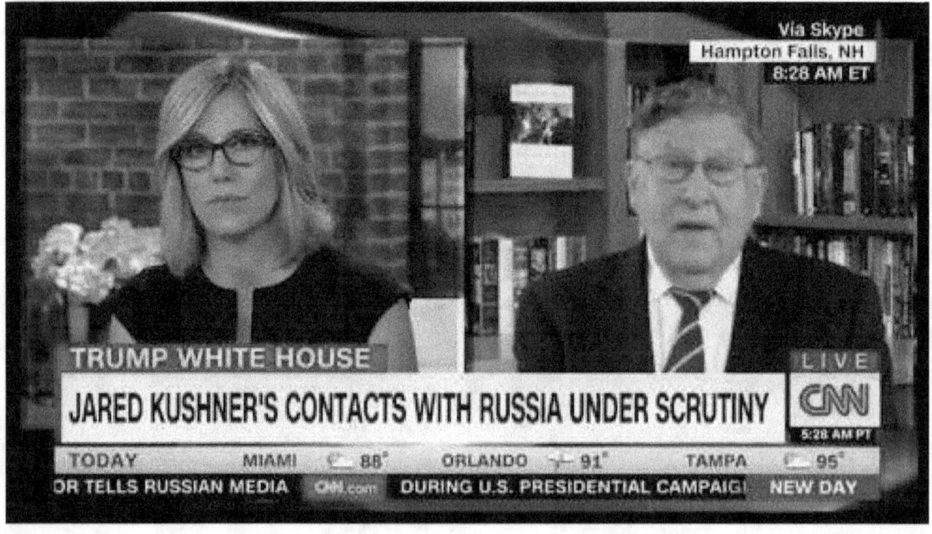

Via Skype
Hampton Falls, NH
8:28 AM ET
TRUMP WHITE HOUSE
JARED KUSHNER'S CONTACTS WITH RUSSIA UNDER SCRUTINY
LIVE
CNN
5:28 AM PT
TODAY   MIAMI   88°   ORLANDO   91°   TAMPA   95°
OR TELLS RUSSIAN MEDIA   CNN.com   DURING U.S. PRESIDENTIAL CAMPAIG   NEW DAY

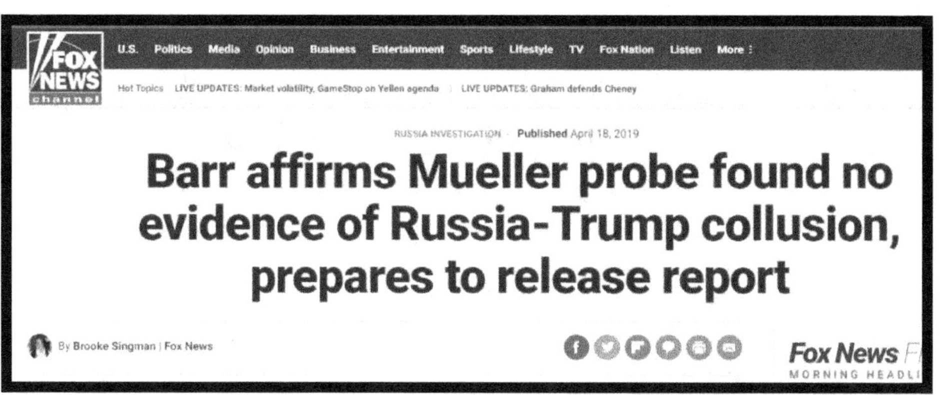

FOX NEWS channel
U.S.   Politics   Media   Opinion   Business   Entertainment   Sports   Lifestyle   TV   Fox Nation   Listen   More
Hot Topics   LIVE UPDATES: Market volatility, GameStop on Yellen agenda   LIVE UPDATES: Graham defends Cheney
RUSSIA INVESTIGATION · Published April 18, 2019
Barr affirms Mueller probe found no evidence of Russia-Trump collusion, prepares to release report
By Brooke Singman | Fox News
Fox News
MORNING HEADLI

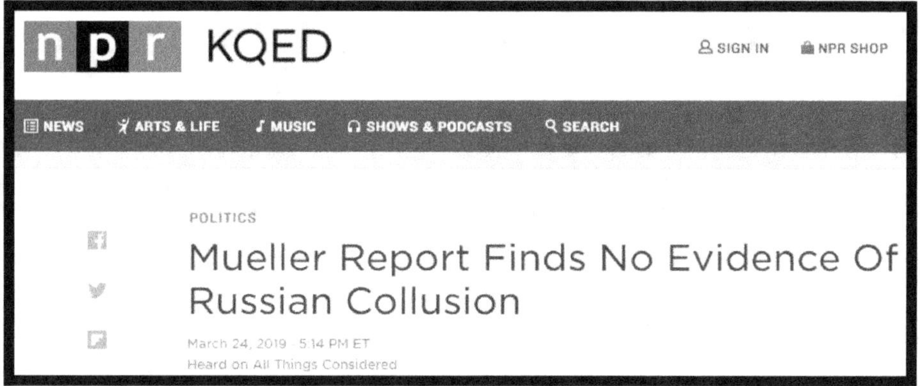

npr   KQED
SIGN IN   NPR SHOP
NEWS   ARTS & LIFE   MUSIC   SHOWS & PODCASTS   SEARCH
POLITICS
Mueller Report Finds No Evidence Of Russian Collusion
March 24, 2019 · 5:14 PM ET
Heard on All Things Considered

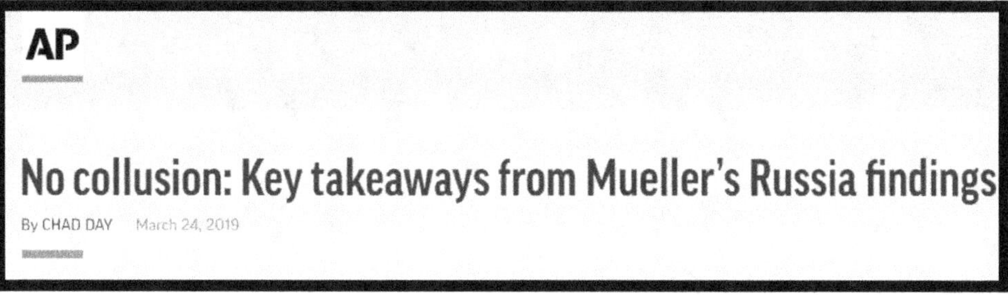

AP
No collusion: Key takeaways from Mueller's Russia findings
By CHAD DAY   March 24, 2019

THE "BLACK LIVES MATTER" PARAMILITARY ORGANIZATION IS MOTIVATED BY POLITICAL REASONS AND ARE NOT *ACTUALLY* FIGHTING FOR RACIAL JUSTICE AS THEY FALSELY CLAIM?

IS NOTHING SACRED?

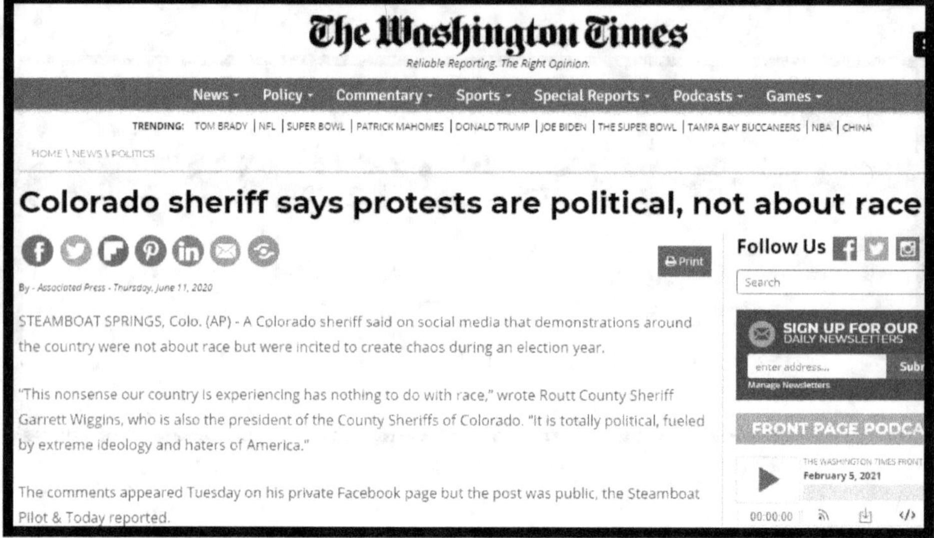

The Washington Times

Reliable Reporting. The Right Opinion.

News ▾   Policy ▾   Commentary ▾   Sports ▾   Special Reports ▾   Podcasts ▾   Games ▾

TRENDING: TOM BRADY | NFL | SUPER BOWL | PATRICK MAHOMES | DONALD TRUMP | JOE BIDEN | THE SUPER BOWL | TAMPA BAY BUCCANEERS | NBA | CHINA

HOME \ NEWS \ POLITICS

Colorado sheriff says protests are political, not about race

🖨 Print

Follow Us

Search

By - Associated Press - Thursday, June 11, 2020

STEAMBOAT SPRINGS, Colo. (AP) - A Colorado sheriff said on social media that demonstrations around the country were not about race but were incited to create chaos during an election year.

"This nonsense our country is experiencing has nothing to do with race," wrote Routt County Sheriff Garrett Wiggins, who is also the president of the County Sheriffs of Colorado. "It is totally political, fueled by extreme ideology and haters of America."

The comments appeared Tuesday on his private Facebook page but the post was public, the Steamboat Pilot & Today reported.

SIGN UP FOR OUR DAILY NEWSLETTERS

enter address...   Subr

Manage Newsletters

FRONT PAGE PODCA

THE WASHINGTON TIMES FRONT
February 5, 2021

00:00:00

"STEAMBOAT SPRINGS, Colo. (AP) - A Colorado sheriff said on social media that demonstrations around the country were not about race but were incited to create chaos during an election year.

"'This nonsense our country is experiencing has nothing to do with race,' wrote Routt County Sheriff Garrett Wiggins, who is also the president of the County Sheriffs of Colorado. 'It is totally political, fueled by extreme ideology and haters of America.'"

IT DOES NOT MATTER IF THE OPINION IS ACCURATE OR NOT (ALTHOUGH IT CLEARLY IS) – ALL SPEECH IS PROTECTED BY THE UNITED STATES CONSTITUTION.

(OF COURSE, BESIDES THE "YELLING 'FIRE' IN A CROWDED THEATER")

REGARDLESS, "BLACK LIVES MATTER" RIOTERS HAVE DESTROYED MINORITY-OWNED BUSINESSES AND NEIGHBORHOODS, AND THEY HAVE *MURDERED* PEOPLE:

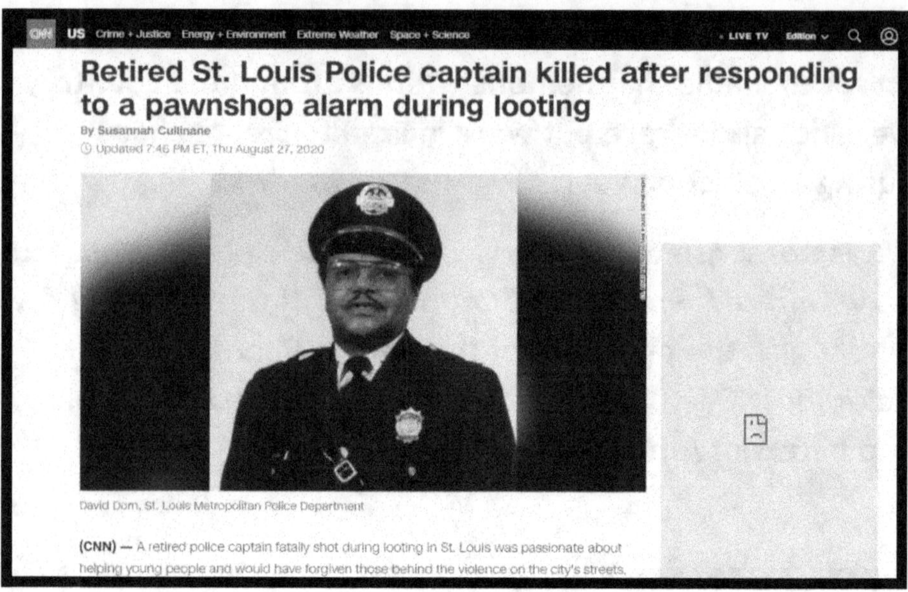

US Crime + Justice Energy + Environment Extreme Weather Space + Science
LIVE TV Edition
Retired St. Louis Police captain killed after responding to a pawnshop alarm during looting
By Susannah Cullinane
Updated 7:46 PM ET, Thu August 27, 2020
David Dorn, St. Louis Metropolitan Police Department
(CNN) — A retired police captain fatally shot during looting in St. Louis was passionate about helping young people and would have forgiven those behind the violence on the city's streets.

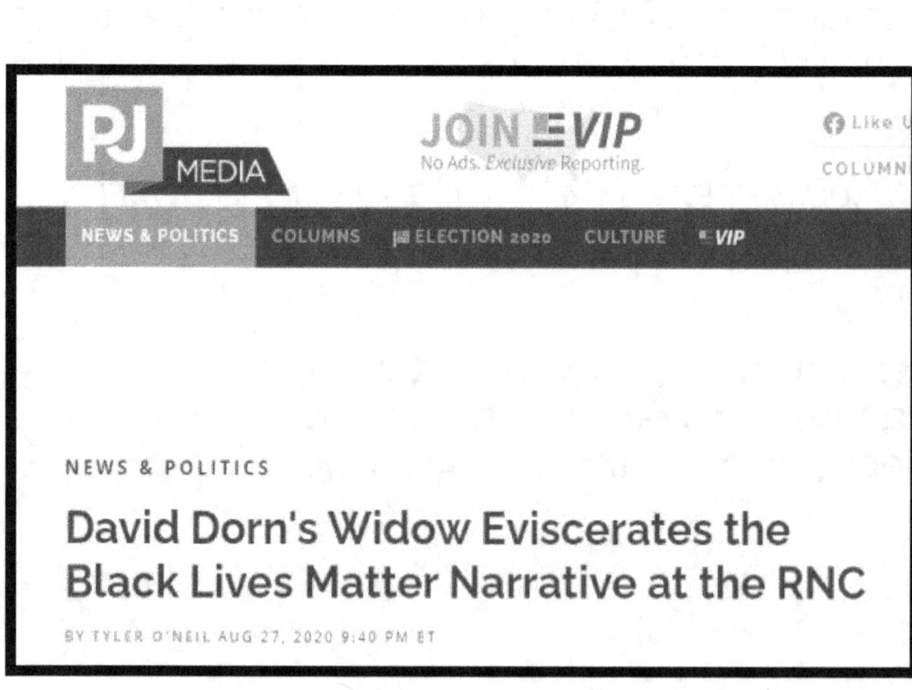

PJ MEDIA
JOIN VIP
No Ads. Exclusive Reporting.
Like
COLUMN
NEWS & POLITICS COLUMNS ELECTION 2020 CULTURE VIP
NEWS & POLITICS
David Dorn's Widow Eviscerates the Black Lives Matter Narrative at the RNC
BY TYLER O'NEIL AUG 27, 2020 9:40 PM ET

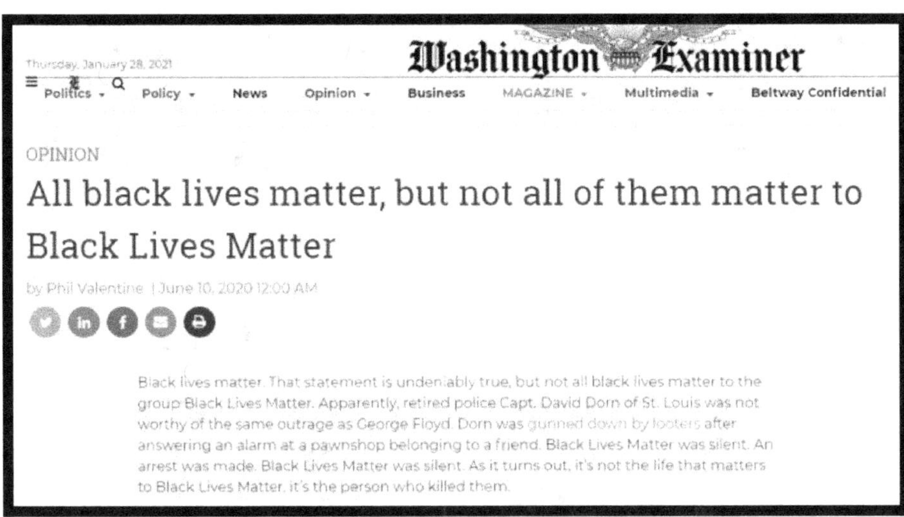

Washington Examiner

Politics ▾   Policy ▾   News   Opinion ▾   Business   MAGAZINE ▾   Multimedia ▾   Beltway Confidential

OPINION

All black lives matter, but not all of them matter to Black Lives Matter

by Phil Valentine | June 10, 2020 12:00 AM

Black lives matter. That statement is undeniably true, but not all black lives matter to the group Black Lives Matter. Apparently, retired police Capt. David Dorn of St. Louis was not worthy of the same outrage as George Floyd. Dorn was gunned down by looters after answering an alarm at a pawnshop belonging to a friend. Black Lives Matter was silent. An arrest was made. Black Lives Matter was silent. As it turns out, it's not the life that matters to Black Lives Matter, it's the person who killed them.

IT IS ESPECIALLY IMPORTANT TO RECOGNIZE THAT THERE IS NO EPIDEMIC OF POLICE BRUTALITY AGAINST BLACK PEOPLE

THE NARRATIVE EXPRESSED BY "BLACK LIVES MATTER" IS A POLITICAL LIE DRIVEN BY THE CORRUPT "MAINSTREAM MEDIA" MANIPULATING THE EMOTIONS OF INDIVIDUALS CREATING SOLIDARITY AGAINST FALSIFIED SCAPEGOATS

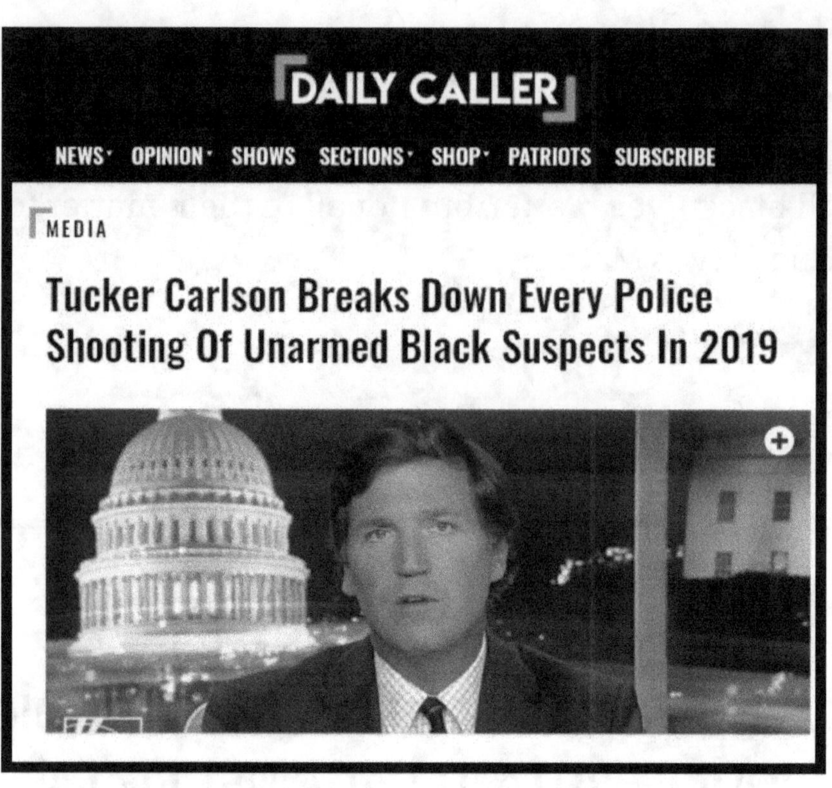

"...Tucker Carlson deconstructed the ongoing narrative of police committing "genocide" against black people by detailing the specifics of all *TEN* unarmed blacks killed by police last year."

10

TEN UNARMED BLACKS WERE KILLED BY POLICE IN 2019.

(THAT IS NOT TO SAY THAT THOSE UNFORTUNATE KILLINGS WERE UNWARRANTED)

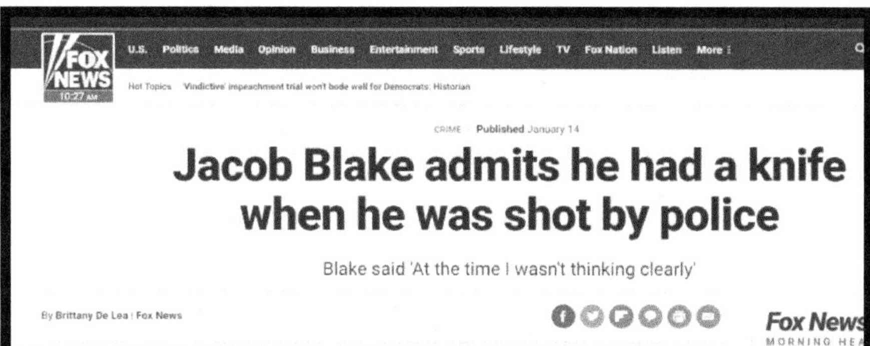

FOX NEWS
10:27 AM
U.S. Politics Media Opinion Business Entertainment Sports Lifestyle TV Fox Nation Listen More
Hot Topics 'Vindictive' impeachment trial won't bode well for Democrats: Historian
CRIME · Published January 14
Jacob Blake admits he had a knife when he was shot by police
Blake said 'At the time I wasn't thinking clearly'
By Brittany De Lea | Fox News
Fox News
MORNING HEA

Donations to Black Lives Matter Go to 'ActBlue' - The Activist Arm of the Democrat Party

By Elizabeth Vaughn | Jun 12, 2020 7:50 AM ET

Share   Tweet

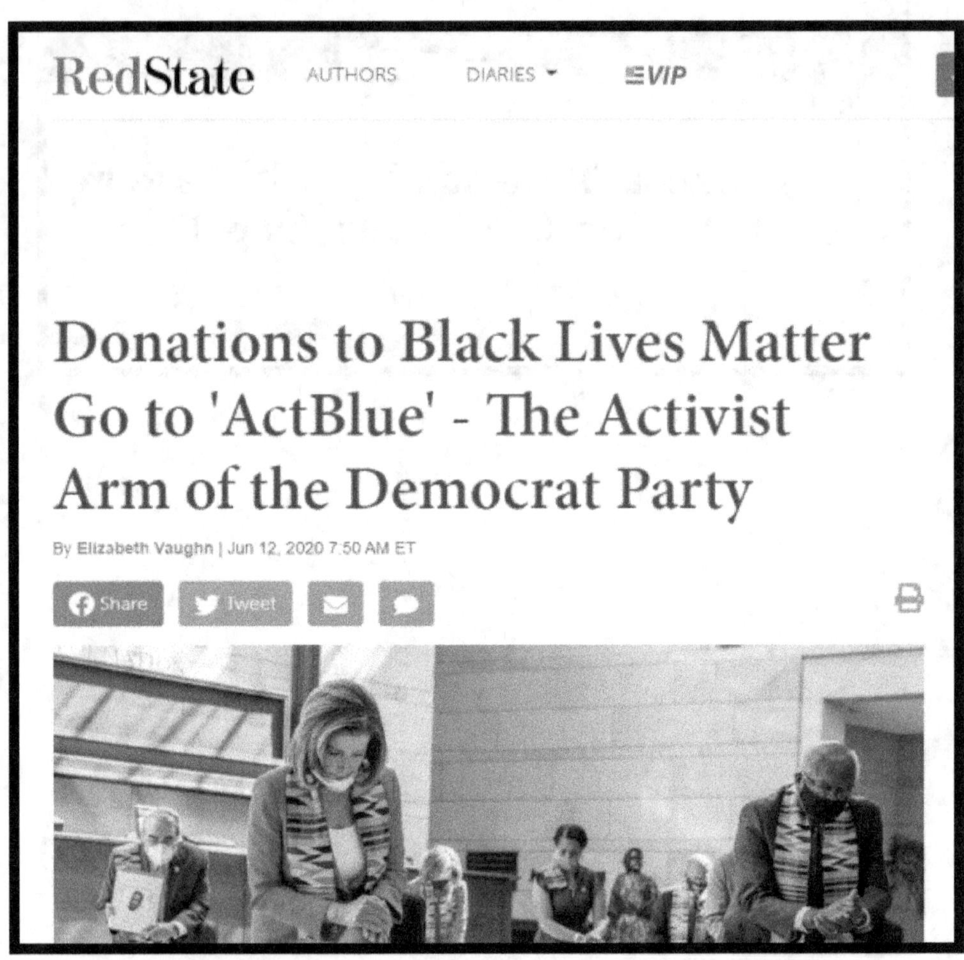

"…if a campaign or a committee doesn't cash an ActBlue check within 60 days or a contribution is refused, the donation "will be re-designated as a contribution to ActBlue."

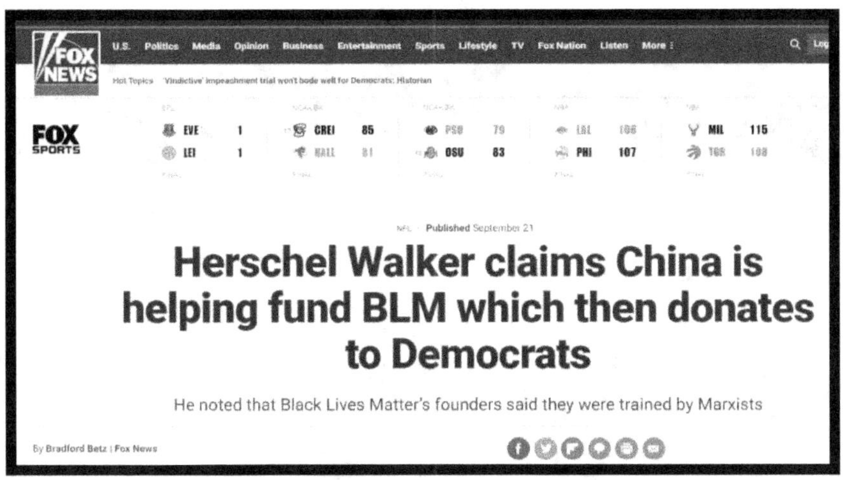

Herschel Walker claims China is helping fund BLM which then donates to Democrats

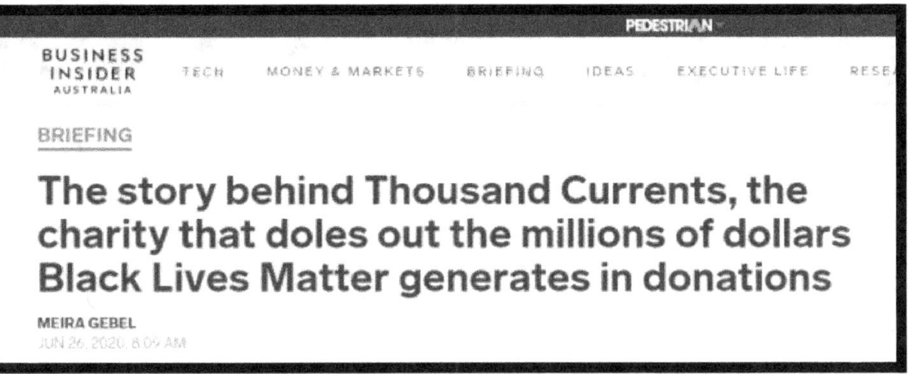

The story behind Thousand Currents, the charity that doles out the millions of dollars Black Lives Matter generates in donations

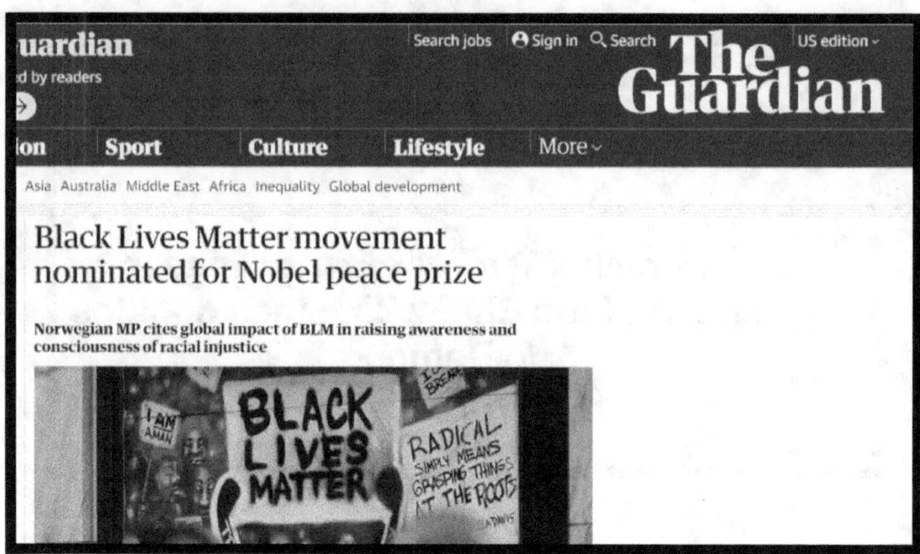
uardian
d by readers
Search jobs   Sign in   Search
The Guardian
US edition
ion   Sport   Culture   Lifestyle   More
Asia Australia Middle East Africa Inequality Global development
Black Lives Matter movement
nominated for Nobel peace prize
Norwegian MP cites global impact of BLM in raising awareness and
consciousness of racial injustice
I AM A MAN
BLACK LIVES MATTER
RADICAL
SIMPLY MEANS
GRASPING THINGS
AT THE ROOTS

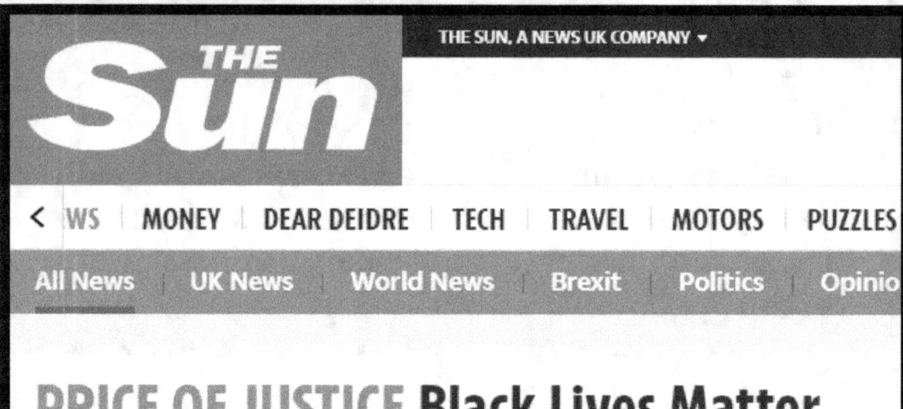
THE SUN, A NEWS UK COMPANY
THE SUN
WS   MONEY   DEAR DEIDRE   TECH   TRAVEL   MOTORS   PUZZLES
All News   UK News   World News   Brexit   Politics   Opinio
PRICE OF JUSTICE Black Lives Matter
protests and 'riots' after George
Floyd's death did as much as $2BILLION
worth of damage
Mollie Mansfield
17 Sep 2020, 16:53

Exclusive: $1 billion-plus riot damage is most expensive in insurance history

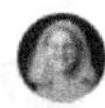 Jennifer A. Kingson

Reproduced from Insurance Information Institute; Table: Axios Visuals

The vandalism and looting following the death of George Floyd at the hands of the Minneapolis police will cost the insurance industry more than any other violent demonstrations in recent history, Axios has learned.

Why it matters: The protests that took place in 140 U.S. cities this spring were mostly peaceful, but the arson, vandalism and looting that did occur will result in at least $1 billion to $2 billion of paid insurance claims — eclipsing the record set in Los Angeles in 1992 after the acquittal of the police officers who brutalized Rodney King.

"The protests that took place in 140 U.S. cities this spring were mostly peaceful, but the arson, vandalism and looting that did occur will result in at least $1 billion to $2 billion of paid insurance claims..."

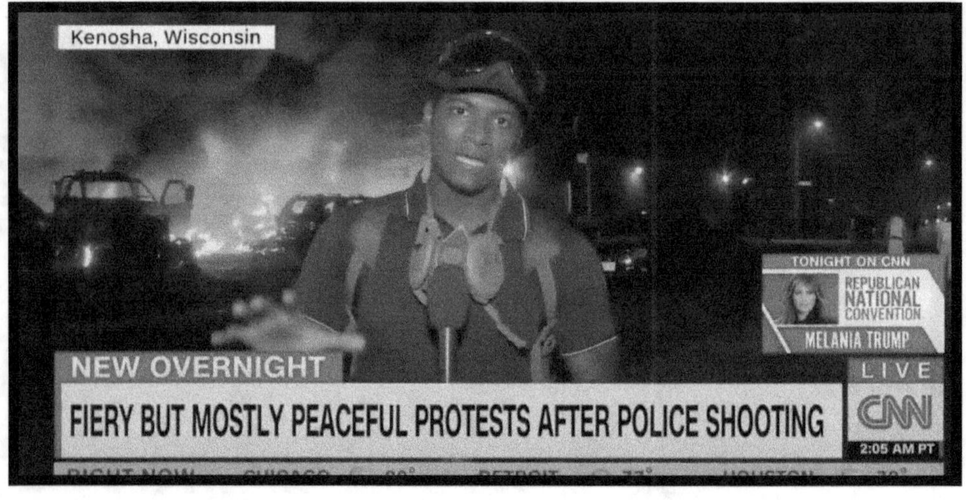

*"**Revolver News** drew attention to the ominous similarities between the strategies and tactics the United States government employs in so-called **'Color Revolutions'** and the coordinated efforts of government bureaucrats, NGOs, and the media to oust President Trump."*

"A 'Color Revolution' in this context refers to a specific type of coordinated attack that the United States government has been known to deploy against foreign regimes, particularly in Eastern Europe deemed to be 'authoritarian' and hostile to American interests. Rather than using a direct military intervention to effect regime change as in Iraq, ***Color Revolutions attack a foreign regime by contesting its electoral legitimacy, organizing mass protests and acts of civil disobedience, and leveraging media contacts to ensure favorable coverage to their agenda***..."

revolver

← Front page / Exclusive

Transition Integrity Project: Is this Soros Linked Group Plotting a "Color Revolution" Against President Trump?

September 4, 2020 (5mo ago)   💬 73

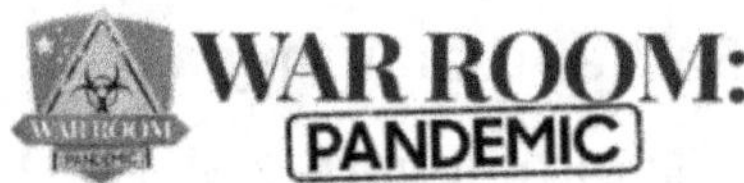

LISTEN LIVE   HOME   PODCAST ⌄   SHOW NOTES   NEWSROOM   MEDIA   TIMELINE   ▶ AGGREGATOR   ▶▶▶ JOIN

Raheem Kassam: Transition Integrity Project Linked to George Soros, Bill Gates, and the Chinese Communist Party

September 3, 2020 by Staff Writer

NO SURPRISE: The Transition "Integrity" Project Is Working to Remove President Trump from Office No Matter What – Has Connections to China, Soros, Obama and Hunter Biden

By Joe Hoft
Published September 15, 2020 at 8:48am
191 Comments

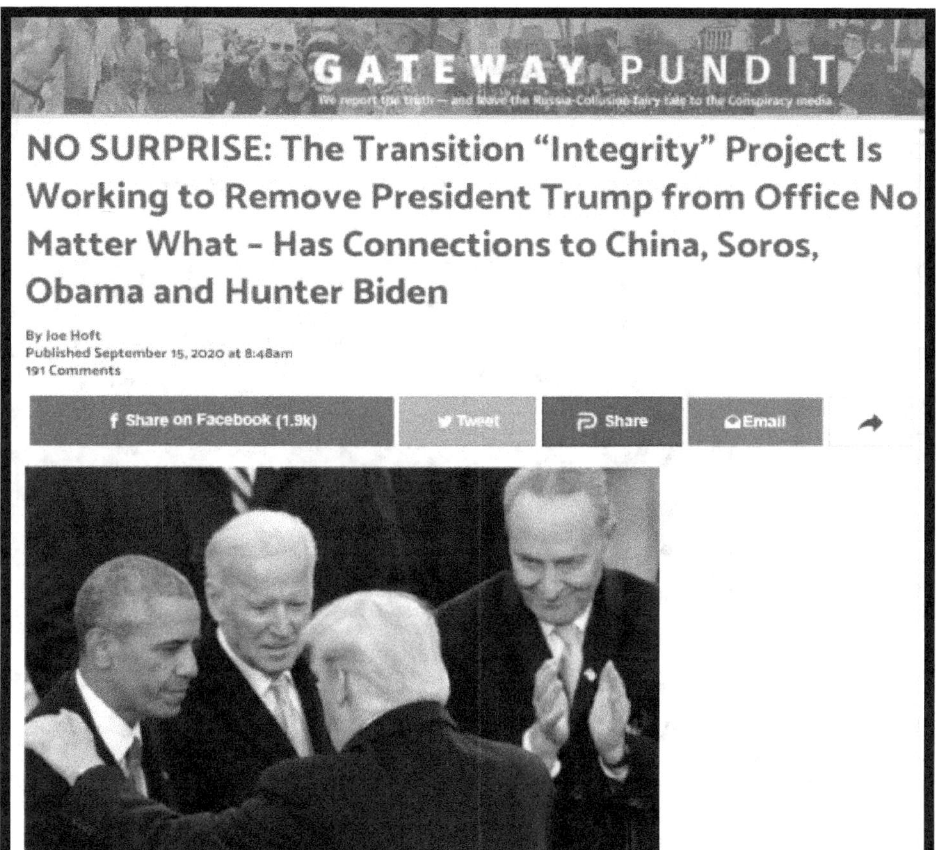

HERE IS THE MEDIA MANIPULATION:

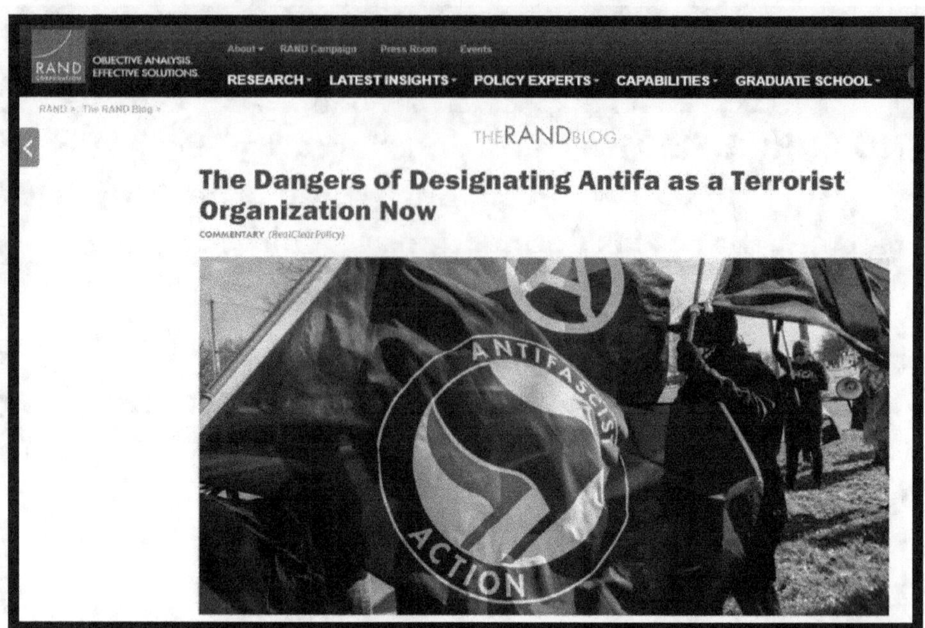

RECEIVER OF DONATION = RAND CORPORATION = RESULTING MANIPULATED MEDIA MESSAGE

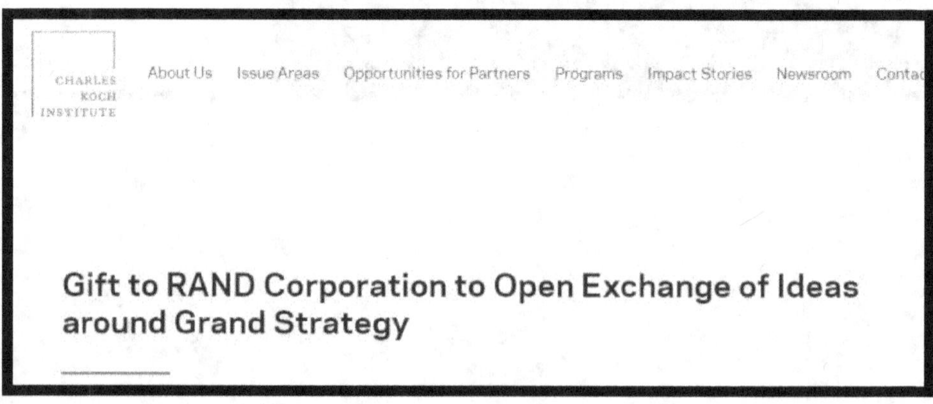

GIVER OF THE DONATION = "THE KOCH INSTITUTE,"
CERTAINLY NOT A FAN OF THE TRUMP ADMINISTRATION
(ALTHOUGH SUPPOSEDLY "REPUBLICAN")

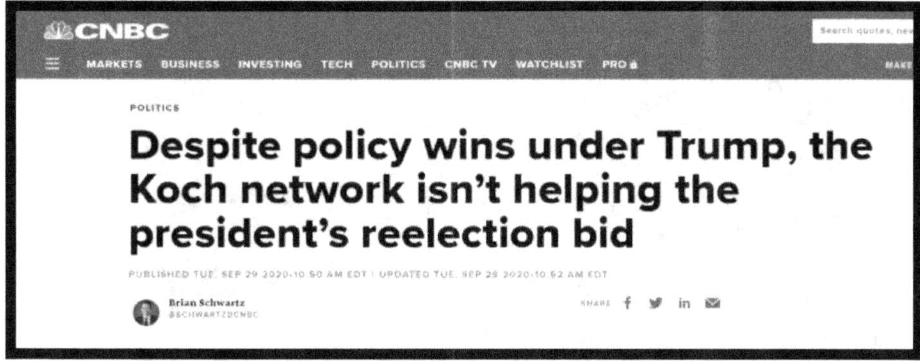

(SEE HOW IT WORKS?)

PLEASE OBSERVE THE FOLLOWING FRAUD PUBLISHED IN THE
HEADLINES OF THE "MAINSTREAM MEDIA"

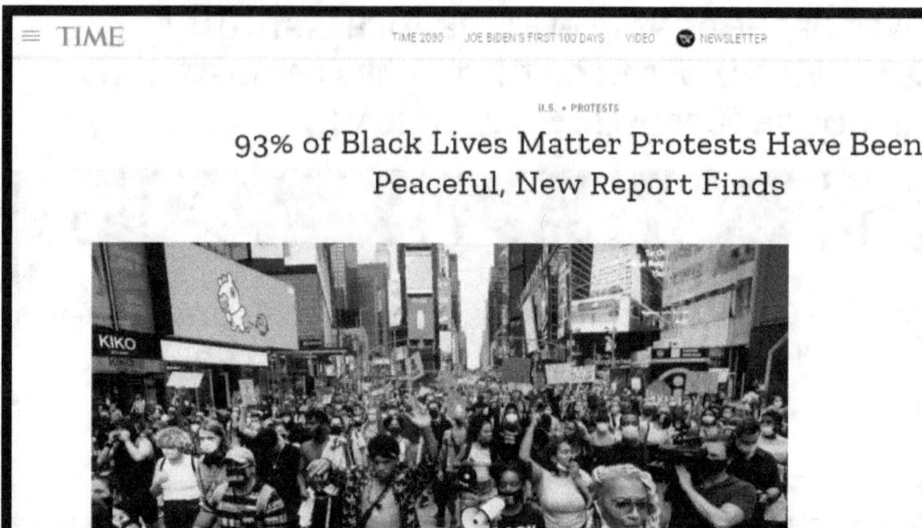

93% of Black Lives Matter Protests Have Been Peaceful, New Report Finds

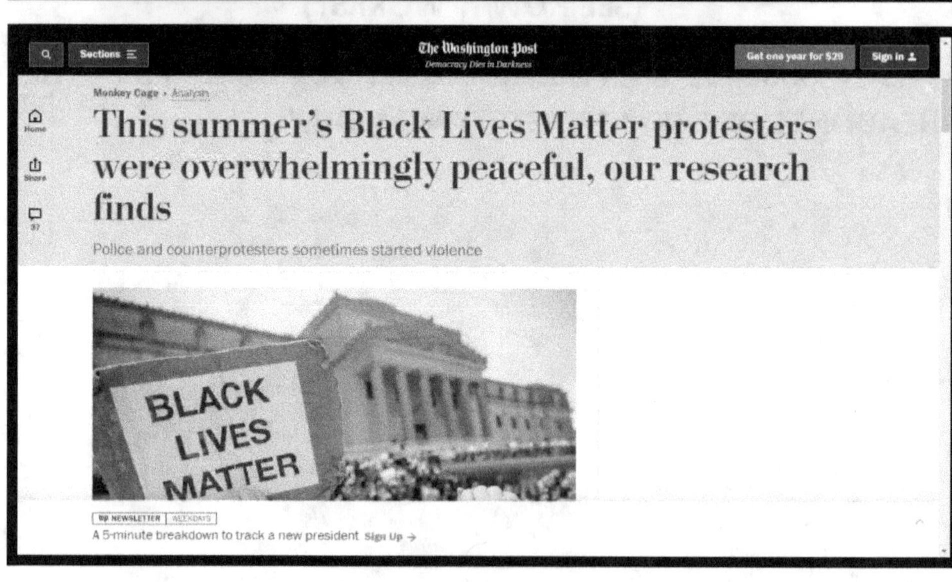

This summer's Black Lives Matter protesters were overwhelmingly peaceful, our research finds

Police and counterprotesters sometimes started violence

HOWEVER, THE REALITY OF THESE GROUPS ARE ALL THE SAME, DOMESTIC MILITARIZED INSURGENTS INCLUDING "BLACK LIVES MATTER" AND "ANTIFA" AND "THE WEATHERMEN" AND THE MILITANT GERMAN COMMUNIST GROUP **"Antifaschistische Aktion"** – SOUND FAMILIAR?

–

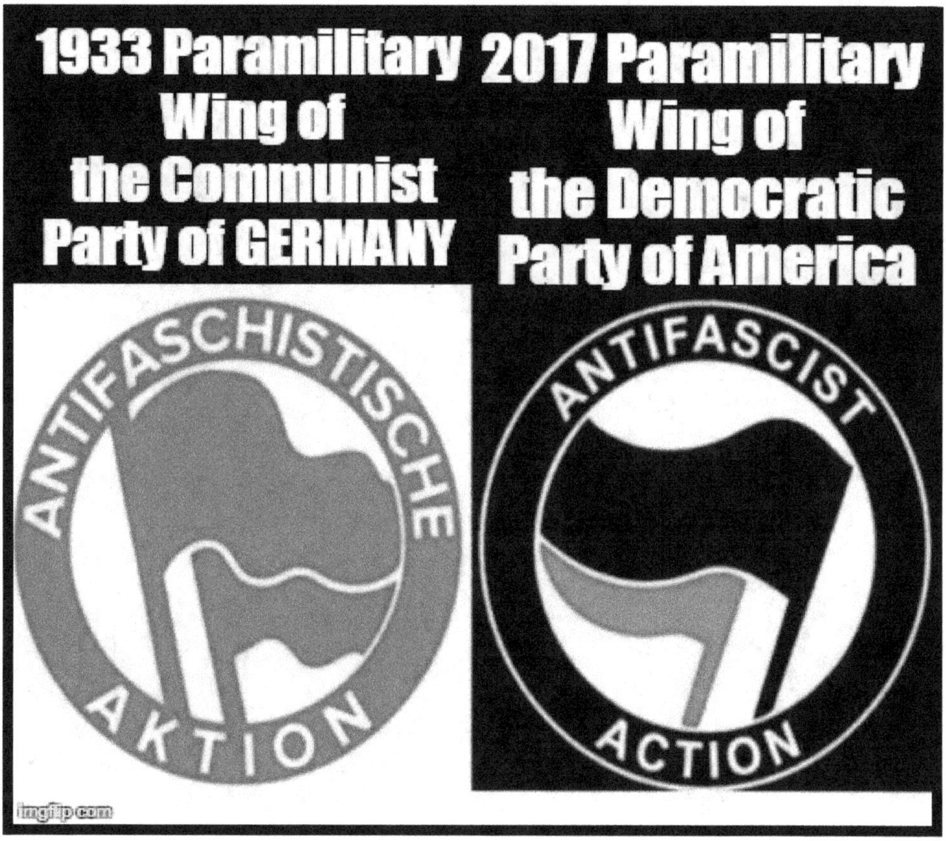

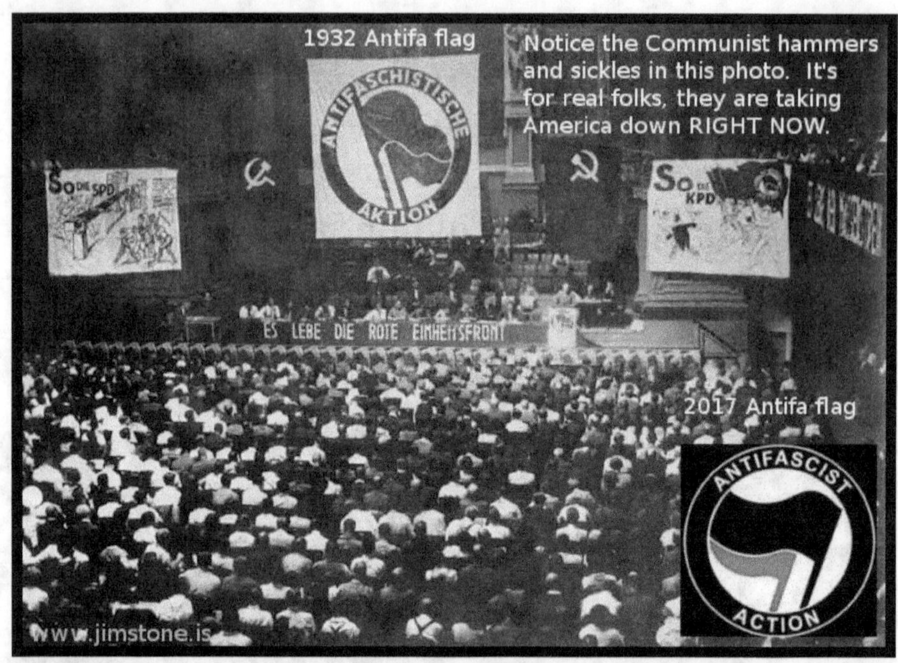

1932 Antifa flag
Notice the Communist hammers and sickles in this photo. It's for real folks, they are taking America down RIGHT NOW.
ANTIFASCHISTISCHE AKTION
So DIE SPD
So DIE KPD
ES LEBE DIE ROTE EINHEITSFRONT
2017 Antifa flag
ANTIFASCIST ACTION
www.jimstone.is

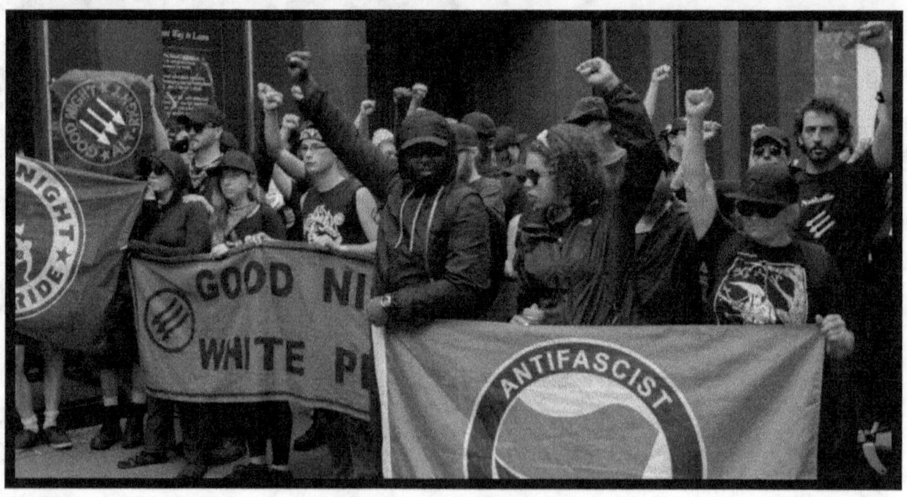

GOOD NIGHT
WHITE P
GOOD NIGHT PRIDE
ANTIFASCIST

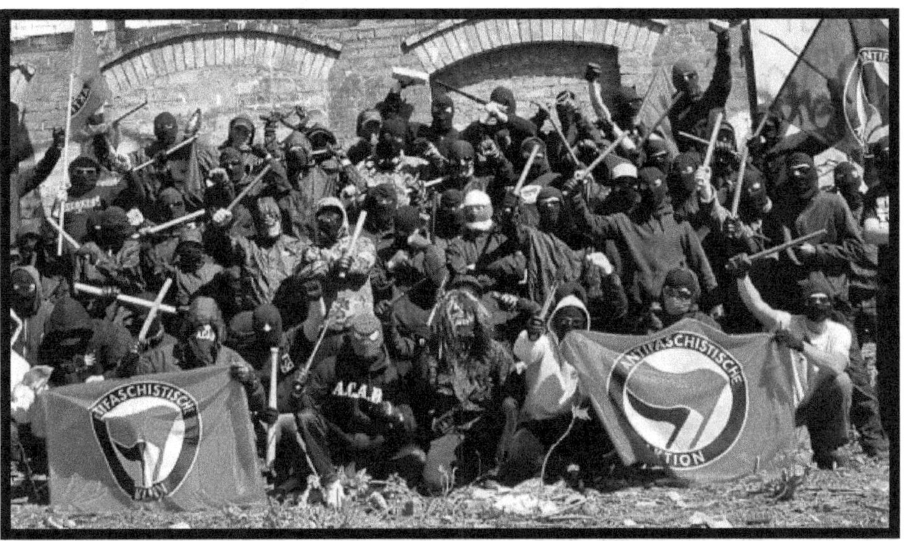

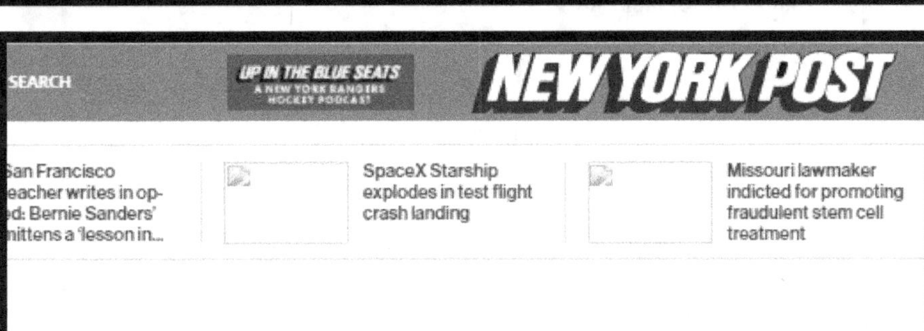

Two known Antifa members posed as pro-Trump to infiltrate Capitol riot: sources

By Larry Celona

January 7, 2021 | 12:40am | Updated

Townhall COLUMNISTS TIPSHEET CARTOONS PODCASTS 2020 Election VIP SECTIONS SITES JOIN VIP LOGIN

Townhall · Tipsheet · Katie Pavlich VIOLENCE

Report: Armed Antifa Members Violently Took Over a Hotel

Katie Pavlich | @KatiePavlich | Posted: Feb 01, 2021 3:30 PM

Share Tweet

CHANNEL 411 NEWS
RIGHT NEWS, RIGHT NOW

US News World News Weird & Bizarre Politics Sports Entertainment Business

Horoscope Weather Special Offers Uncategorized

Home / Antifa activists take over hotel near Seattle as owner begs authorities for help

US News December 30, 2020

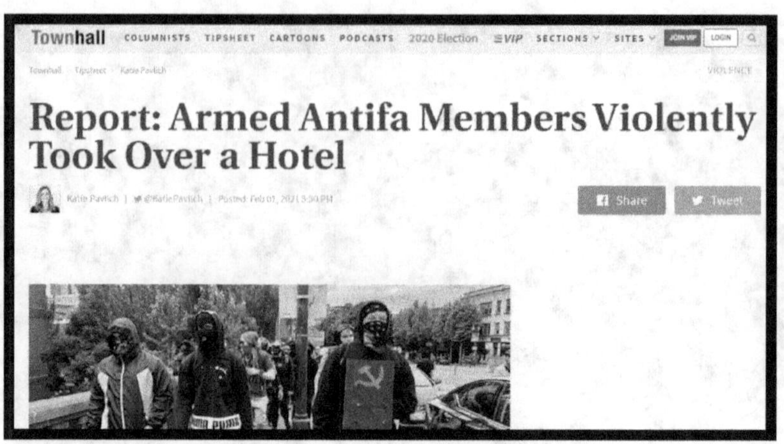

Antifa activists take over hotel near Seattle as owner begs authorities for help

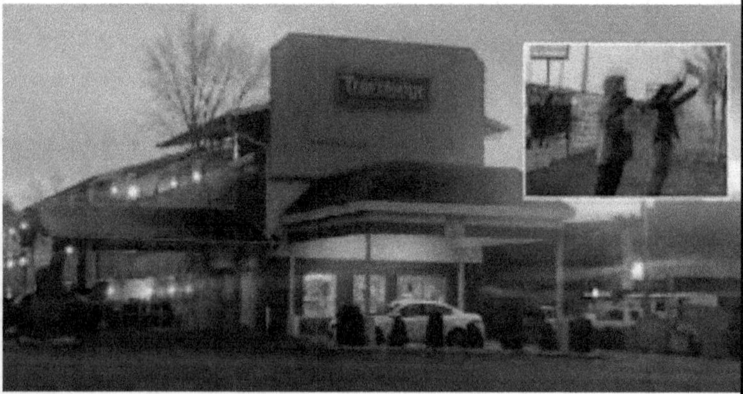

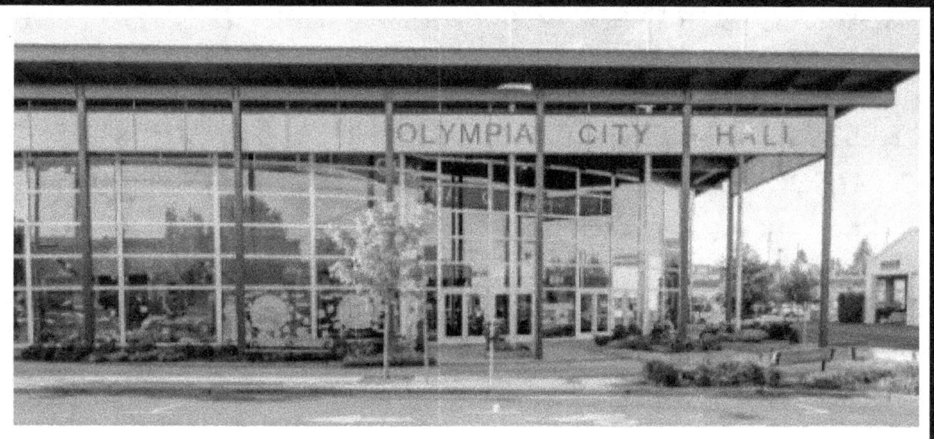

Statement on Red Lion Occupation

The Olympia Police Department (OPD) is in the process of clearing the Downtown Olympia Red Lion Hotel after it was forcibly occupied by a group identified as Oly Housing Now, a homeless activist group. Employees of the hotel have been safely escorted out of the occupied hotel after sheltering in the basement through the afternoon and part of the evening.

At about 11 a.m. today, people inside the Red Lion began calling 911 to report a group was attempting to forcibly take over the hotel. OPD received reports that the employees felt under threat from the group, and that an employee was allegedly assaulted.

Employees reported that some members of the activist group inside the hotel were armed with items such as hatchets, batons, knives and had gasmasks, helmets and goggles apparently in preparation for a confrontation. OPD estimated about 45 members of the group inside and outside of the hotel.

"BLACK LIVES MATTER" AND "ANTIFA" ARE NOT "PEACEFUL PROTEST" GROUPS

THESE ARE DOMESTIC TERRORISTS – THE COMMUNIST-CONTROLLED "MEDIA" WANTS YOU TO THINK OTHERWISE – JUST LOOK AT WHAT THEY DID:

WATCH: ANTI-POLICE PROTEST TURNS VIOLENT AFTER DARK IN ROCHESTER, NY

f   270   ✉ EMAIL   ⅂ PARLER   🐦 TWEET

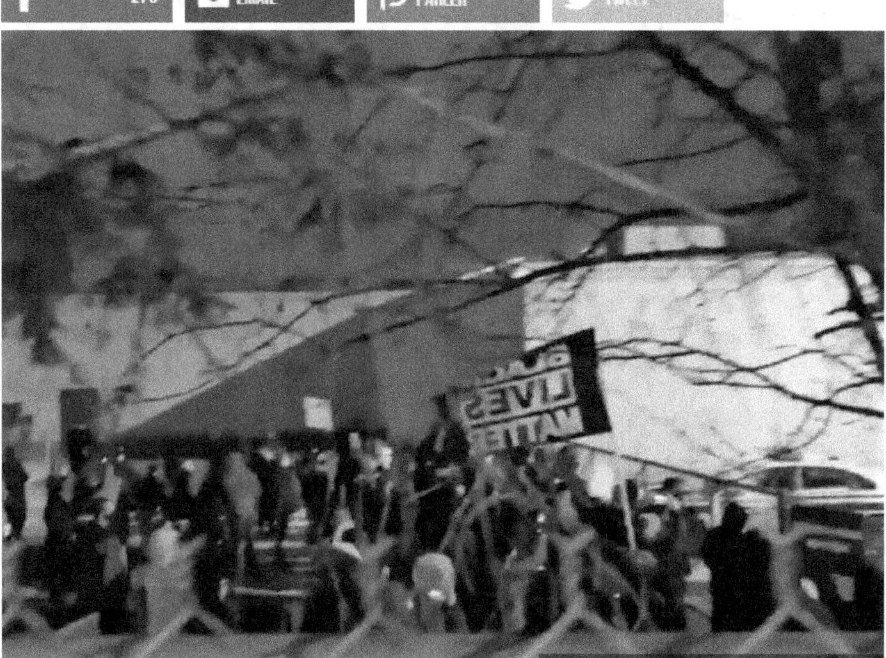

Twitter Video Screenshot/Jack Watson, News 8

by BOB PRICE | 1 Feb 2021 | 620

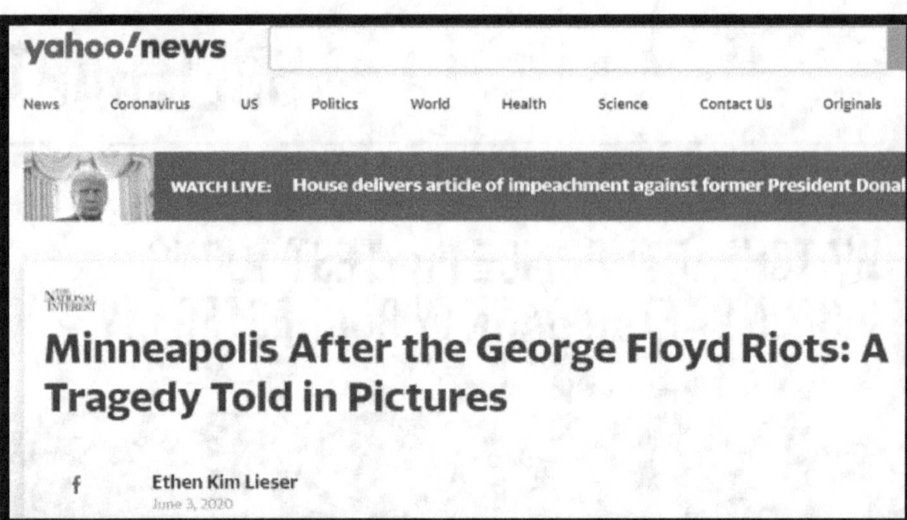

yahoo!news
News   Coronavirus   US   Politics   World   Health   Science   Contact Us   Originals
WATCH LIVE: House delivers article of impeachment against former President Donal
THE NATIONAL INTEREST
Minneapolis After the George Floyd Riots: A Tragedy Told in Pictures
f   Ethen Kim Lieser
June 3, 2020

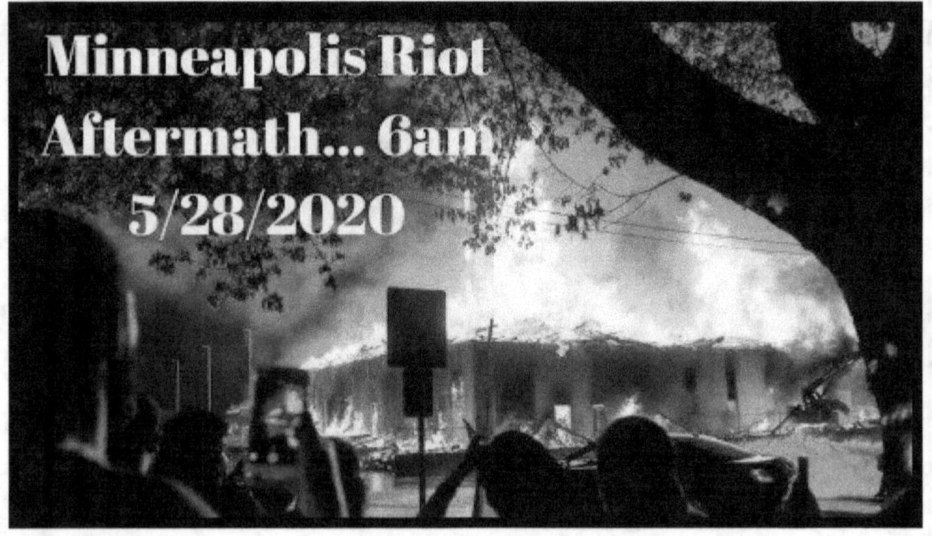

Minneapolis Riot Aftermath... 6am 5/28/2020

Home | U.K. | News | Sports | U.S. Showbiz | Australia | Femail | Health | Science | Money

Latest Headlines | Covid-19 | Royal Family | Crime | Boris Johnson | Prince Harry | World News | Headlines |

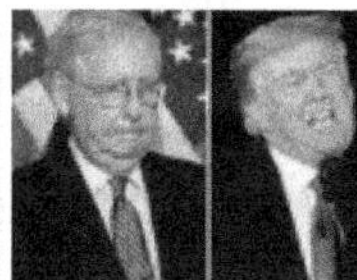

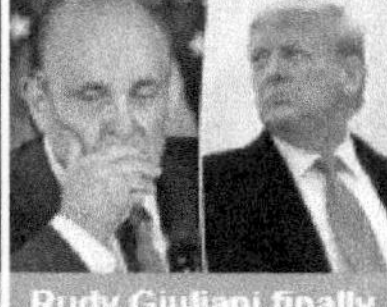

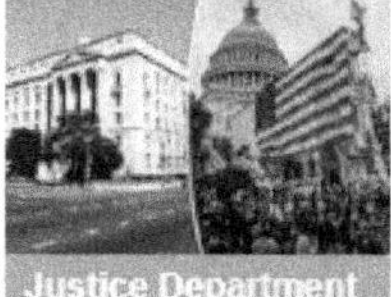

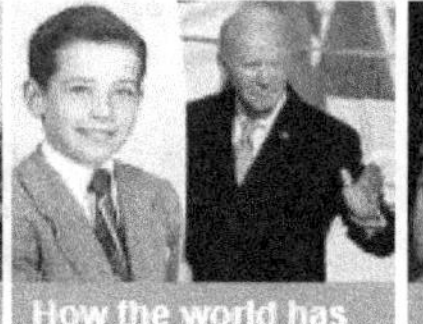

PICTURED: Portland police identify suspect, 25, behind vicious attack on truck driver who was kicked unconscious on the street when 'BLM protesters chased his vehicle' after he tried to stop a trans woman being robbed

- Police are searching for for 25-year-old Marquise Love, known by friends as 'Keese Love', for his apparent involvement in the vicious attack on Sunday
- Police say they have left Love a number of messages, urging him to hand himself in, but have so far received no response from the suspect
- The victim was trying to help a transgender woman who had some of her belongings stolen at the scene
- The incident took place before 10:30pm Sunday, just blocks away from a Black Lives Matter demonstration outside of the federal courthouse
- Police received a 911 call from a bystander who reported that a group of

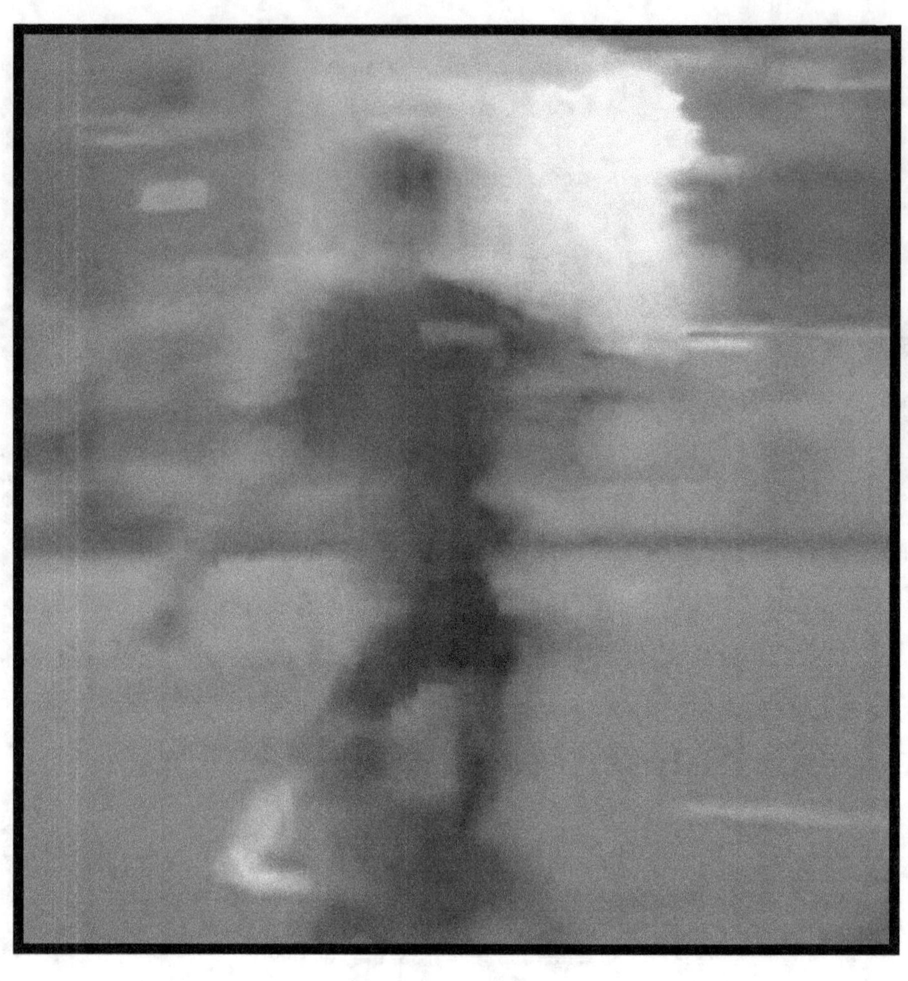

Portland police identify man suspected of assaulting driver during Black Lives Matter protest

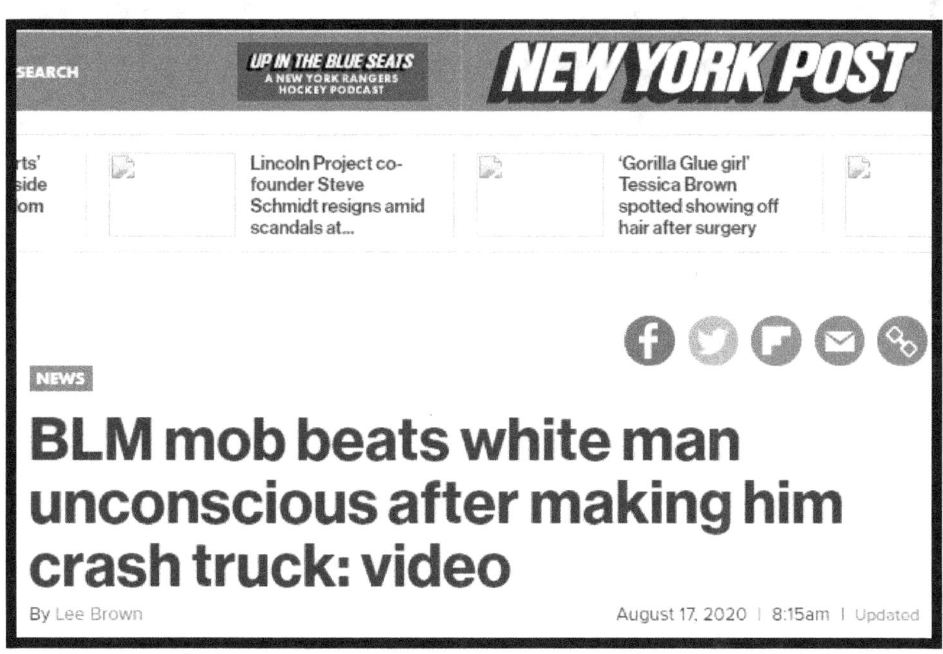

BLM mob beats white man unconscious after making him crash truck: video

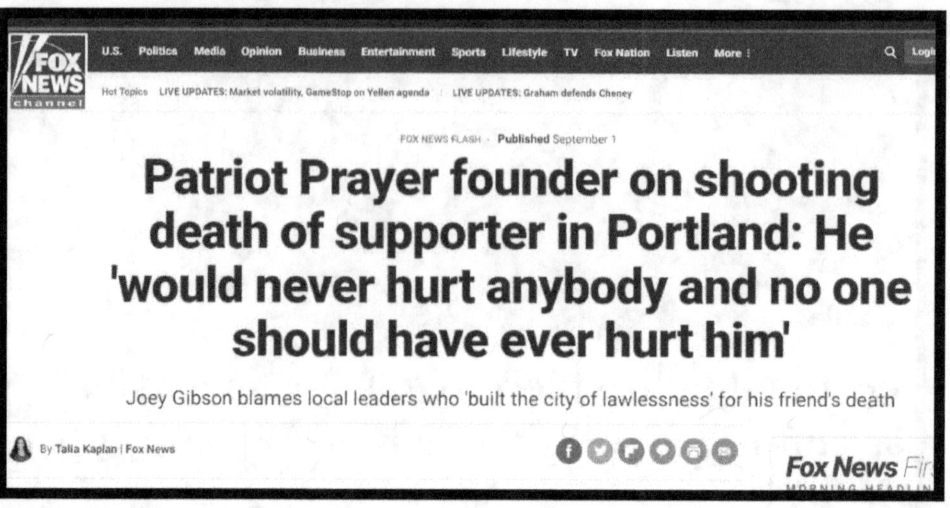

FOX NEWS
channel
U.S.   Politics   Media   Opinion   Business   Entertainment   Sports   Lifestyle   TV   Fox Nation   Listen   More :
Hot Topics   LIVE UPDATES: Market volatility, GameStop on Yellen agenda   LIVE UPDATES: Graham defends Cheney
FOX NEWS FLASH · Published September 1
Patriot Prayer founder on shooting death of supporter in Portland: He 'would never hurt anybody and no one should have ever hurt him'
Joey Gibson blames local leaders who 'built the city of lawlessness' for his friend's death
By Talia Kaplan | Fox News
Fox News Fir
MORNING HEADLIN

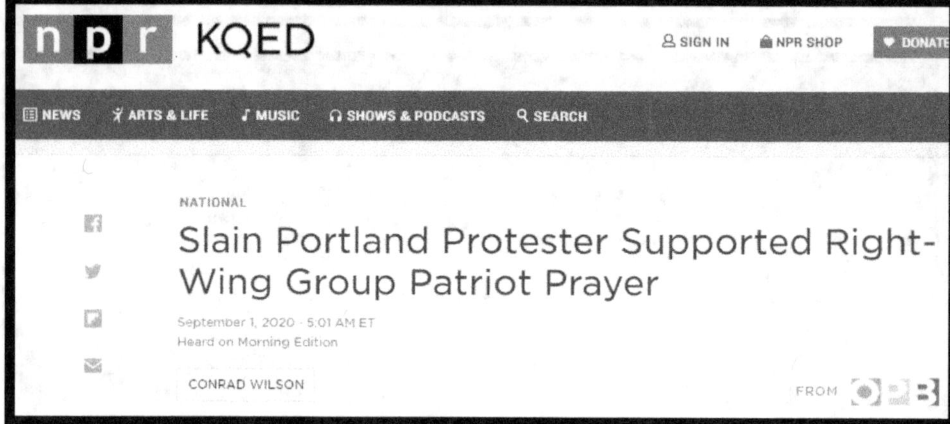

npr   KQED
SIGN IN   NPR SHOP   DONATE
NEWS   ARTS & LIFE   MUSIC   SHOWS & PODCASTS   SEARCH
NATIONAL
Slain Portland Protester Supported Right-Wing Group Patriot Prayer
September 1, 2020 · 5:01 AM ET
Heard on Morning Edition
CONRAD WILSON
FROM

Patriot Prayer is the creation of conservative activist and former Washington Senate candidate Joey Gibson, who has led protests in Portland and other cities since 2016.

The man who was fatally shot in Portland as supporters of President Trump skirmished with Black Lives Matter protesters was a supporter of right-wing Patriot Prayer, which doesn't have a big national footprint but is well known in the Pacific Northwest.

'I AM NOT SAD THAT A F*ING FASCIST DIED TONIGHT' OVERHEARD AT ANTIFA GATHERING IN PORTLAND AFTER PATRIOT PRAYER BACKER WAS SHOT TO DEATH**

The shooting victim was identified by Gibson as Aaron "Jay" Danielson of Portland. Photos taken of the body show he was wearing a Patriot Prayer hat.

"We love Jay and he had such a huge heart," Gibson wrote on Facebook on Sunday. "God bless him and the life he lived."

NEW YORK POST

Rochester cops suspended after girl pepper-sprayed

New whale species identified in Gulf of Mexico is critically endangered,...

John Durham probe largely focused on FBI: report

 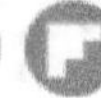 

Video captures deadly shooting of man in Patriot Prayer cap during Portland protests

By Elizabeth Rosner and Lee Brown

August 30, 2020 | 9:41am | Updated

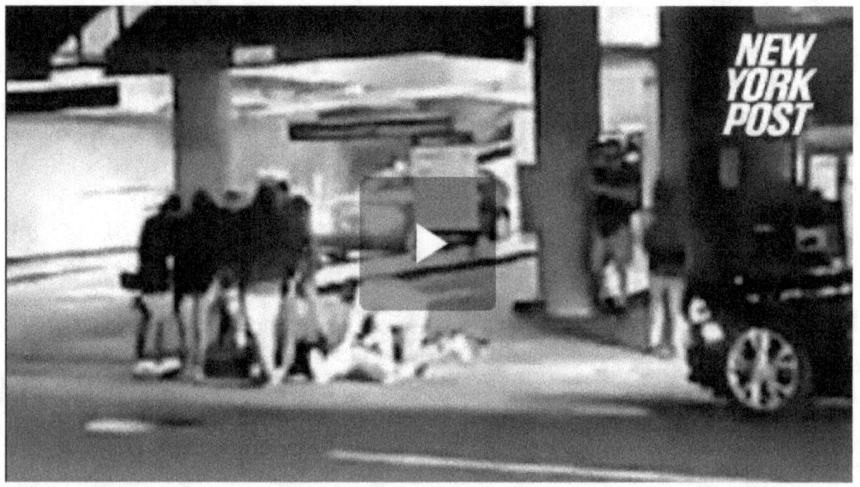

MORE ON:
PORTLAND PROTESTS

Video shows wild confrontation between

Shocking video captured the moment a man in a right-wing Patriot Prayer cap was shot dead in Portland after a day of violent clashes between President Trump supporters and Black Lives Matter protesters.

THIS IS PLAIN EVIL, AND THE INDIVIDUALS INVOLVED WITH THESE ORGANIZATIONS ARE EVIL THEMSELVES

HOW MUCH MORE EVIL IS IT TO PROVIDE PROTECTION FOR SUCH DESTRUCTIVE AND HATEFUL INDIVIDUALS?

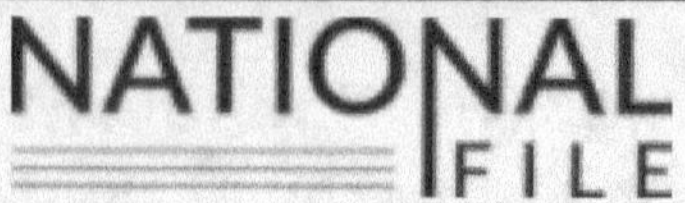

REVEALED: Anti-White, Pro-BLM Social Media Posts Of Black Woman Charged In White Child's Death After Jan 6 Capitol Protest

Ariel Robinson obsessively tweeted about white privilege, BLM, and Donald Trump days before being charged in the death of 3-year-old Victoria Rose Smith

GK *by* GABRIEL KEANE — January 25, 2021   💬 63

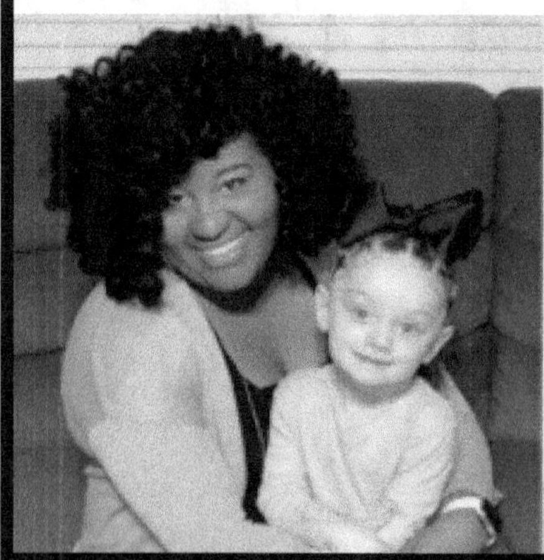
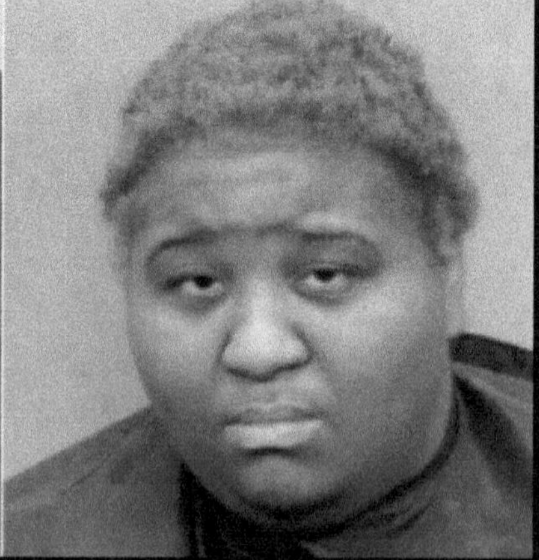

On January 20, black adoptive parents Ariel Robinson and Jerry Robinson were charged in the blunt force homicide of their adopted white daughter, 3-year-old Victoria Rose Smith. Smith's death was discovered just days after a deluge of anti-white, pro-Black Lives Matter social media posts by Ariel Robinson in response to pro-Trump protests at the Capitol on Jan. 6.

Ariel Robinson, 29, achieved a meager amount of notoriety after winning Season 20 of the Food Network show Worst Cooks In America. She leveraged that modest following to advocate for BLM and leftist politics on social media, and attempted to jumpstart a career in standup comedy.

TMZ found footage from one of Ariel Robinson's standup routines where she "jokes" about punching her children in the throat and locking them up in cages. Robinson also frequently referred to the 3-year-old Smith as a nuisance in social media posts, which frequently featured pictures of her children.

January 6's pro-Trump protests at the Capitol elicited a strong reaction from Ariel Robinson. She reposted a slew of tweets from Democrat celebrities that ranted about white privilege and praised BLM, and even wrote some political posts of her own on her @arifunnycomedy Twitter and Instagram pages.

THE COLOR BEING USED FOR THE "COLOR REVOLUTION"
STRATEGY OF THE FOREIGN-SUPPORTED ORGANIZATION
KNOWN AS "BLACK LIVES MATTER" IS OBVIOUS

"BLUE VS. RED"

"WOMEN VS. MEN"

"BLACK VS. WHITE"

WHATEVER IT TAKES TO DIVIDE AND CONQUER, AND THE
MEDIA IS COMPLICIT, ALSO SUPPORTED AND ORGANIZED BY
FOREIGN COMPANIES, INCLUDING ENEMIES TO THE PEOPLE
OF THE UNITED STATES

THESE SIX COMPANIES ARE:

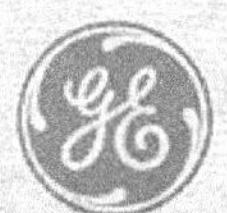
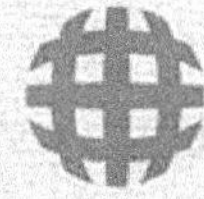
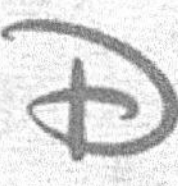
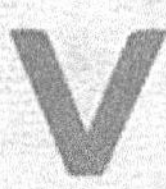
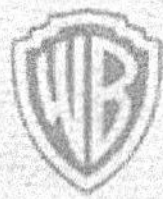
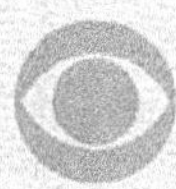

GE
Notable Properties:
COMCAST
NBC
UNIVERSAL PICTURES
FOCUS FEATURES

NEWS-CORP
Notable Properties:
FOX
WALL STREET JOURNAL
NEW YORK POST

DISNEY
Notable Properties:
ABC
ESPN
PIXAR
MIRAMAX
MARVEL STUDIOS

VIACOM
Notable Properties:
MTV
NICK JR
BET
CMT
PARAMOUNT PICTURES

TIME WARNER
Notable Properties:
CNN
HBO
TIME
WARNER BROS

CBS
Notable Properties:
SHOWTIME
SMITHSONIAN CHANNEL
NFL.COM
JEOPARDY
60 MINUTES

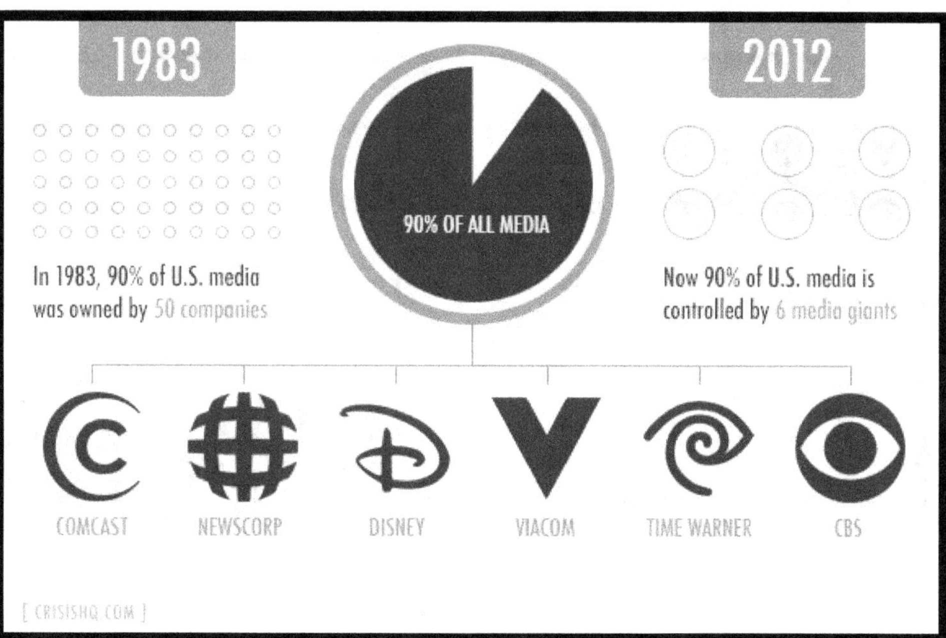
1983
2012
90% OF ALL MEDIA
In 1983, 90% of U.S. media was owned by 50 companies
Now 90% of U.S. media is controlled by 6 media giants
COMCAST
NEWSCORP
DISNEY
VIACOM
TIME WARNER
CBS
[CRISISHQ.COM]

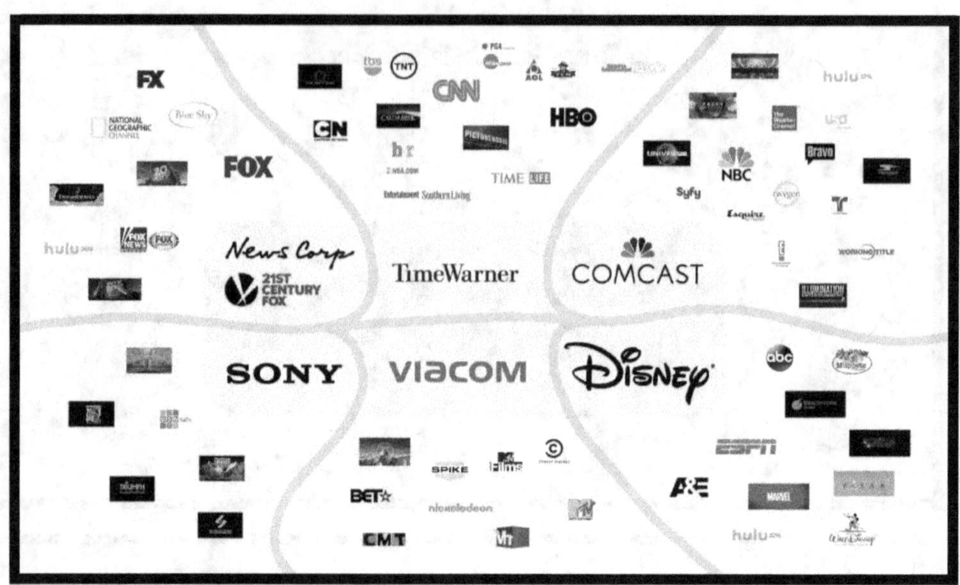

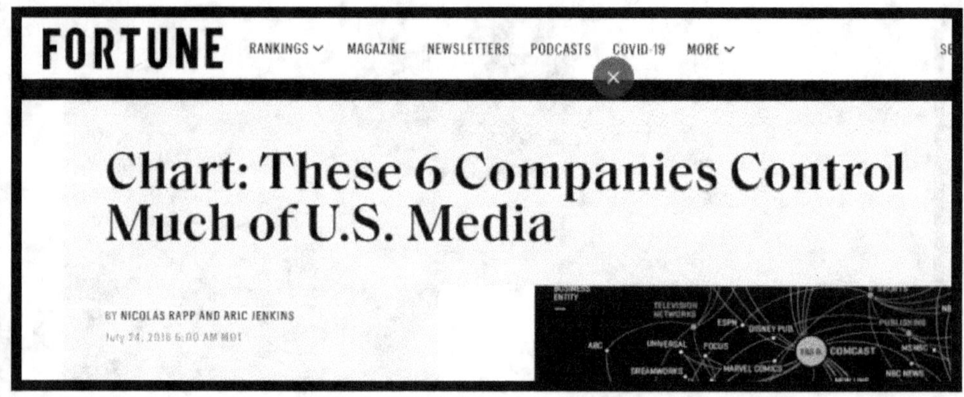

Chart: These 6 Companies Control Much of U.S. Media

(WHO OWNS "DISNEY?")

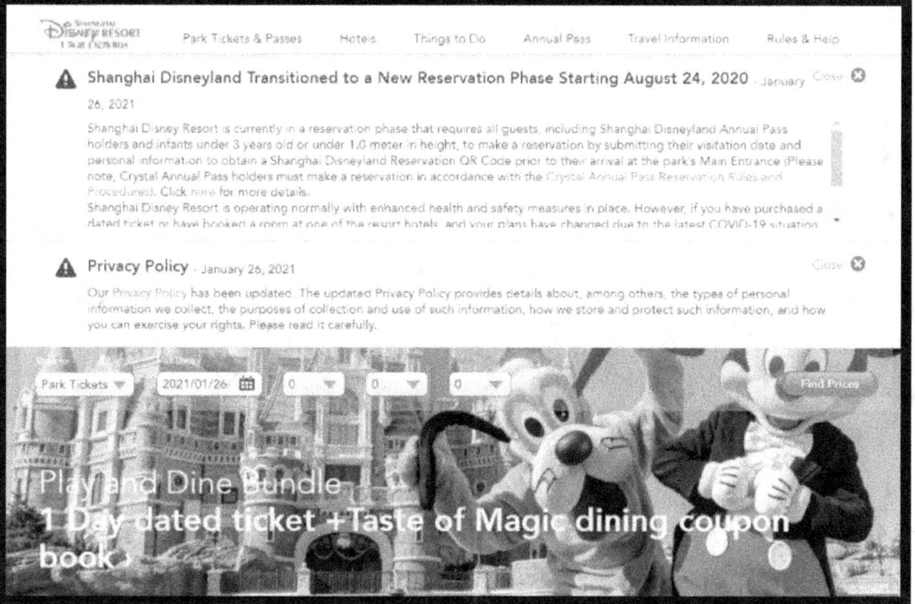

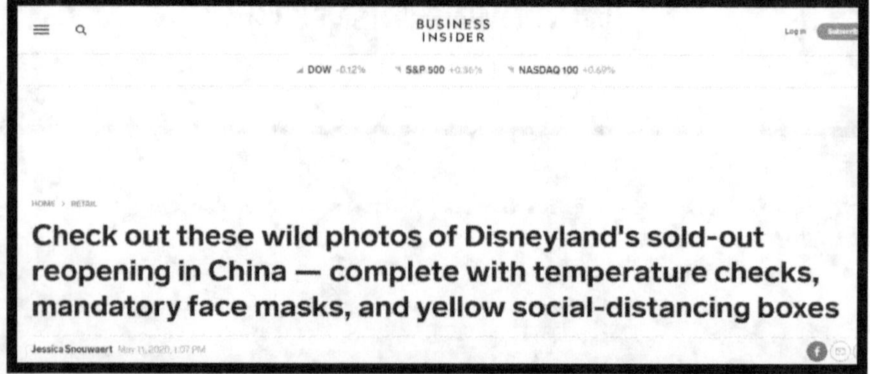

BUSINESS
INSIDER
DOW -0.12%   S&P 500 +0.36%   NASDAQ 100 +0.69%
Log in   Subscribe
HOME > RETAIL
Check out these wild photos of Disneyland's sold-out reopening in China — complete with temperature checks, mandatory face masks, and yellow social-distancing boxes
Jessica Snouwaert   May 11, 2020, 1:07 PM

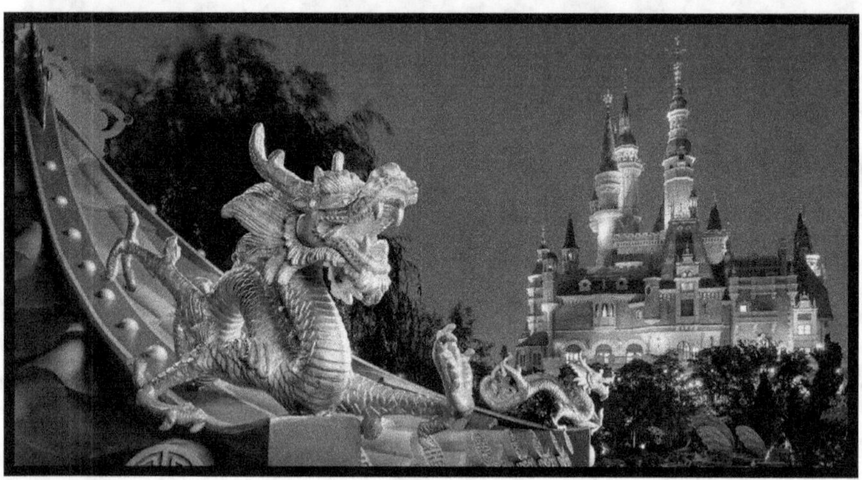

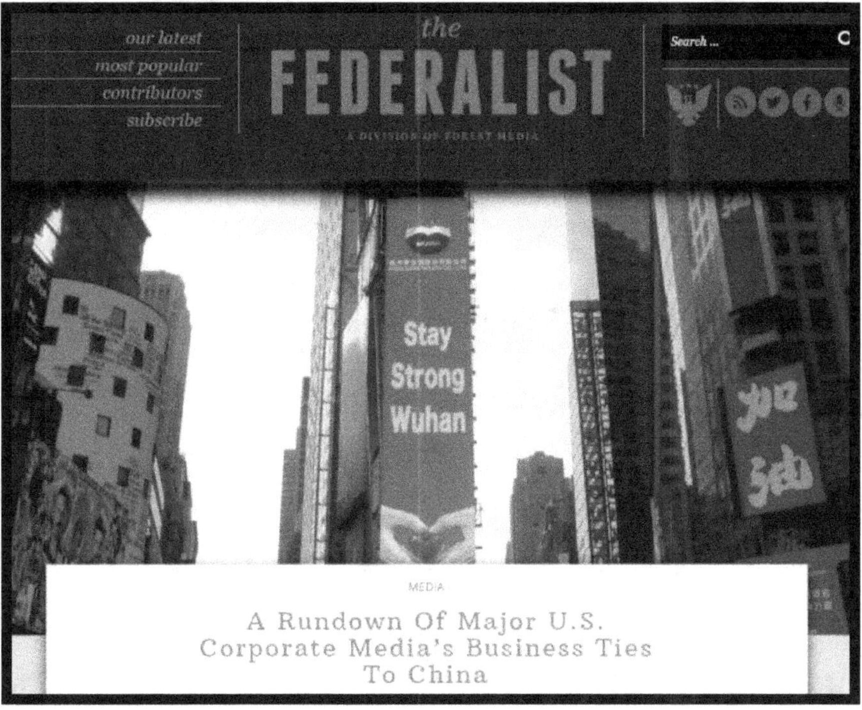

"Despite the Chinese Communist Party's (CCP) record of oppression, corporate media outlets are parroting the authoritarian government's propaganda, even in the midst of an outbreak the CCP worsened through a cover-up. Many of those media outlets have financial ties to Chinese companies with intense oversight from the CCP."

"'You often see representatives from American companies with financial ties to China naturally become defenders of the CCP's policies and spreading the CCP's propaganda,' said Helen Raleigh, an author and senior contributor at The Federalist who emigrated from China. 'The financial tie means these Americans will be much less likely to challenge China's human rights record or unacceptable demand such as technology transfer.'"

(INCIDENTALLY, "THE FEDERALIST" IS NOT OWNED BY ONE OF THE SIX MEGA-CORPORATIONS THAT OWN THE MAJORITY OF ALL MEDIA – HOWEVER, THOSE "OWNED" MEDIA ORGANIZATIONS CALL THE READERS OF "THE FEDERALIST" DISPARAGING NAMES LIKE "CONSPIRACY THEORIST" AND "WHITE SUPREMACIST")

SEE HOW IT WORKS?

ARE YOU BEGINNING TO UNDERSTAND WHAT HAS BEEN HAPPENING?

NEW YORK POST

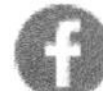  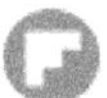  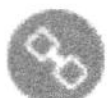

NEWS

Chinese virologist claims COVID was made in lab — but US studies don't agree

By Natalie Musumeci

September 11, 2020 | 5:30pm | Updated

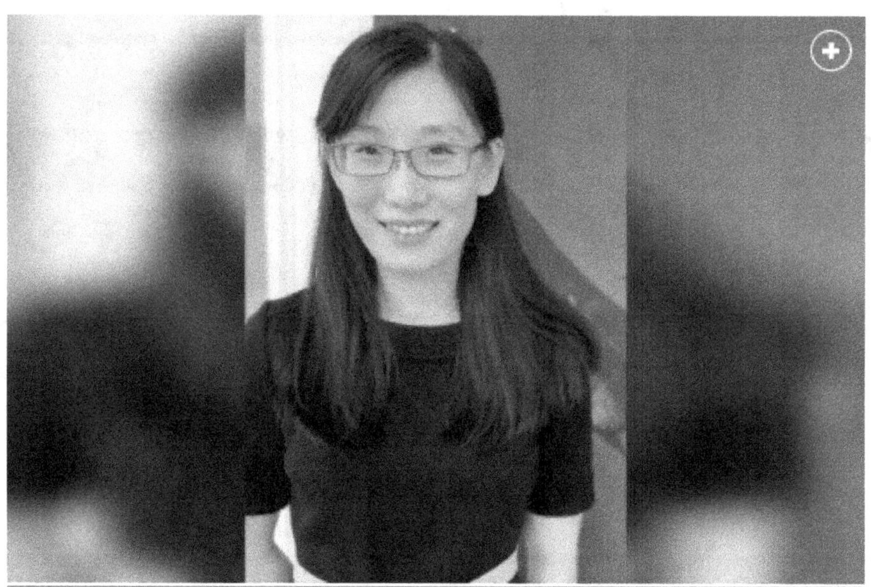

Dr. Li-Meng Yan

Handout

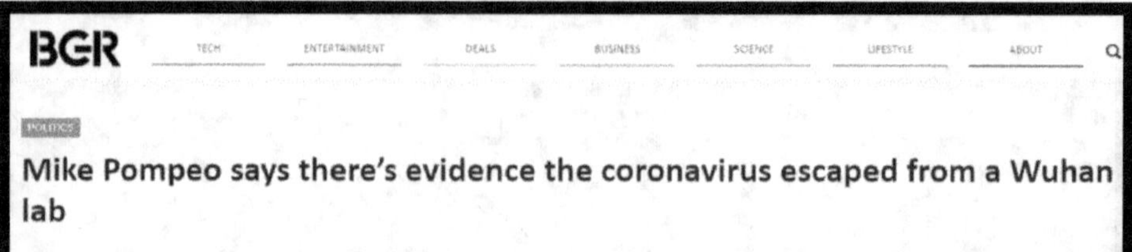

POLITICS

Mike Pompeo says there's evidence the coronavirus escaped from a Wuhan lab

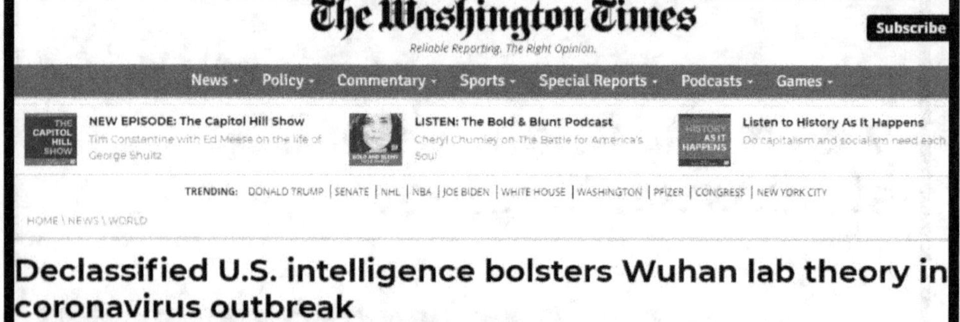

HOME \ NEWS \ WORLD

Declassified U.S. intelligence bolsters Wuhan lab theory in coronavirus outbreak

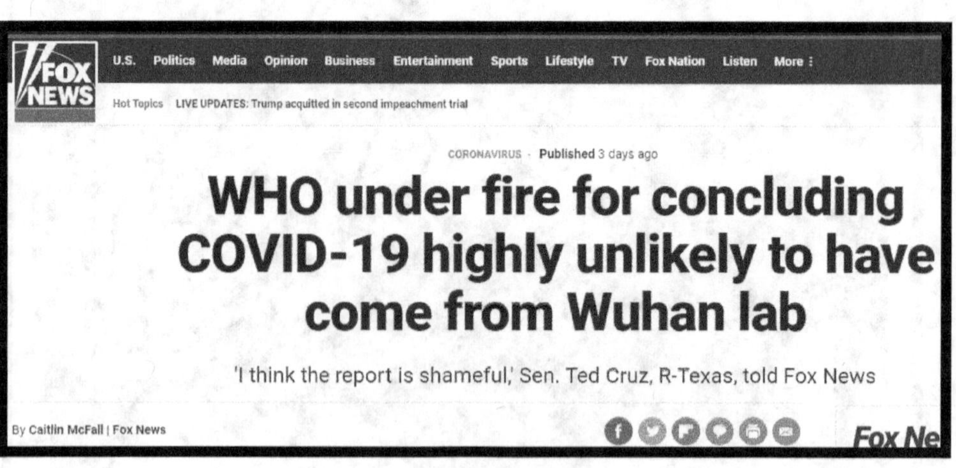

CORONAVIRUS · Published 3 days ago

WHO under fire for concluding COVID-19 highly unlikely to have come from Wuhan lab

'I think the report is shameful,' Sen. Ted Cruz, R-Texas, told Fox News

By Caitlin McFall | Fox News

Why the US Hispanic conservative movement is surging — even without...

Sen. Paul clashes with George Stephanopoulos over 2020 election results

Boosters jump to Joe Biden's defense over coverage of his high-end watches

  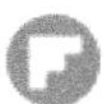  

NEWS

China blasts Mike Pompeo for 'conspiracy theory' about COVID-19's Wuhan lab origins

By Lee Brown

January 18, 2021 | 8:47am | Updated

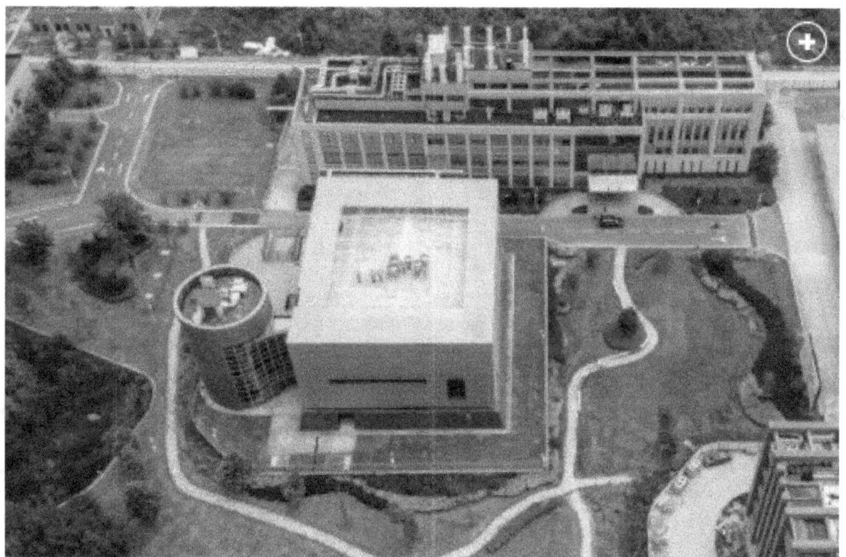

China is denying claims that the coronavirus was created in a Wuhan laboratory.
Getty Images

CHINA IS APPARENTLY UPSET THAT SECRETARY OF STATE MIKE POMPEO EXPOSED THAT THE COMMUNIST CHINESE PARTY (CCP) HAS BEEN SPENDING BILLIONS OF DOLLARS IN MEDIA MANIPULATION IN ATTEMPT TO COVER-UP

FOX NEWS 6:43 PM

U.S. Politics Media Opinion Business Entertainment Sports Lifestyle TV Fox Nation Listen More

Hot Topics

CHINA · **Published** February 8

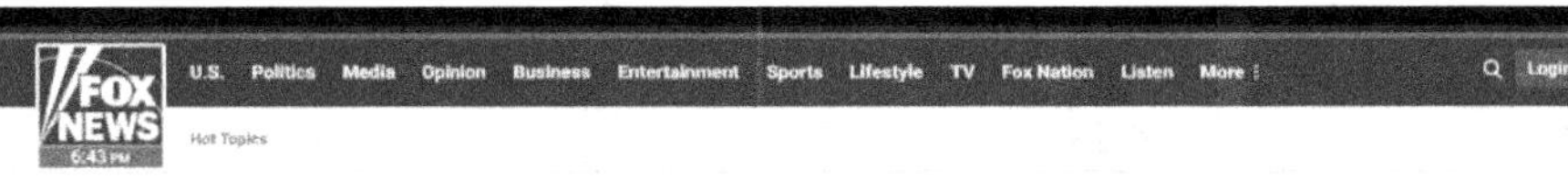

Pompeo warns governors of Chinese infiltration into US: 'It's happening in your state'

By Nick Givas | Fox News

Fox News Fir
MORNING HEADLIN

E A DONATION

THE EPOCH TIMES

POLITICS CHINA WORLD OPINION BUSINESS SCIENCE LIFE MIND & BODY ARTS ENTERTAINMENT VIDE

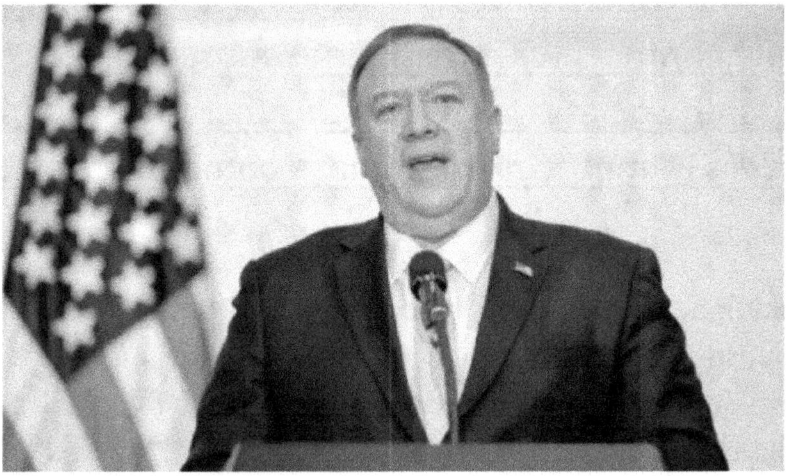

US Secretary of State Mike Pompeo speaks during the III Hemispheric Ministerial Conference of Fight Against Terrorism, in Bogota on Jan. 20, 2020. (Raul Arboleda/AFP via Getty Images)

CHINA-US NEWS

Pompeo Warns US Governors About Chinese Influence

BY FRANK FANG | February 9, 2020 Updated: February 9, 2020

"In a keynote speech on Feb. 8 at the National Governors' Association (NGA) annual conference, **Secretary of State Mike Pompeo virtually ordered state officials from across the United States to stop pursuing, and cut off, any contacts with the Chinese-American Friendship Society, the Confucius Institutes, Chinese investors in their states, Chinese companies, etc.**

"Speaking peremptorily as he often does, Pompeo instructed the governors that 'China is watching you, working you,' and that the State Department has the documents by which China is 'ranking' them as open and friendly, or not. This was equivalent to saying, 'We are watching you,' we know what you've done and we want no friendly interchanges by you with China."

CHINA HAS BEEN INFILTRATING THE UNITED STATES FOR DECADES, SLOWLY SEIZING CONTROL OF UNIVERSITIES, MEDIA COMPANIES AND TECH COMPANIES, NOT TO MENTION BOUGHT-AND-PAID-FOR POLITICIANS THROUGH BRIBERY AND BLACKMAIL

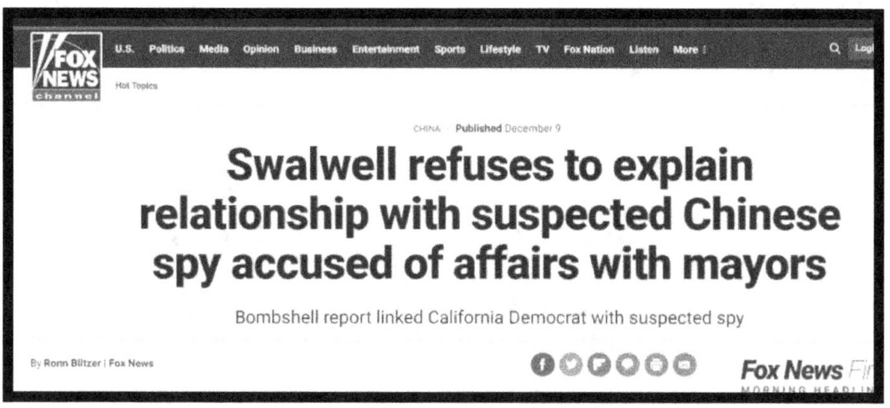

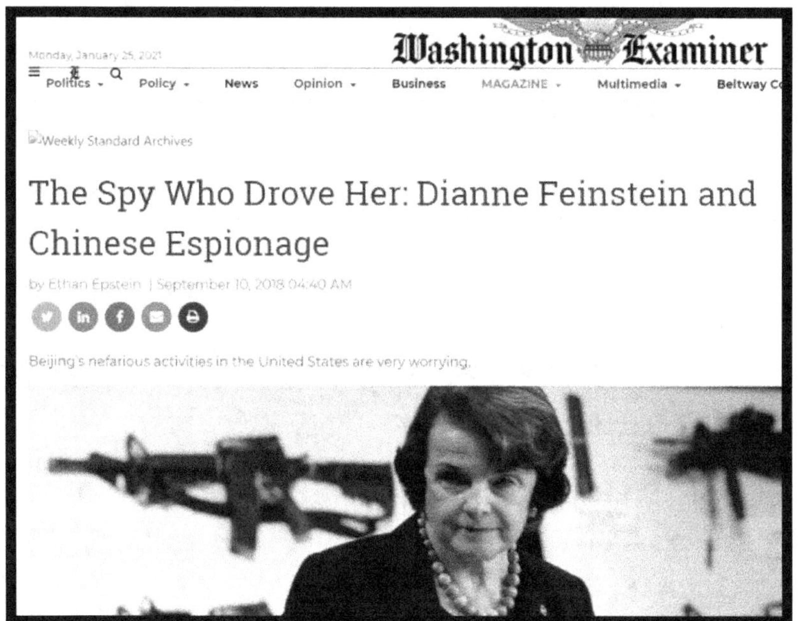

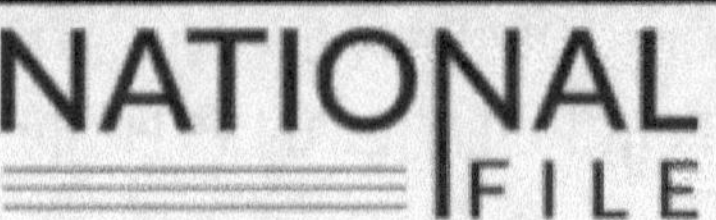

THIS IS NOT A MATTER OF "REPUBLICANS VS. DEMOCRATS" – THAT IS THE STRATEGY OF THE "COLOR REVOLUTION," TO DIVIDE AND CONQUER

THIS IS A MATTER OF "TRAITORS" VS. "PATRIOTS," AND IT IS THAT SIMPLE, AND THE TRAITORS ARE REPUBLICANS AS WELL AS DEMOCRATS, COMPRISING ABOUT 95% OF ALL ELECTED OFFICIALS IN WASHINGTON D.C.

...AND THAT IS EXACTLY WHY THE FOREIGN ENTITY OF "WASHINGTON D.C." HAS BECOME AN OPEN-AIR PRISON

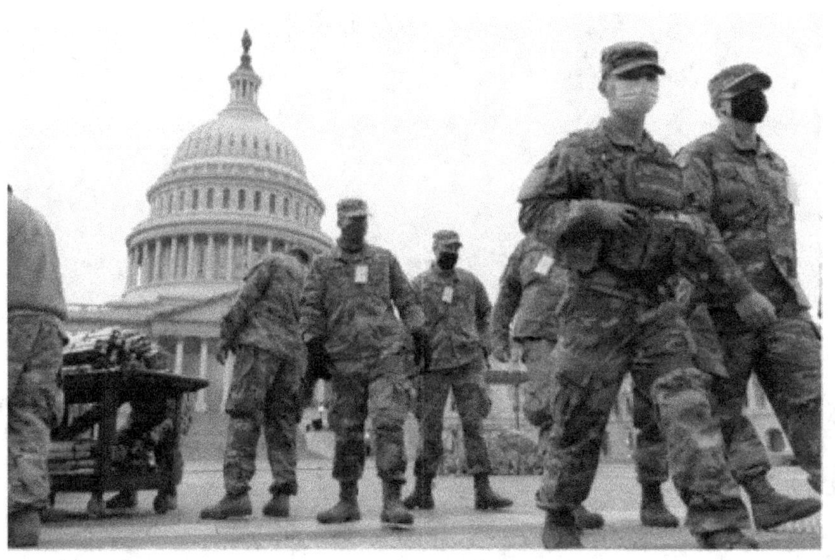

POLITICO

CONGRESS

Impeachment trial to keep National Guard troops at Capitol

There are fears of mass demonstrations.

Federal law enforcement officials told lawmakers the impeachment trial poses a big enough threat to require thousands of National Guard troops to remain in Washington through mid-March. | Jacquelyn Martin/AP Photo

THOSE TROOPS ARE ASSUREDLY NOT IN WASHINGTON D.C. TO PROTECT AGAINST SO-CALLED *"CONSERVATIVE DOMESTIC TERRORISTS,"* WHICH ARE A MEDIA FABRICATION

THIS STORY IS MUCH DEEPER – MILITARY TRIBUNALS ARE TAKING PLACE AS THE US CAPITAL BECOMES A MILITARY COURT

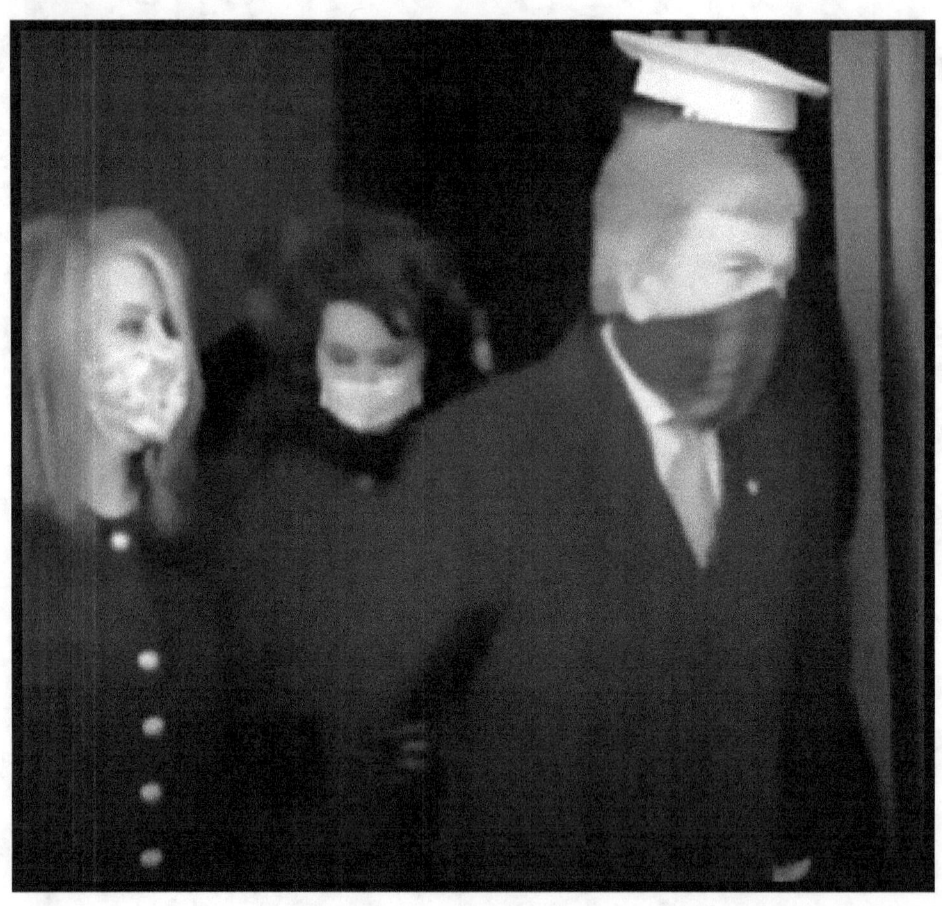

WASHINGTON D.C. IS NOT A PART OF THE UNITED STATES – IT IS A FOREIGN OCCUPYING POWER, AND IT HAS NOW BECOME A PRISONER OF THE US MILITARY, ALONG WITH THE MAJORITY OF POLITICIANS WHO HAVE BEEN COMMITTING TREASON TO BENEFIT THEMSELVES BY SELLING OUT THEIR OFFICES OF REPRESENTATION FOR THE PEOPLE OF OUR COUNTRY – THEY ARE TRAITORS.

DO YOU UNDERSTAND THE MASSIVE SCOPE OF THIS "COLOR REVOLUTION" AND THOSE WHO ARE INVOLVED?

WHO DO YOU SUPPORT?

THE PEOPLE OF THE UNITED STATES, OR THE COMMUNIST CHINESE PARTY?

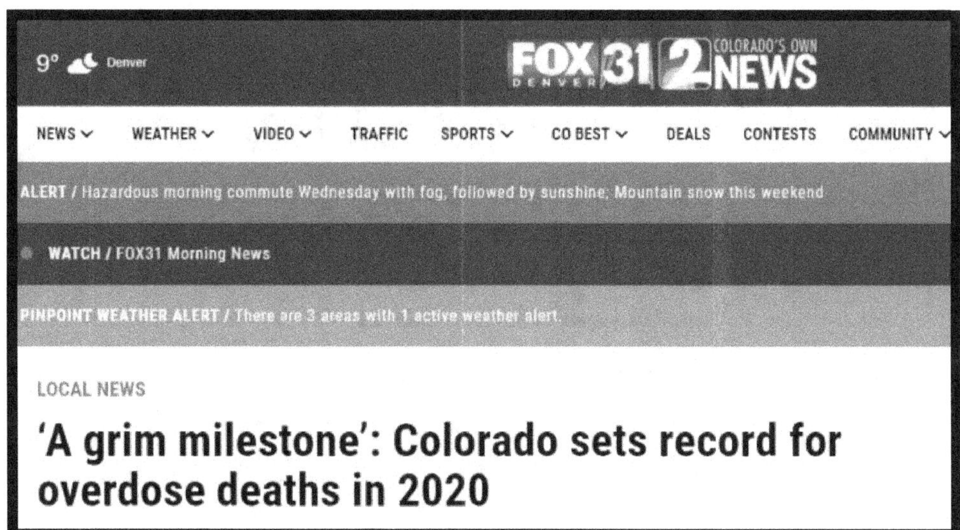

"Statewide, 448 people died from a Fentanyl-related overdose in 2020, more than twice the 2019 total.

"Psychologists say it's likely the COVID-19 pandemic contributed to the spike in numbers.

"'The isolation is driving a lot of it,' says Dr. Liz Chamberlain. 'When we have a lot of stress, a lot of times we want to just get rid of it, or push it away, so a lot of time people will turn to substances to help them do that.'"

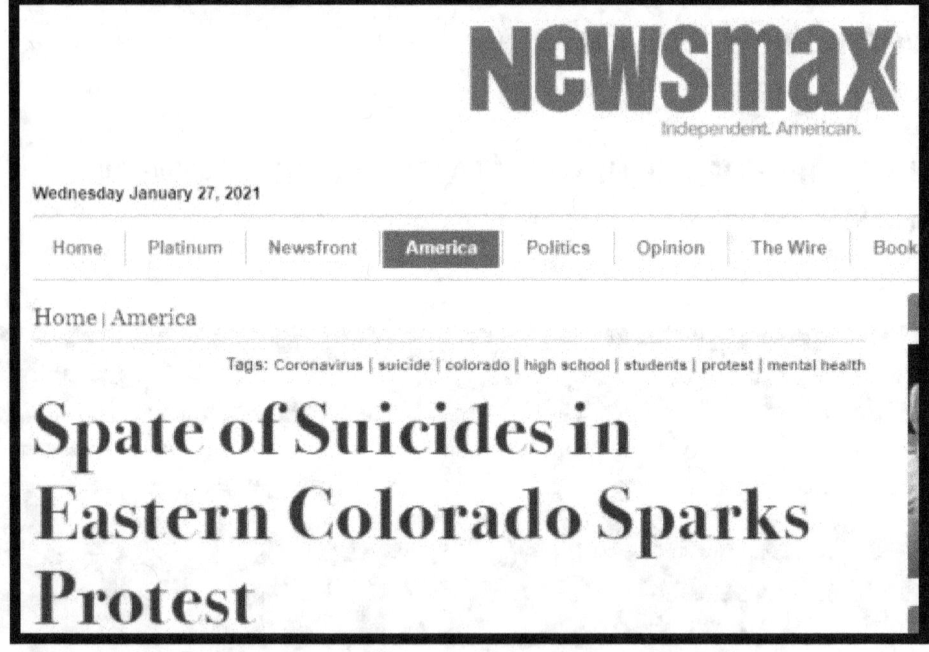

"A series of suicides among high school students in northeastern Colorado has young people protesting the restrictions against activities like school clubs and sports put in place due to the coronavirus pandemic, the Colorado Sun reports.

"At least seven young people have died by suicide over the last few months in one of the state's least populated regions."

—

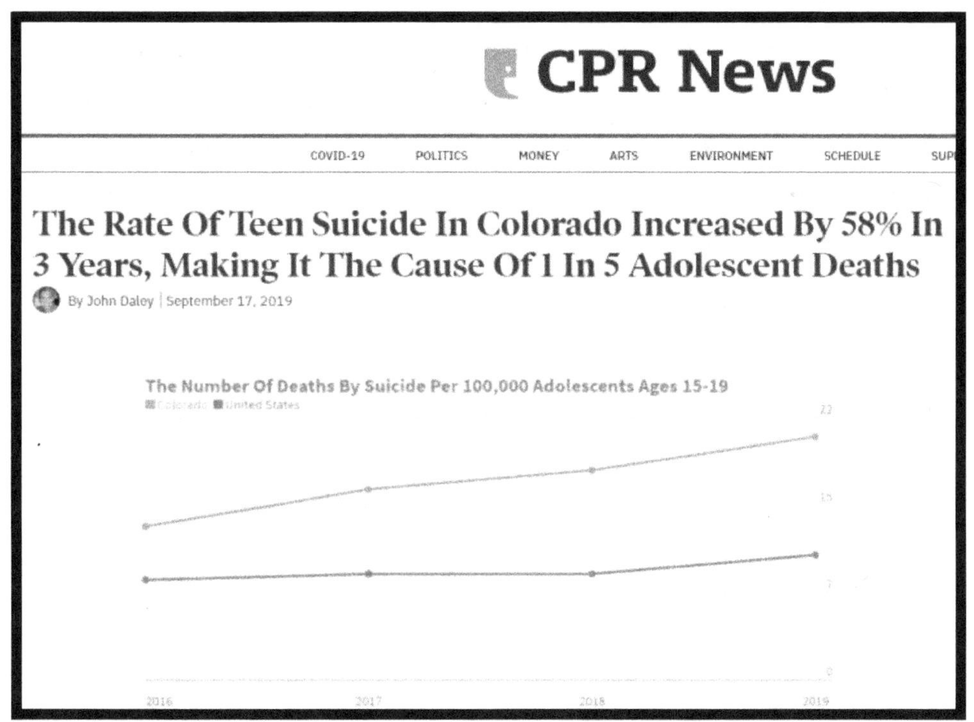

"Male teenagers in Colorado were more than twice as likely to complete suicide than female teens. Most deaths were by white victims."

DO WE CARE ABOUT WHITE, MALE TEENAGE SUICIDE DEATHS, OR DO ONLY "BLACK LIVES MATTER?"

WE DO NOT NEED TO BE CONCERNED ABOUT STUDENT SUICIDES THAT HAVE INCREASED SINCE THE BEGINNING OF GOVERNMENT-MANDATED "COVID" LOCKDOWN RESTRICTIONS.

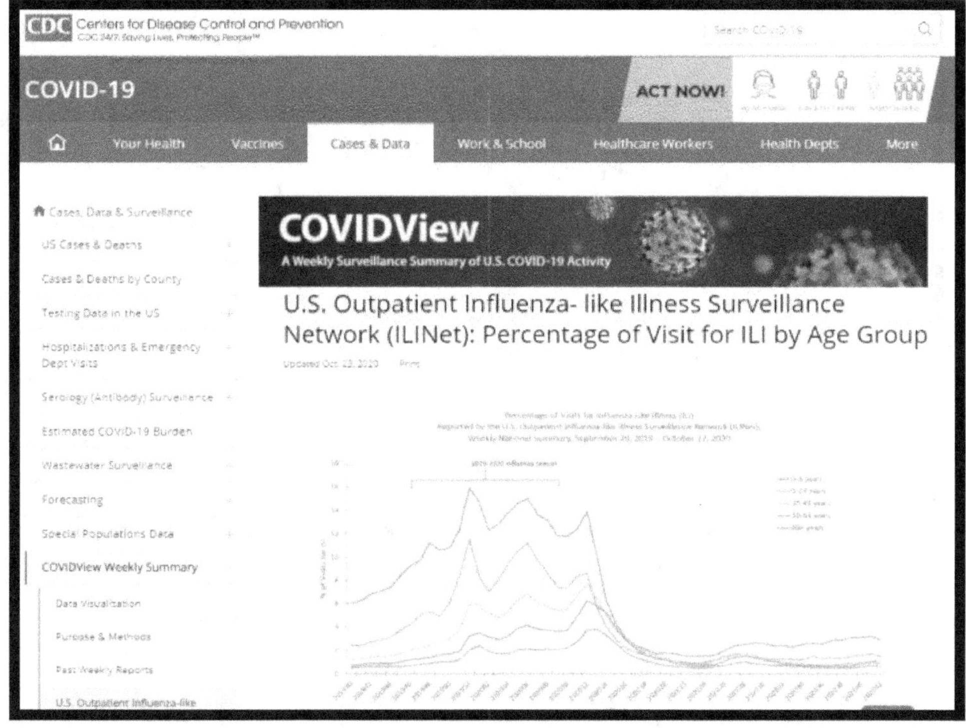

The striking dip in cases of "influenza-like illness" dropped approximately at the time of May, 2020, when the "COVID" cases were supposedly rising.

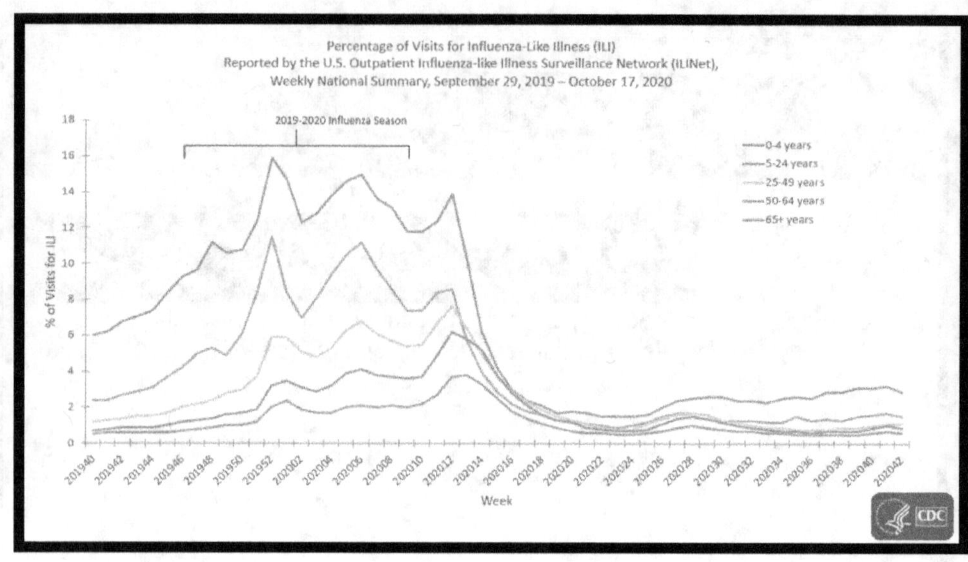

HAVE "COVID" RESTRICTIONS KILLED OFF THE FLU?

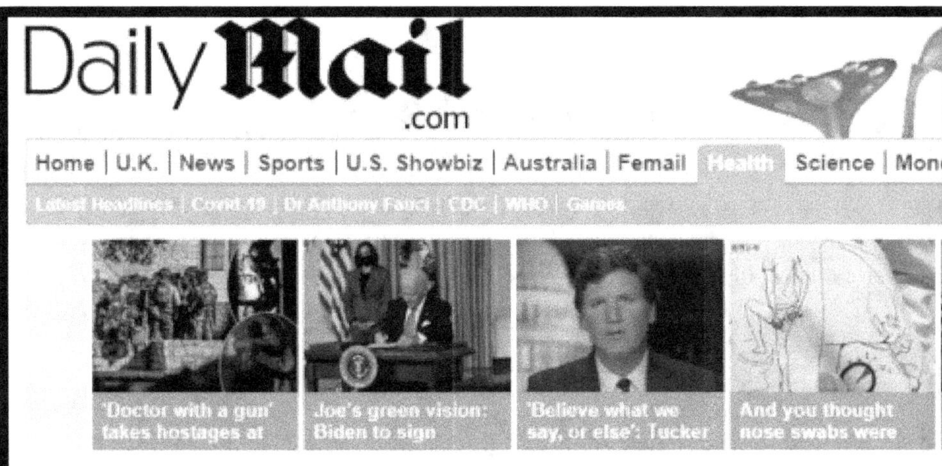

"The disappearing act began as Covid-19 rolled in towards the end of our flu season in March. And just how swiftly rates have plummeted can be observed in 'surveillance' data collected by the World Health Organization (WHO)."

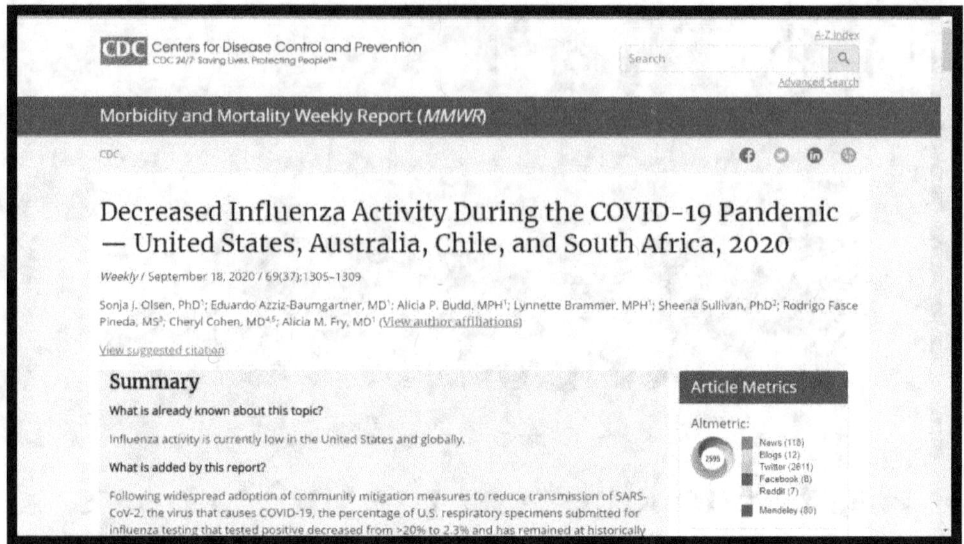

"Following widespread adoption of community mitigation measures to reduce transmission of SARS-CoV-2, the virus that causes COVID-19, the percentage of U.S. respiratory specimens submitted for influenza testing that tested positive decreased from ..."

DUE TO "COVID" MITIGATION EFFORTS, THE NUMBERS OF FLU CASES AND DEATHS HAVE DRASTICALLY REDUCED.

IT IS IMPOSSIBLE THAT THE AVERAGE FLU CASES WERE MISDIAGNOSED AS "COVID."

THE MITIGATION EFFORTS REDUCED THE FLU CASES

THE FLU CASES WERE NOT MISDIAGNOSED BY FALSE-POSITIVE "COVID" TESTS.

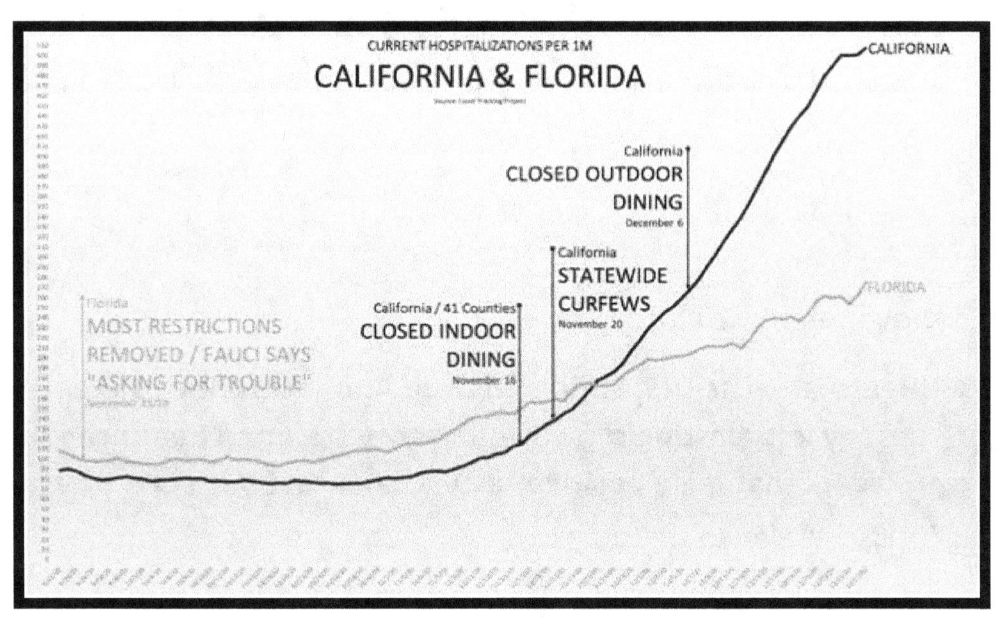

–

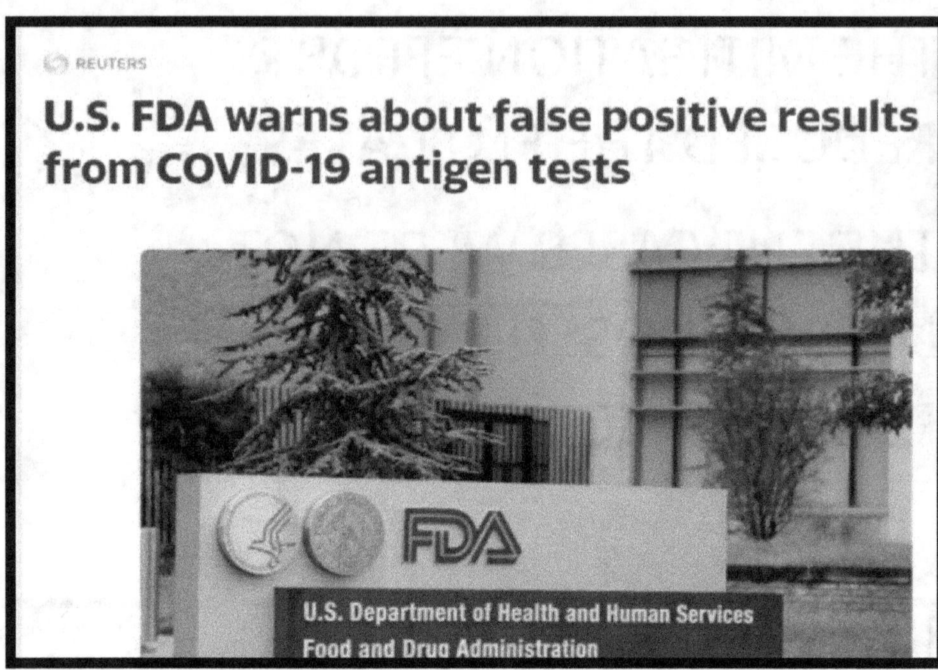

(November 3, 2020)

"(Reuters) – The U.S. Food and Drug Administration said on Tuesday it is alerting clinical laboratory staff and healthcare providers that false positive results can occur with COVID-19 antigen tests."

THE AVERAGE FLU CASES WERE NOT

MISDIAGNOSED AS "COVID" CASES BY

THE FALSE-POSITIVE TEST RESULTS THAT THE US FOOD & DRUG ADMINISTRATION WARNED ABOUT.

THERE WERE NO POLITICAL CONNECTIONS BETWEEN THE TIMING OF THE "COVID" OUTBREAK AND THE MOST CONSEQUENTIAL PRESIDENTIAL ELECTION IN THE HISTORY OF THE UNITED STATES AND THE WORLD.

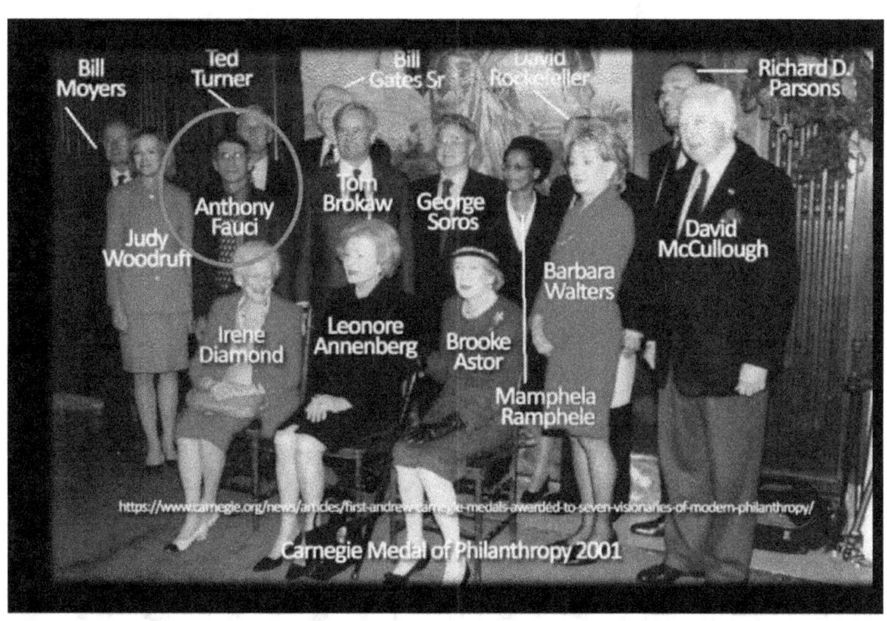

(Young Anthony Fauci, please meet George Soros, Ted Turner, David Rockefeller and Bill Gates' father – Got any plans together?)

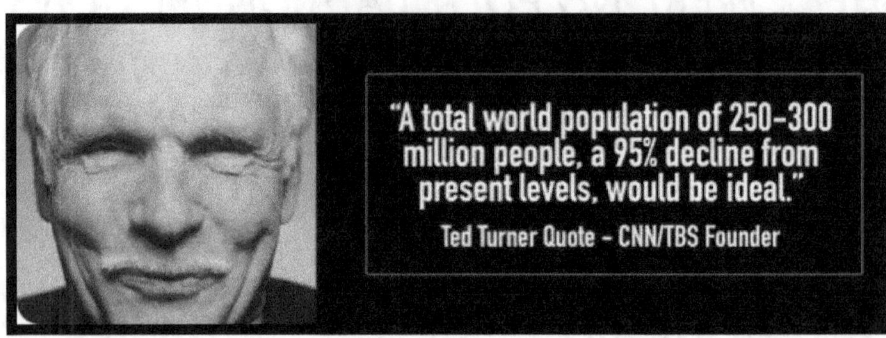

ANTHONY FAUCI:

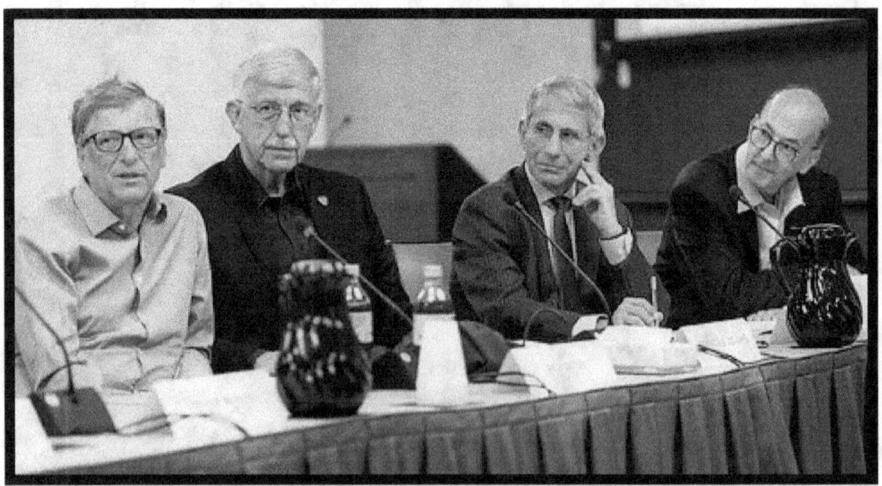

**1). The Highest Paid Employee In The Entire U.S. Federal
Government**

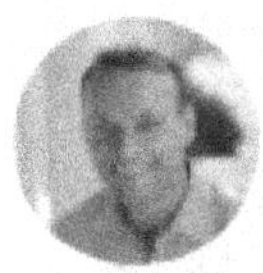

2). Dr. Fauci backed funding for controversial Wuhan lab studying origin of coronavirus

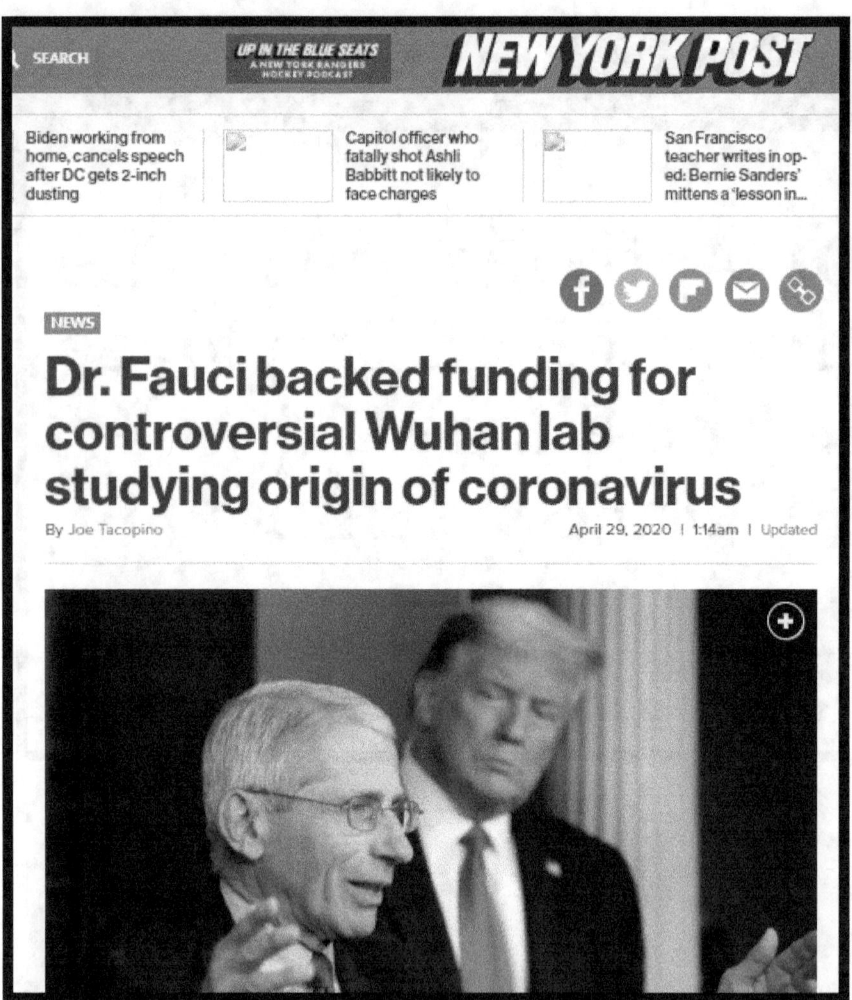

3). Fauci stated that COVID19 is "probably about 10 times more lethal than the seasonal flu," which would mean 300-600,000 coronavirus deaths this year, at the same time in a respected medical journal he compared Covid-19 as similar to seasonal flu in morbidity.

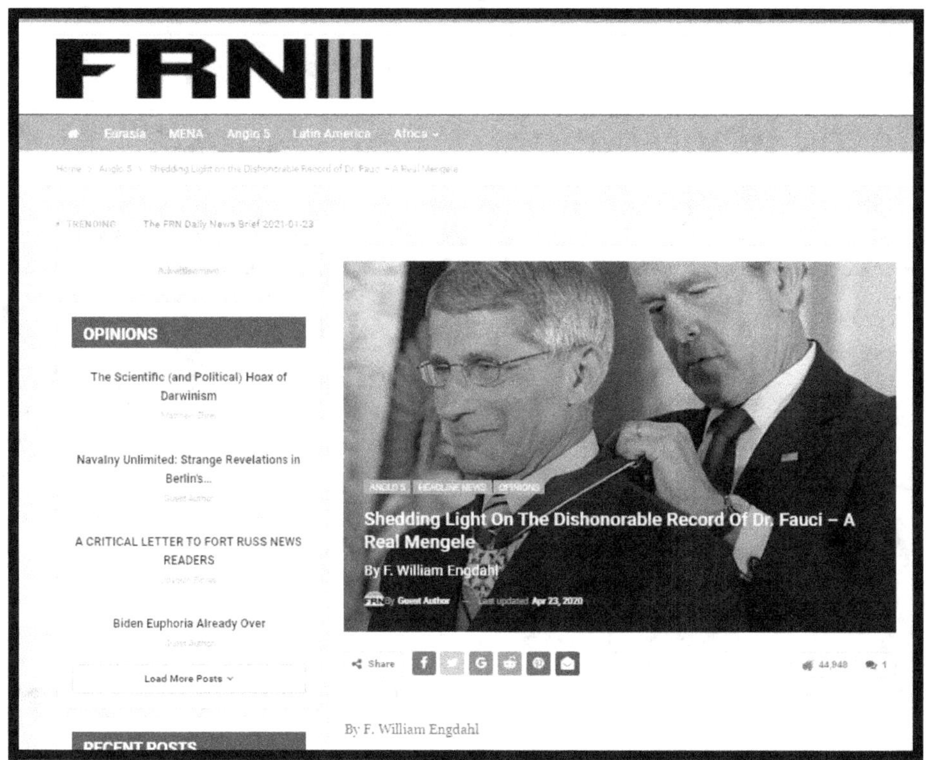

4). The only people who need masks are those who are already infected to keep from exposing others. The masks sold at drugstores aren't even good enough to truly protect anyone, Fauci said.

"If you look at the masks that you buy in a drug store, the leakage around that doesn't really do much to protect you," he said. "People start saying, 'Should I start wearing a mask?' *Now, in the United States,* **there is absolutely no reason whatsoever to wear a mask."**

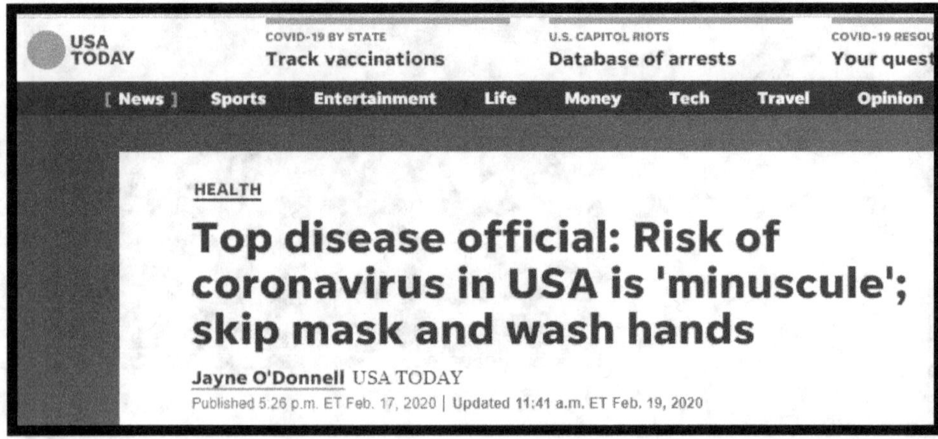

5).

Coronavirus Task Force
VP Pence   -- Debra Birx--   Anthony Fauci
Mark Dybul, worked with Fauci
to establish PEPFAR
The Global Fund
$90 billion est.
TAXPAYER MONEY
PEPFAR
The Global Fund
UN
DP
World Health
Organization

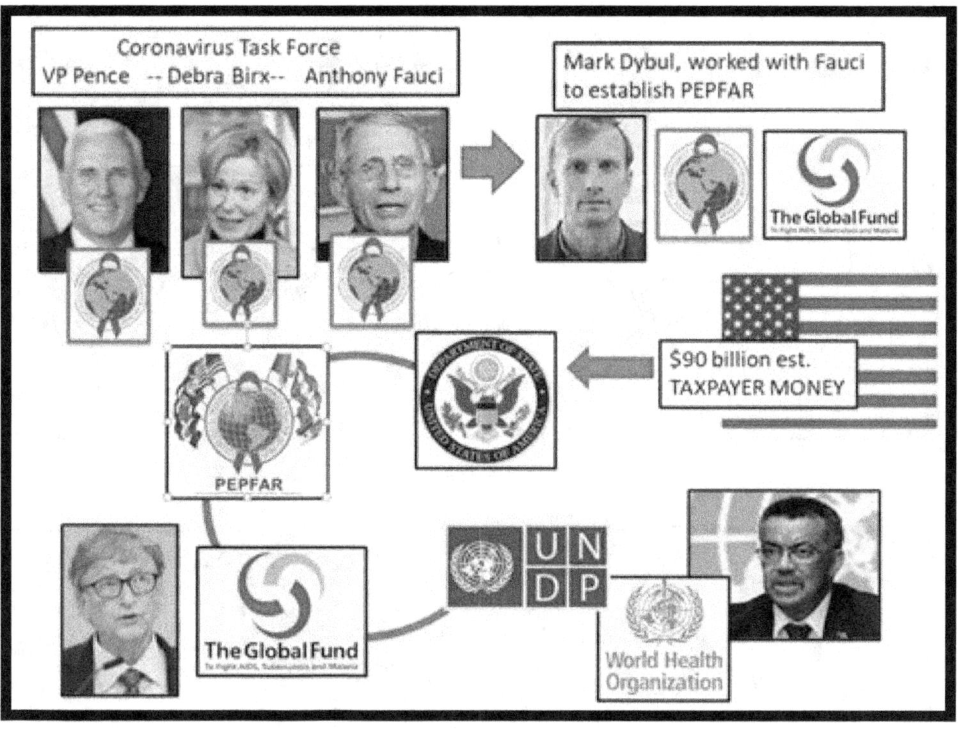

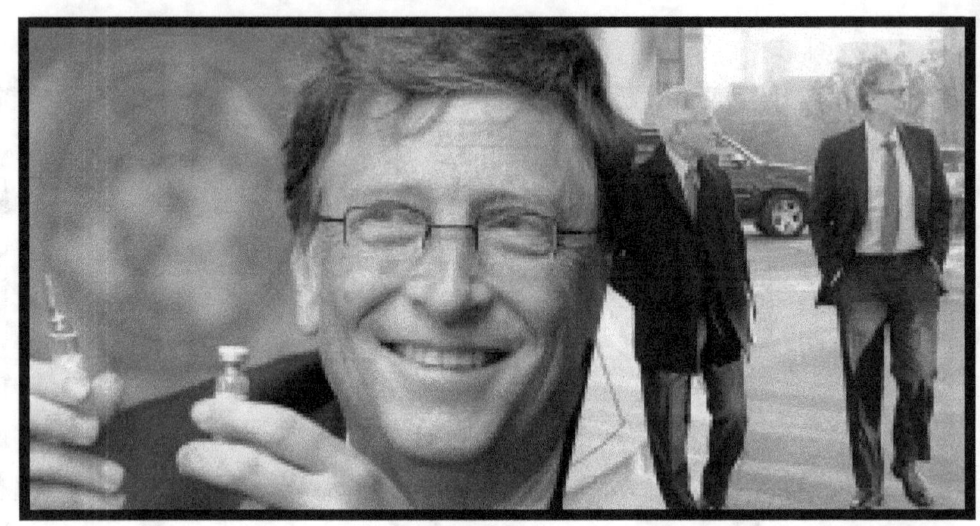

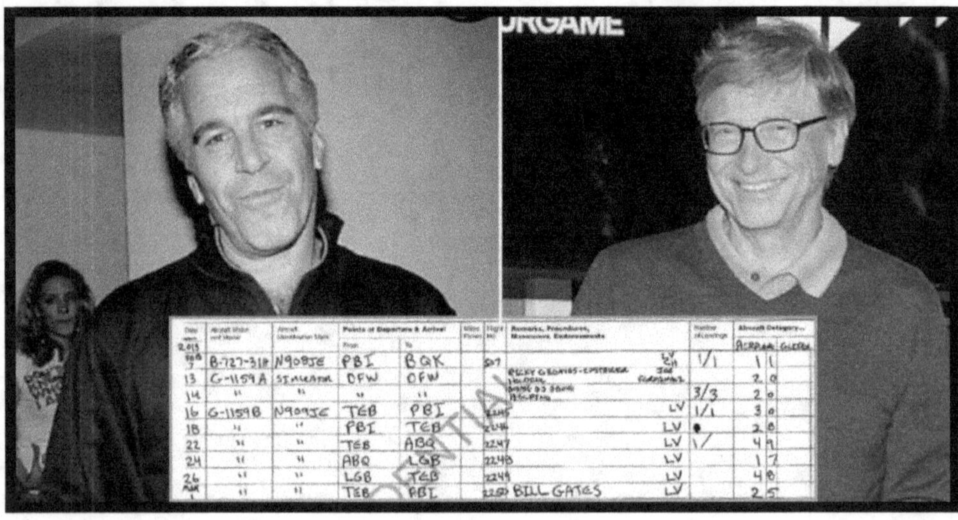

Date 2013	Aircraft Make and Model	Aircraft Identification Mark	Points of Departure & Arrival From	To	Miles Flown	Flight No.	Remarks, Procedures, Maneuvers, Endorsements		Number of Landings	Aircraft Category Airplane	Glider
7	B-727-31P	N908JE	PBI	BGK	207			LV	1/1	1	1
13	G-1159A	SIMUEATM	DFW	DFW			RICKY GERVAIS - EPSTEINER HOLIDAY			2	0
14	"	"	"	"			BOTH GS FROM ABS-PIMS		3/3	2	0
16	G-1159B	N909JE	TEB	PBI	2245			LV	1/1	3	0
18	"	"	PBI	TEB	2246			LV	●	2	0
22	"	"	TEB	ABQ	2247			LV	1/	4	4
24	"	"	ABQ	LGB	2248			LV		1	7
26	"	"	LGB	TEB	2249			LV		4	0
AUG 1	"	"	TEB	PBI	2250		BILL GATES	LV		2	5

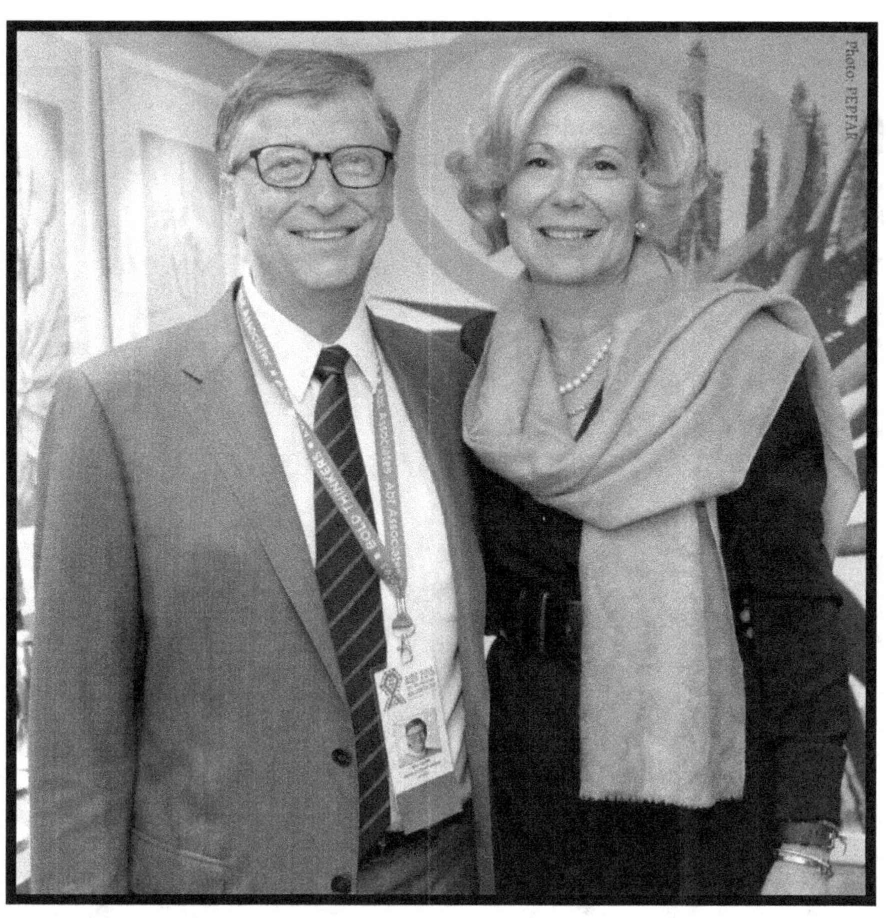

Photo: PEPFAR

Bill Gates Met With Jeffrey Epstein Many Times, Despite His Past

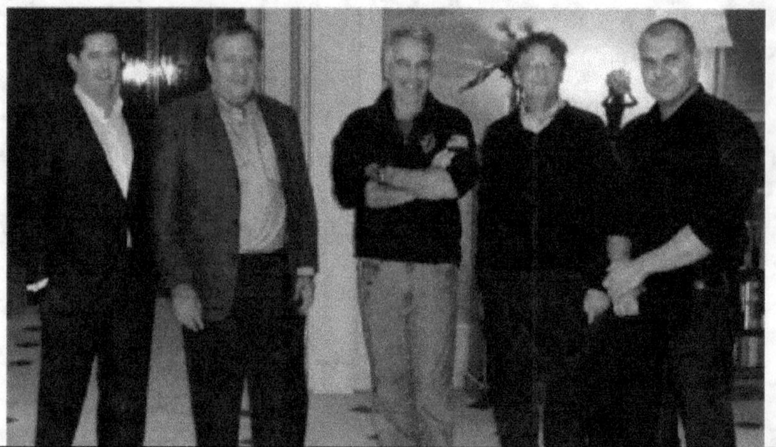

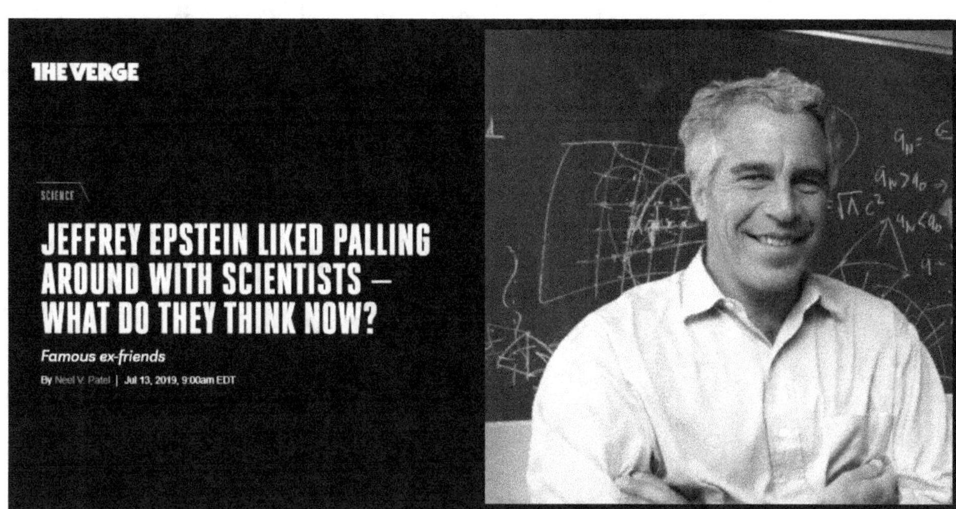
THE VERGE
SCIENCE
JEFFREY EPSTEIN LIKED PALLING AROUND WITH SCIENTISTS —
WHAT DO THEY THINK NOW?
Famous ex-friends
By Neel V. Patel | Jul 13, 2019, 9:00am EDT

WHY DOES BILL GATES AND HIS FATHER, BILL
GATES SR., GET INVOLVED WITH ACTIVITIES
THAT RESULT IN KILLING PEOPLE?

BILL GATES SR. WAS THE FORMER HEAD OF
"PLANNED PARENTHOOD"

THE "VACCINES" FROM BILL GATES KILL PEOPLE

BABIES IN THE WOMB AREN'T PEOPLE?

PEOPLE AREN'T DYING FROM "VACCINES?"

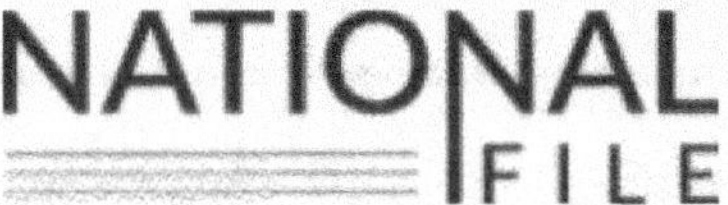

Fauci Photographed With Soros and Bill Gates' Father, Who Was 'Head of Planned Parenthood'

Bill Gates Made A Stunning Family Revelation

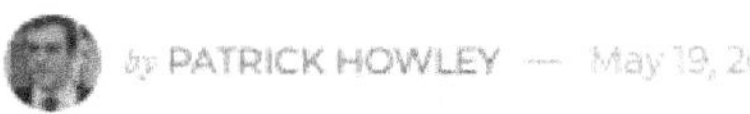

by PATRICK HOWLEY — May 19, 2020   ⊙ 3

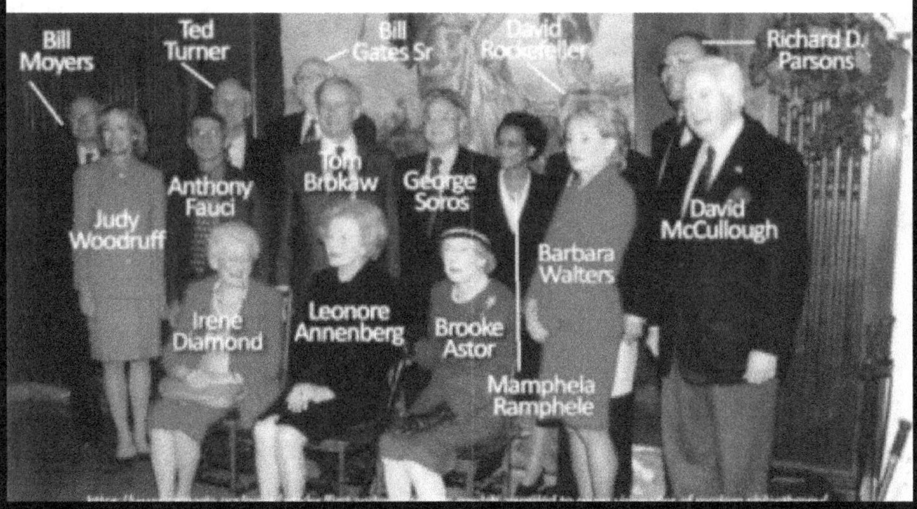

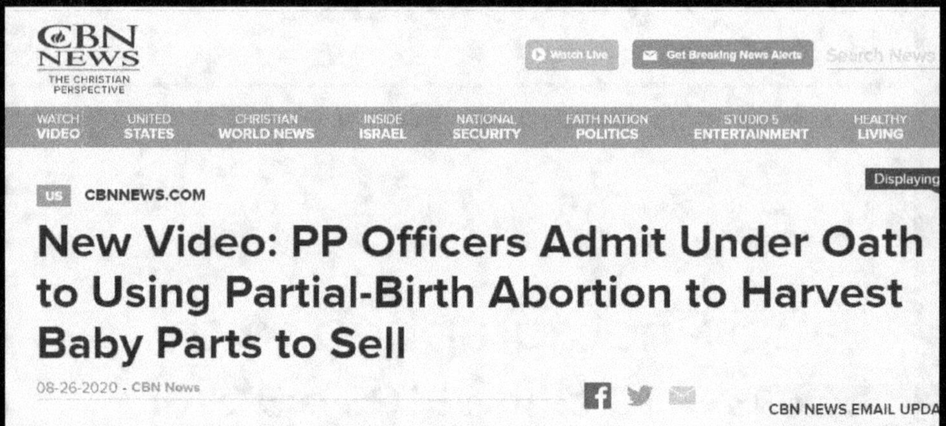

CBN NEWS
THE CHRISTIAN PERSPECTIVE
Watch Live
Get Breaking News Alerts
Search News
WATCH VIDEO
UNITED STATES
CHRISTIAN WORLD NEWS
INSIDE ISRAEL
NATIONAL SECURITY
FAITH NATION POLITICS
STUDIO 5 ENTERTAINMENT
HEALTHY LIVING
Displaying
US   CBNNEWS.COM
New Video: PP Officers Admit Under Oath to Using Partial-Birth Abortion to Harvest Baby Parts to Sell
08-26-2020 - CBN News
CBN NEWS EMAIL UPDA

IS THERE A DEVIOUS CONNECTION BETWEEN BILL GATES JR. AND BILL GATES SR.?

ABORTED BABIES ARE HARVESTED FOR FETAL CELLS AND BODY PARTS

ARE THERE FETAL CELLS IN "VACCINES?"

YES

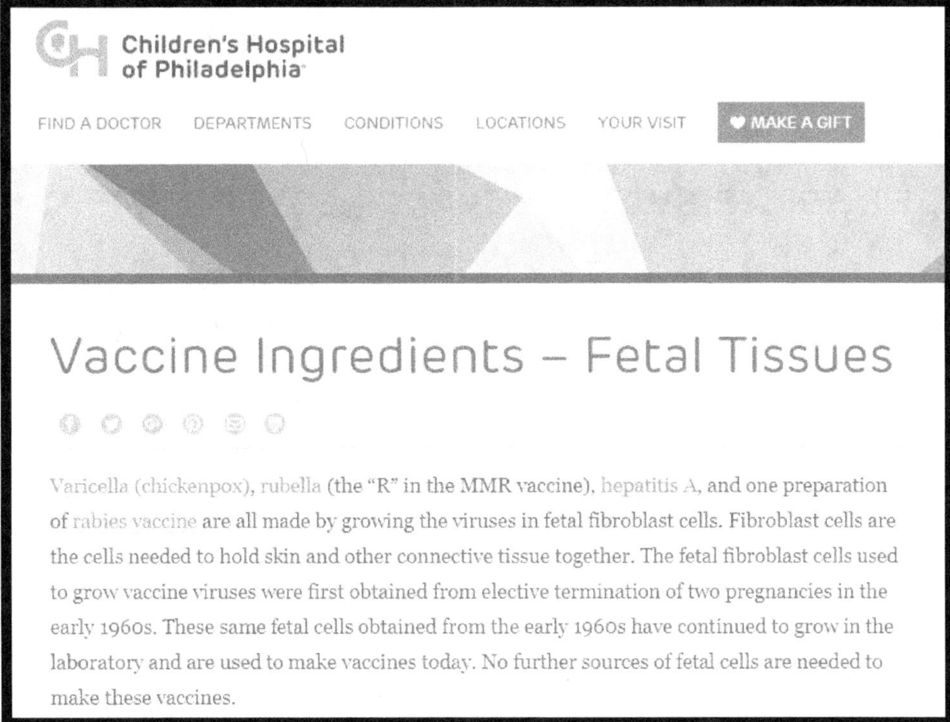

WHY ARE "VACCINES" DISTRIBUTED TO THE
PUBLIC FOR FREE?

ARE PHARMACEUTICAL COMPANIES KNOWN TO
BE ALTRUISTIC ORGANIZATIONS THAT ARE NOT
CONCERNED ABOUT PROFIT?

WHY DO THEY PROVIDE "VACCINES" FOR FREE,
YET CHARGE FIVE-TIMES THE NECESSARY
AMOUNT FOR INSULIN, NOT TO MENTION THE
OVERPRICED DRUGS THAT EVERYBODY KNOWS
ABOUT?

THEY DISTRIBUTE THE "VACCINES" FOR FREE

WHO IS THE LEADING PUSHER OF "VACCINES?"

BILL GATES

DOES BILL GATES HAVE A LOT OF MONEY?

YES

DOES THE BILL GATES FOUNDATION GIVE "CHARITABLE DONATIONS" TO PHARMACEUTICAL COMPANIES FOR THE DEVELOPMENT OF VACCINES?

YES

WAS BILL GATES' FATHER THE HEAD OF PLANNED PARENTHOOD, THE ORGANIZATION THAT KILLS UNBORN BABIES?

YES

ARE THERE FETAL CELLS FROM UNBORN BABIES IN THE "VACCINES" DEVELOPED BY BILL GATES?

YES

ARE WE IDIOTS?

Under Sworn Testimony, Planned Parenthood Officials Admit Infanticide Occurs In Organ Harvesting

JUNE 30, 2020 By Madeline Osburn

WHO ELSE IS INTERESTED IN ORGAN HARVESTING, AS WELL AS THE DESTRUCTION OF THE UNITED STATES?

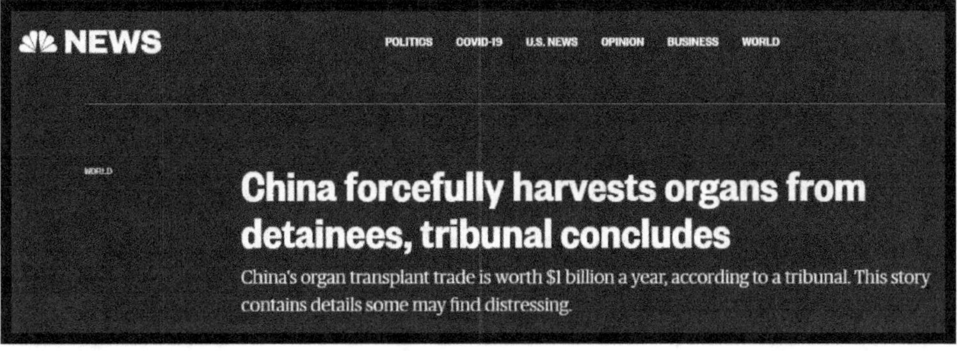

IS THERE A CONNECTION BETWEEN "DR. FAUCI," BILL GATES, AND THE COMMUNIST PARTY OF CHINA (CCP)?

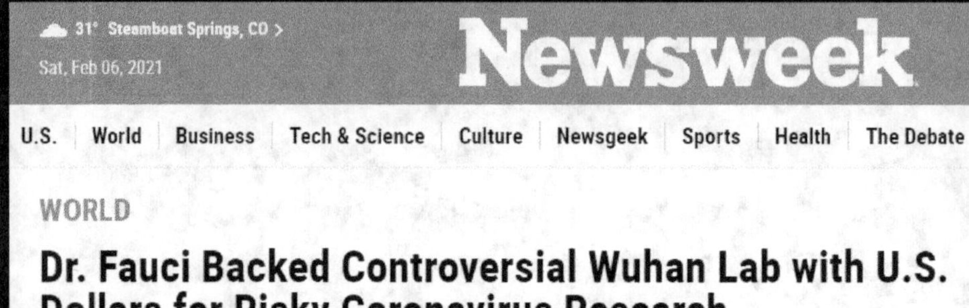

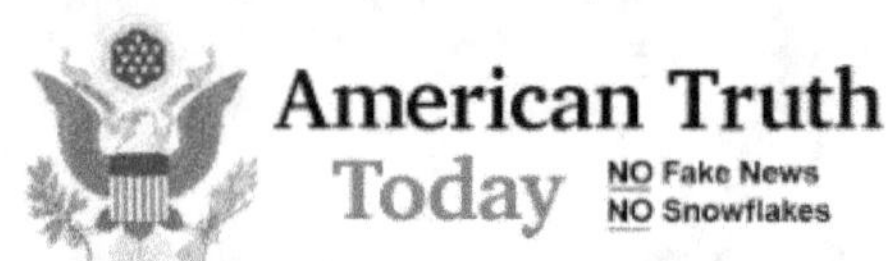

WHAT IS "EUGENICS?"

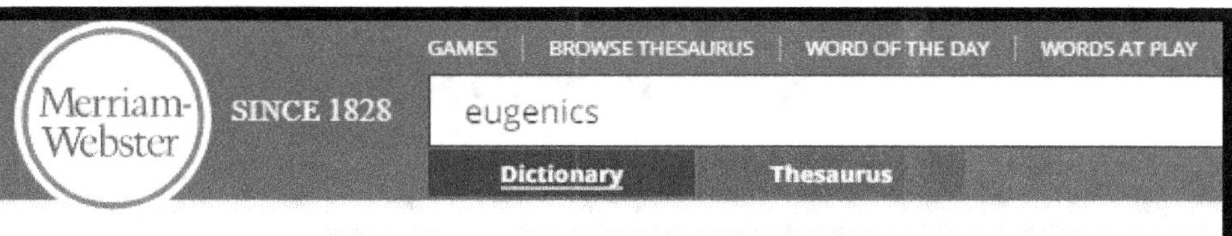

eugenics noun, plural in form but singular in construction

Save Word

eu·gen·ics | \ yü- je-niks \

Definition of *eugenics*

: the practice or advocacy of controlled selective breeding of human populations (as by sterilization) to improve the population's genetic composition

// In 1883 Francis Galton, in England, coined the term "*eugenics*" to encompass the idea of modification of natural selection through selective breeding for the improvement of humankind ...
— Jeremiah A. Barondess

// A half-century ago, *eugenics* became associated with Hitler, genocide and master-race theories, and its reputation has never recovered.
— Dan Seligman

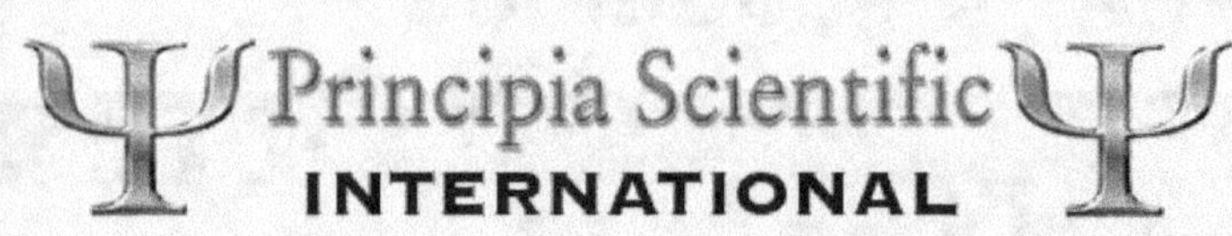

Head Of Pfizer Research: Covid Vaccine Is Female Sterilization

Published on December 10, 2020

Written by healthandmoneynews.wordpress.com

"EUGENICS" IS INTERESTED IN STERILIZATION OF THE PUBLIC AND GLOBAL POPULATION REDUCTION

HOW TO BEST STERILIZE PEOPLE AND "REDUCE THE POPULATION" (KILL PEOPLE)?

ARE "VACCINES" MEANT TO HELP PEOPLE?

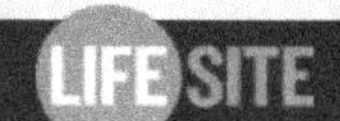

Norway reviewing deaths of frail and elderly patients vaccinated against Covid-19

By Ivana Kottasová, Sarah Dean and Amanda Sealy, CNN
Updated 6:01 AM ET, Tue January 19, 2021

NEWS

At least 271 deaths, 9,845 adverse events after COVID vaccination so far: CDC data

The data indicates that the deaths, reported by the vaccine injury tracking system for the U.S. Centers for Disease Control, mostly occurred within 48 hours of the vaccine being administered

Mon Feb 1, 2021 - 11:39 am EST

Doctor's Death After Covid Vaccine Is Being Investigated

A Florida physician developed an unusual blood disorder shortly after he received the Pfizer vaccine. It is not yet known if the shot is linked to the illness.

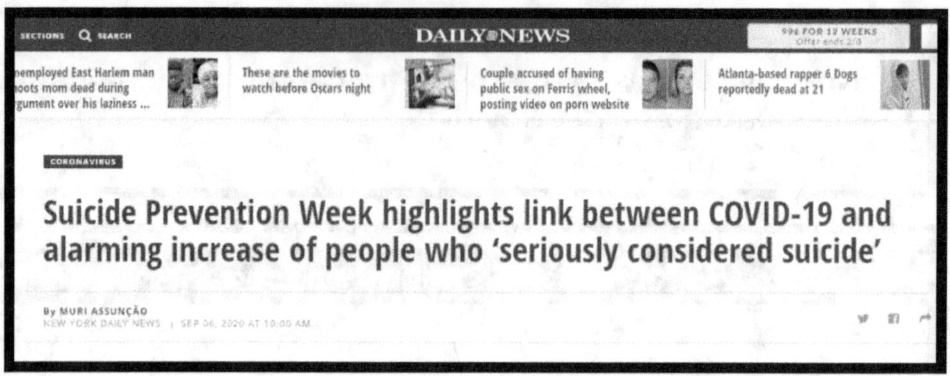

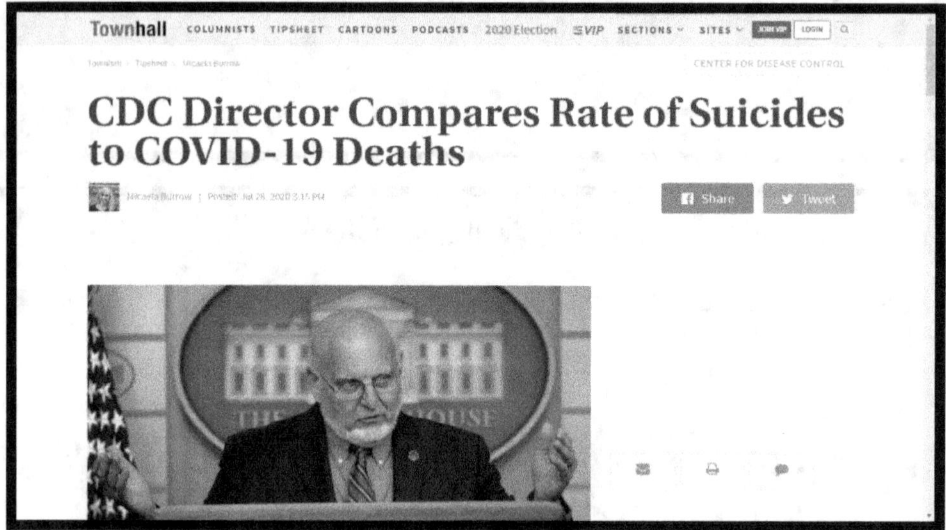

"Center for Disease Control Director Robert Redfield said in a Buck Institute webinar that suicides and drug overdoses have surpassed the death rate for COVID-19 among high school students."

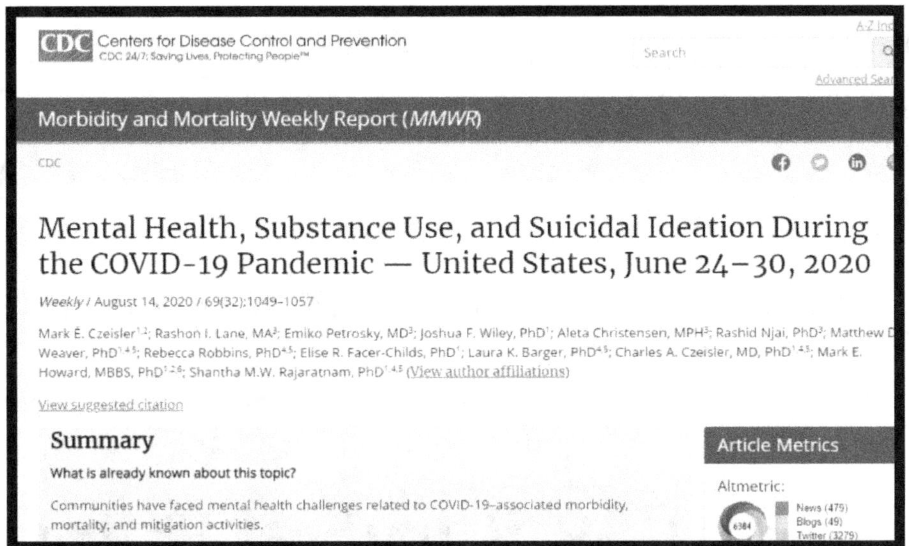

Mental Health, Substance Use, and Suicidal Ideation During the COVID-19 Pandemic — United States, June 24–30, 2020

Weekly / August 14, 2020 / 69(32);1049–1057

Mark É. Czeisler[1,2]; Rashon I. Lane, MA[3]; Emiko Petrosky, MD[3]; Joshua F. Wiley, PhD[1]; Aleta Christensen, MPH[3]; Rashid Njai, PhD[3]; Matthew D. Weaver, PhD[1,4,5]; Rebecca Robbins, PhD[4,5]; Elise R. Facer-Childs, PhD[1]; Laura K. Barger, PhD[4,5]; Charles A. Czeisler, MD, PhD[1,4,5]; Mark E. Howard, MBBS, PhD[1,2,6]; Shantha M.W. Rajaratnam, PhD[1,4,5] (View author affiliations)

View suggested citation

Summary

What is already known about this topic?

Communities have faced mental health challenges related to COVID-19–associated morbidity, mortality, and mitigation activities.

"During June 24–30, 2020, U.S. adults reported considerably elevated adverse mental health conditions associated with COVID-19. Younger adults, racial/ethnic minorities, essential workers, and unpaid adult caregivers reported having experienced disproportionately worse mental health outcomes, increased substance use, and elevated suicidal ideation."

COVID-19 Survival Rates

- Age 0-19: 99.997%
- Age 20-49: 99.98%
- Age 50-69: 99.5%
- Age 70+: 94.6%

"For the overall non-institutionalized population in Indiana, the IFR came out to be 0.26 percent. In other words, for every 1000 people in the community who had gotten infected, an estimated 2.6 ended up dying. *The average age at death was 76.9 years*."

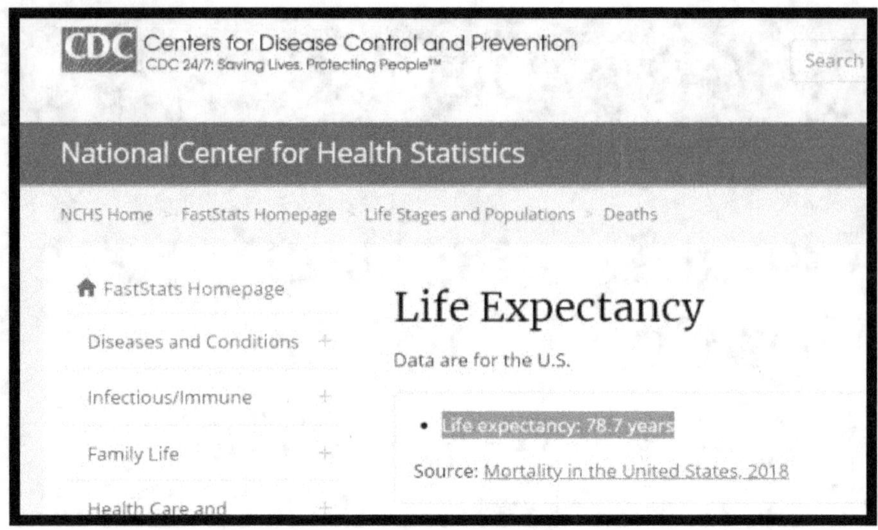

Average American life expectancy: <u>78.7 years</u>

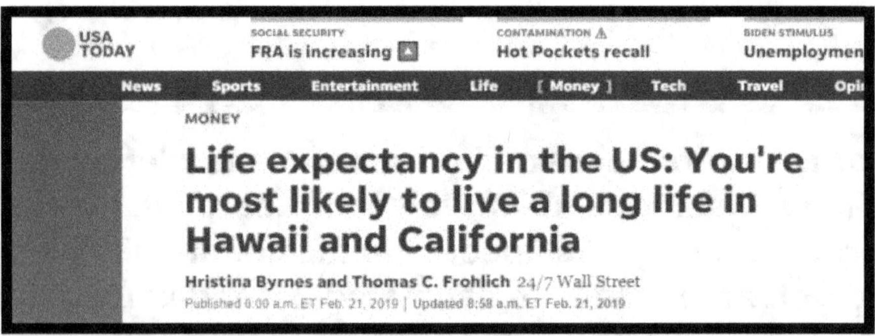

"According to the latest available data, a baby born in 2016 in the United States can be expected to live 78.6 years on average."

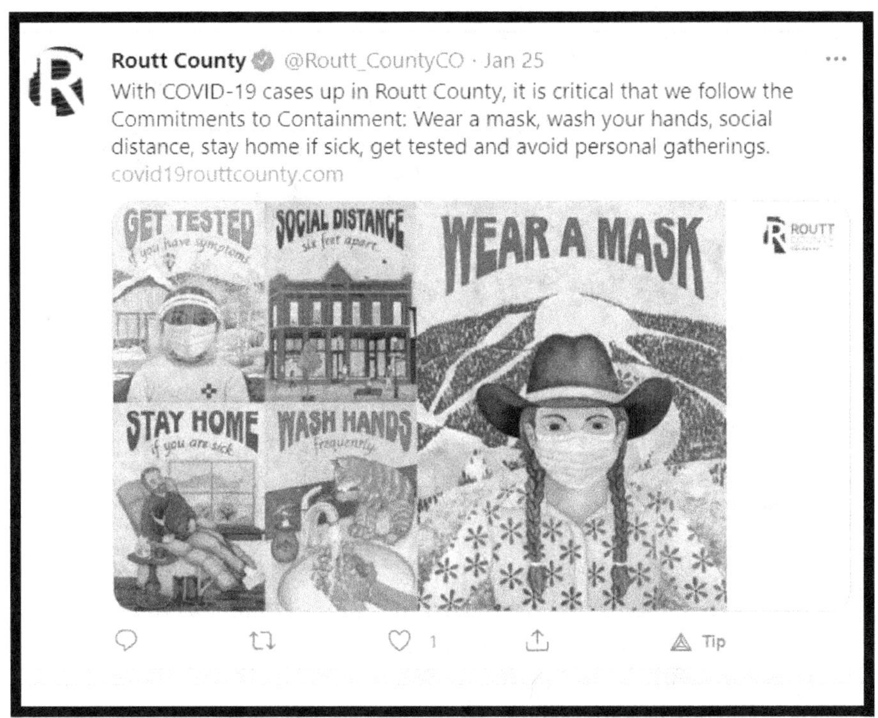

THE *"COMMITMENTS TO CONTAINMENT"* ARE DOING NOTHING TO IMPROVE THE HEALTH OF THE COMMUNITY, AND INSTEAD CONTRIBUTES TO GREATER SUBSTANCE ABUSE, DEPRESSION, DEATHS BY DRUG OVERDOSE AND SUICIDE

GET TESTED
if you have symptoms
SOCIAL DISTANCE
six feet apart.
WEAR A MASK
STAY HOME
if you are sick
WASH HANDS
frequently

SAME =

Wählt
Liste
10
10 10 10
Der Schlag
muss sitzen!
Nationalsozialistische –
Deutsche Arbeiterpartei
(HITLER-BEWEGUNG)

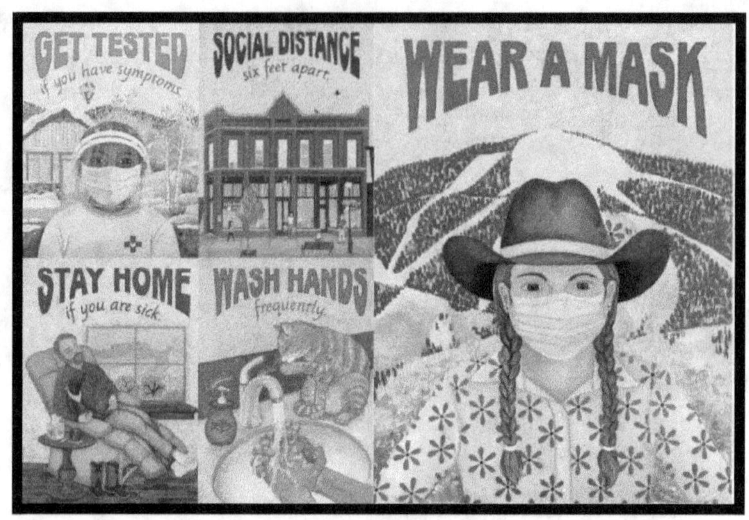

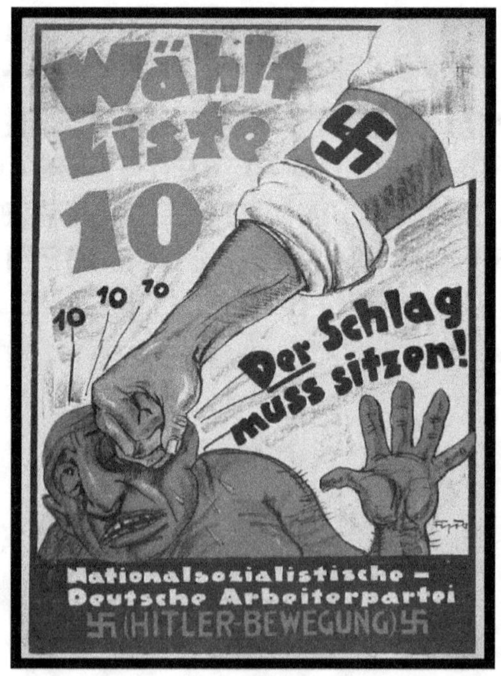

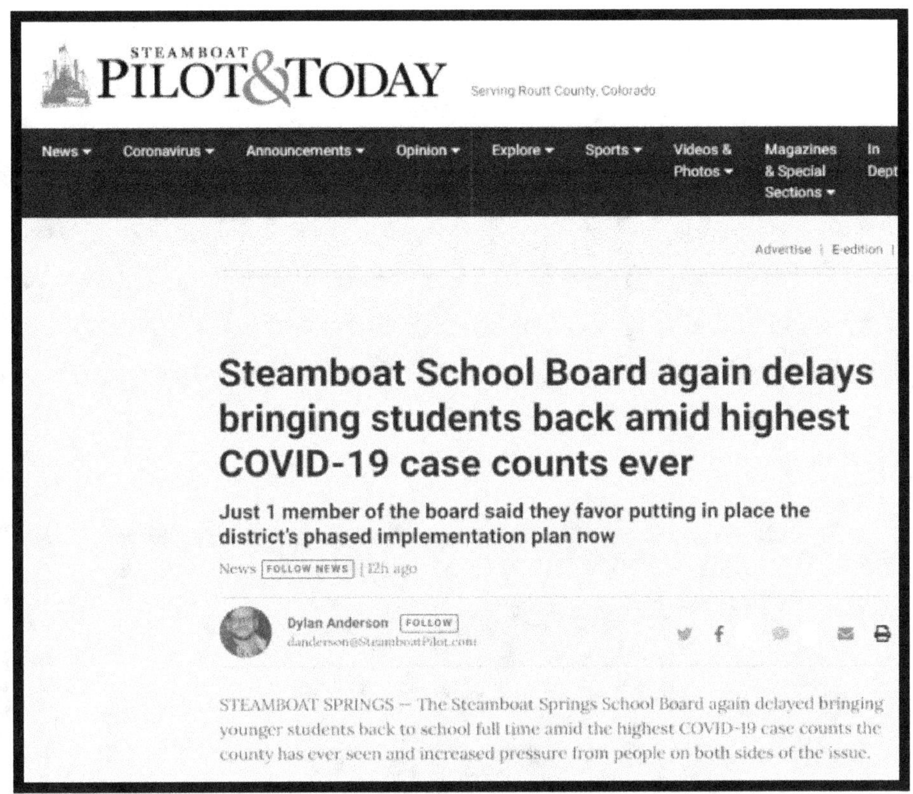

"Routt County recorded **309 cases in the past two weeks**, the highest it has ever been."

HOW MANY WERE

FALSE POSITIVE TEST RESULTS?

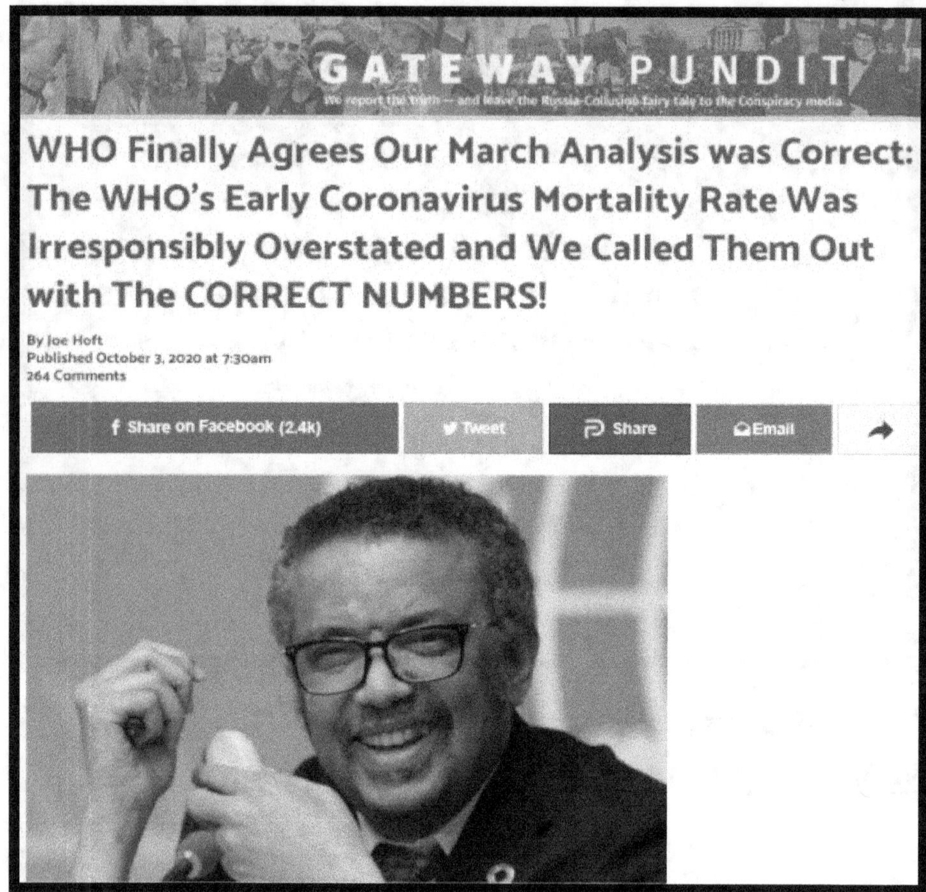

GATEWAY PUNDIT
We report the truth — and leave the Russia-Collusion Fairy tale to the Conspiracy media

WHO Finally Agrees Our March Analysis was Correct: The WHO's Early Coronavirus Mortality Rate Was Irresponsibly Overstated and We Called Them Out with The CORRECT NUMBERS!

By Joe Hoft
Published October 3, 2020 at 7:30am
264 Comments

f Share on Facebook (2.4k)   Tweet   Share   Email

RedState   AUTHORS   DIARIES ▾   ☰VIP

TOTAL COINCIDENCE ALERT: C19 Diagnostic Criteria Tightened by WHO on Biden Inauguration Day!

By Michael Thau | Jan 20, 2021 6:15 PM ET

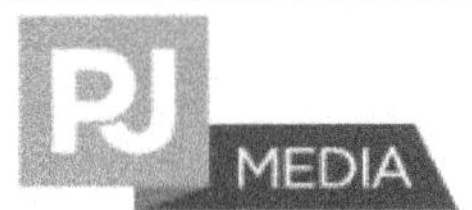

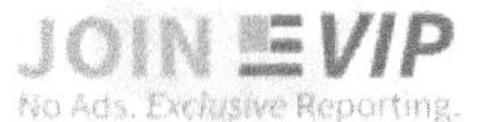

PJ MEDIA

NEWS & POLITICS   COLUMNS   ELECTION 2020   CULTURE   ★ VIP

COLUMNS

The WHO Finally Updates Its COVID-19 Testing Policy... One Hour After Biden's Inauguration

BY STACEY LENNOX JAN 20, 2021 9:22 PM ET

yahoo!news

News Coronavirus US Politics World Health Science Contact Us Originals

NATIONAL REVIEW

Student Suicides Drive Las Vegas Schools to Reopen

Zachary Evans
Mon, January 25, 2021, 8:31 AM

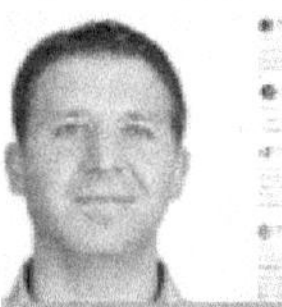
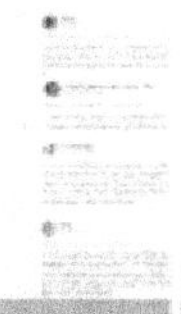
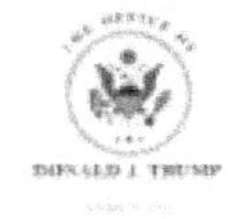
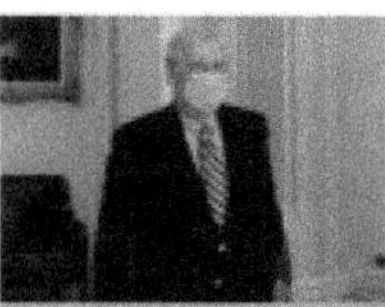
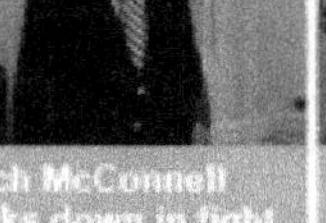
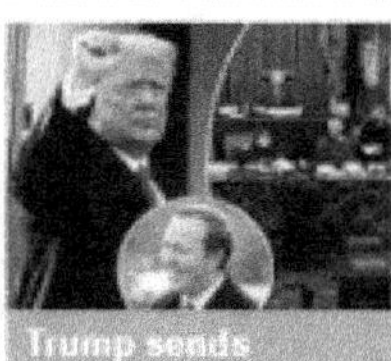

Spate of suicides among Las Vegas students prompts schools to reopen: 18 youngsters - the youngest just nine-years-old - killed themselves during nine-month studying from home period

- Surge in student suicides during final nine months of 2020 has led to Clark County School District Board to approve reopening of schools for vulnerable
- Youngest student to commit suicide in the county was nine years old
- The 18 student suicides recorded in nine months during which schools were closed is double the number recorded in 2019

By RACHAEL BUNYAN FOR MAILONLINE

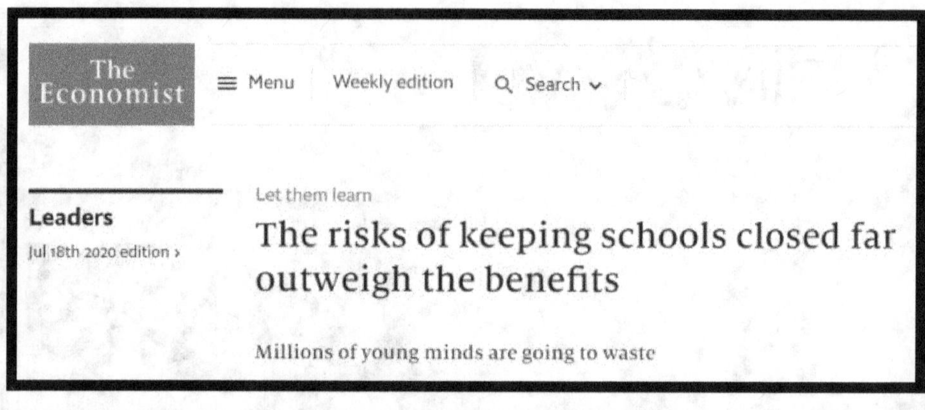

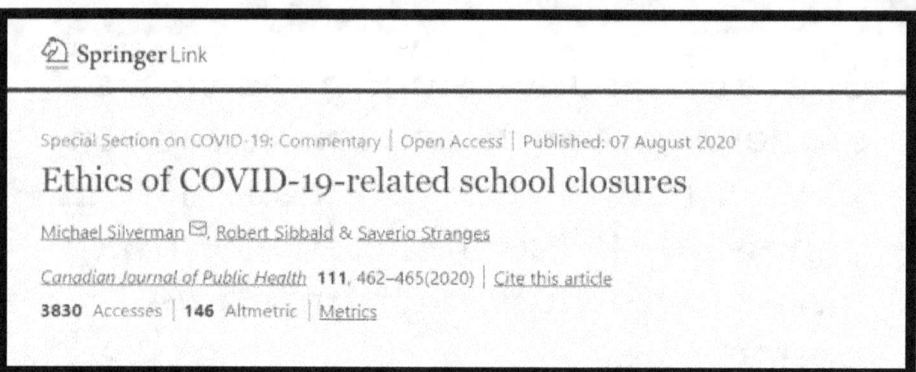

"An argument was made that _**school closures were necessary to prevent harm to vulnerable adults**_, especially the elderly. Although data are still accumulating, the recently described complication, pediatric multisystem inflammatory syndrome, is extremely rare and children remain remarkably unaffected by COVID-19."

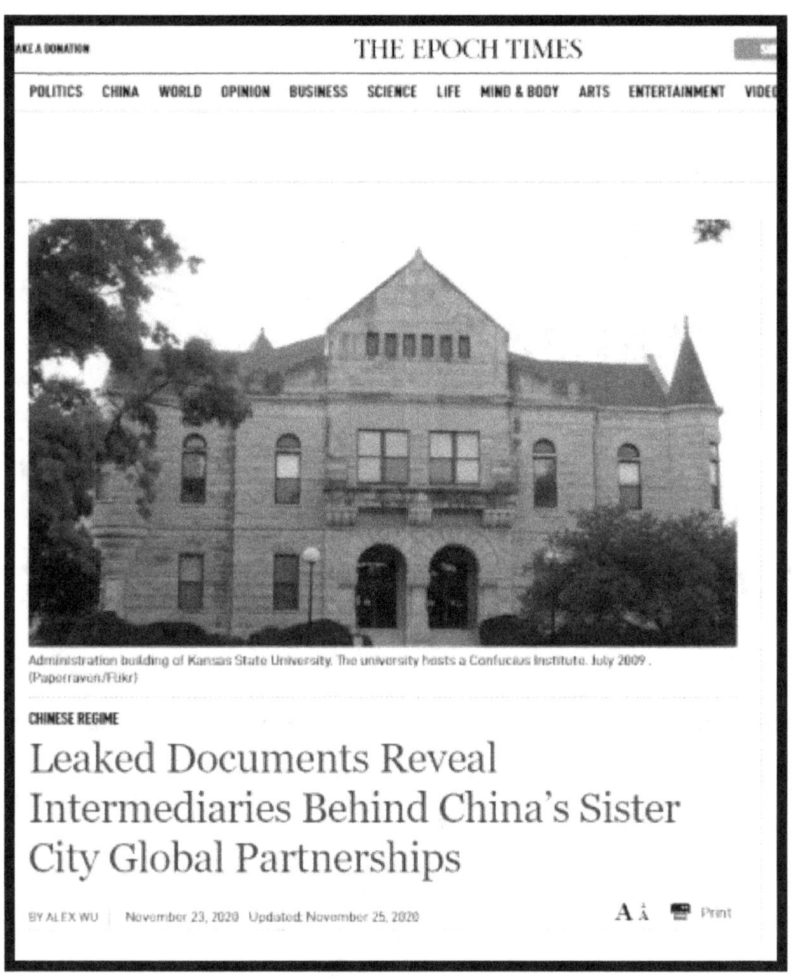

THE EPOCH TIMES

Administration building of Kansas State University. The university hosts a Confucius Institute. July 2009 . (Paperraven/Flikr)

CHINESE REGIME

Leaked Documents Reveal Intermediaries Behind China's Sister City Global Partnerships

BY ALEX WU | November 23, 2020 Updated: November 25, 2020

A Å   Print

"On Feb. 8, during his speech at the National Governors Association meeting, he warned, '**Chinese Communist Party officials, too, are cultivating relationships with county school board members and local politicians**—often through what are known as sister cities programs.'"

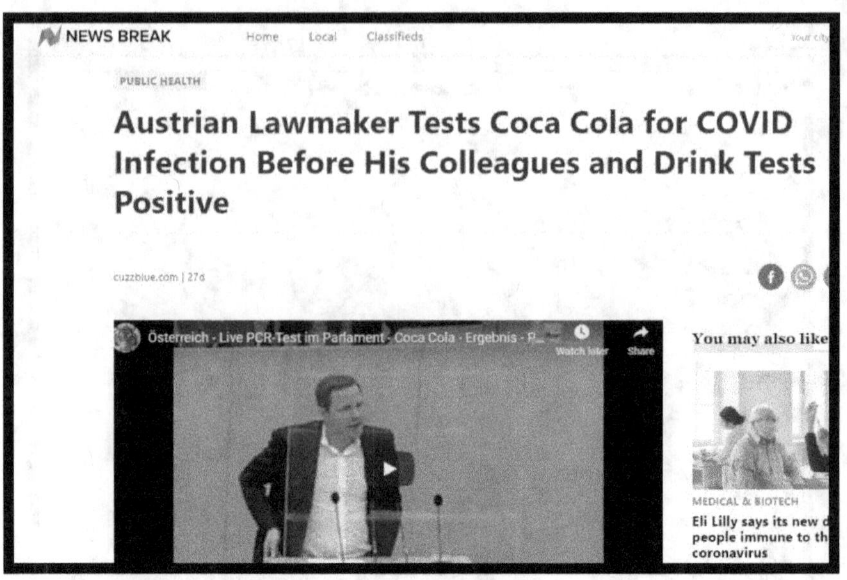
NEWS BREAK
Home   Local   Classifieds
PUBLIC HEALTH
Austrian Lawmaker Tests Coca Cola for COVID Infection Before His Colleagues and Drink Tests Positive
cuzzblue.com | 27d
Österreich · Live PCR-Test im Parlament · Coca Cola · Ergebnis · P...
Watch later   Share
You may also like
MEDICAL & BIOTECH
Eli Lilly says its new
people immune to th
coronavirus

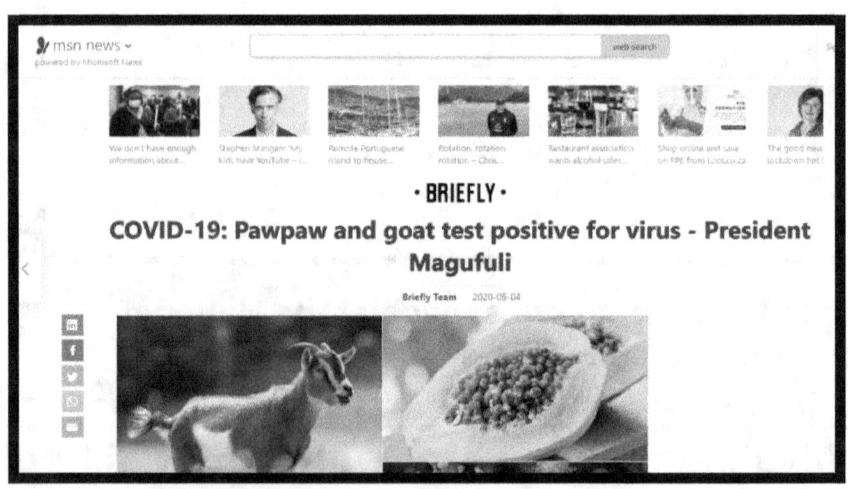
msn news
powered by Microsoft News
web search
We don't have enough information about...
Stephen Mangan: My kids have YouTube – i...
Remote Portuguese island to house...
Rotation, rotation, rotation – Chris...
Restaurant association wants alcohol sales...
Shop online and save on PPE from LootLu.za
The good new lockdown has
· BRIEFLY ·
COVID-19: Pawpaw and goat test positive for virus - President Magufuli
Briefly Team   2020-05-04

Portuguese Court Rules That The PCR Test "Is Unable To Determine" A COVID-19 Infection

November 24, 2020

👁 924   💬 0

 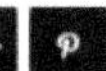  

by Arjun Walia, Collective Evolution:

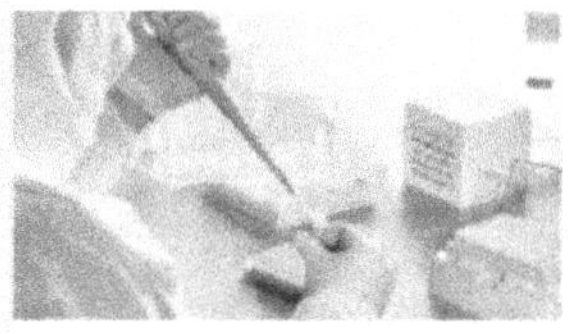

- The Facts: A Portuguese court has determined that the PCR tests used to detect COVID-19 are not able to prove an infection beyond a reasonable doubt, and thus determined that the detainment of four individuals was unlawful and illegal.
- Reflect On: With no clear cut answer, and many doctors and scientists contradicting each other, should governments be allowed to take measures that restrict our freedoms? Instead of force, should they provide the science and simply make recommendations?

BUY
Property **CLICK HERE**
NOW

THE PORTUGAL
News

Casa Verde

Tue, 26 Jan 2021

HOME   NEWS ⌄   ALGARVE ⌄   BUSINESS ⌄   PROPERTY ⌄   WORLD ⌄   SPORT ⌄   LIFESTYLE ⌄   CO

Covid PCR test reliability doubtful – Portugal judges

in News · 27-11-2020 17:50:00 · 14 Comments

NEW YORK POST

China reportedly lying about Pfizer's COVID-19 vaccine to deflect study

Earthquake in Antarctica sparks panic in Chile

Elderly woman who 'died' of COVID-19 reappears at nursing home after 10 days

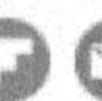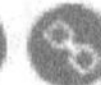

TECH

Elon Musk continues to cast doubt about 'bogus' COVID-19 test results

By Nicolas Vega

November 13, 2020 | 10:37am | Updated

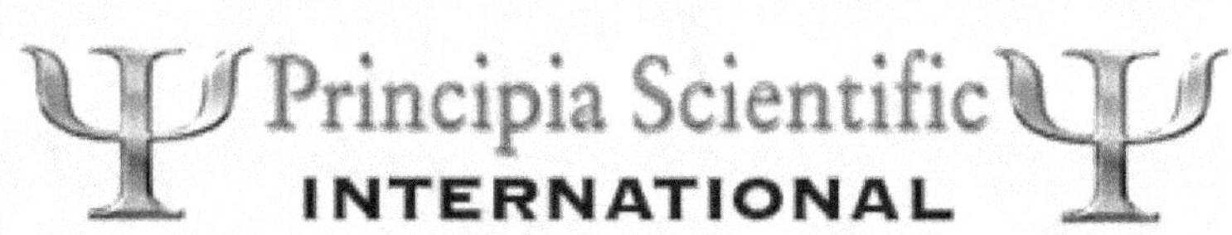

The COVID-19 PCR Test Is Key To The Pandemic Fraud

Published on September 8, 2020

Written by John O'Sullivan

"The PCR test is so well known for giving inaccurate results that the CDC warns not to give the test to asymptomatic persons 'because of the increased likelihood of false-positive results.' In fact, there is a famous Chinese paper that stated if you're testing asymptomatic people with PCR, up to 80% of positives could be false positives."

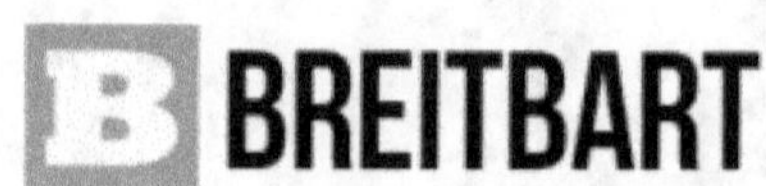

BREITBART

The New American

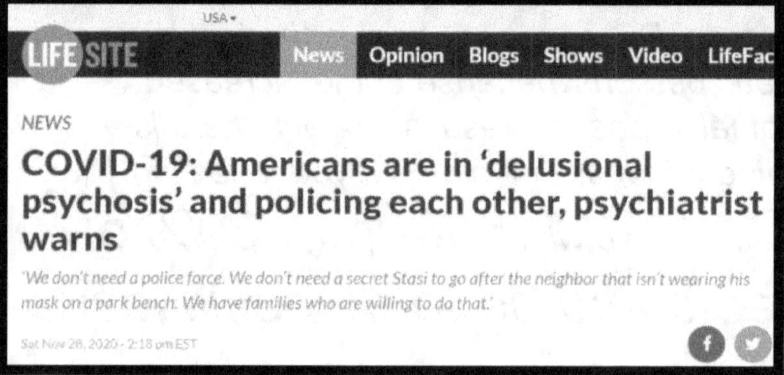

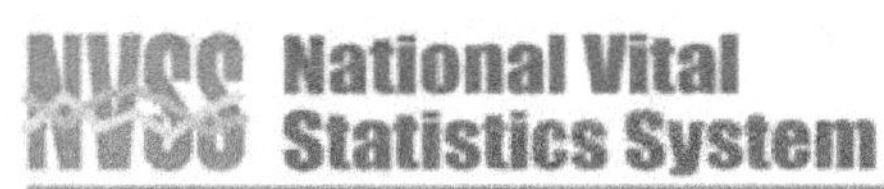

COVID-19 Alert No. 2
March 24, 2020

New ICD code introduced for COVID-19 deaths
This email is to alert you that a newly-introduced ICD code has been implemented to accurately capture mortality data for Coronavirus Disease 2019 (COVID-19) on death certificates.

Please read carefully and forward this email to the state statistical staff in your office who are involved in the preparation of mortality data, as well as others who may receive questions when the data are released.

What is the new code?

"COVID-19 should be reported on the death certificate for all decedents where the disease caused or is *assumed* to have caused or contributed to death."

Should "COVID-19" be reported on the death certificate only with a confirmed test?
COVID-19 should be reported on the death certificate for all decedents where the disease caused **or is assumed to have caused or contributed to death**. Certifiers should include as much detail as possible based on their knowledge of the case, medical records, laboratory testing, etc. If the decedent had other chronic conditions such as COPD or asthma that may have also contributed, these conditions can be reported in Part II. (See attached Guidance for Certifying COVID-19 Deaths)

Steven Schwartz, PhD
Director – Division of Vital Statistics
National Center for Health Statistics
3311 Toledo Rd | Hyattsville, MD 20782

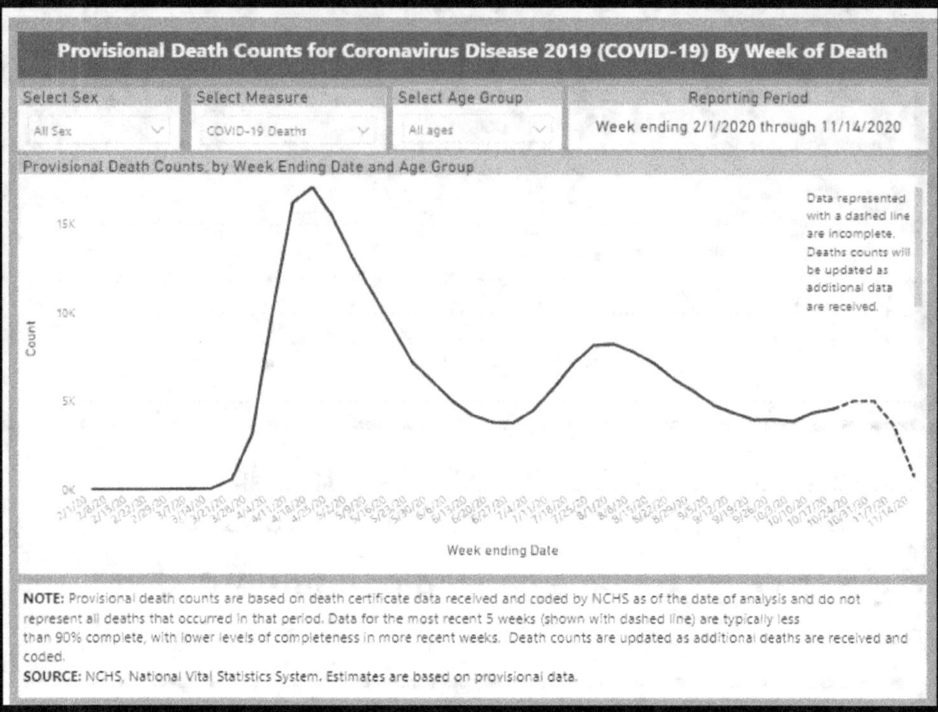

NOTE: Provisional death counts are based on death certificate data received and coded by NCHS as of the date of analysis and do not represent all deaths that occurred in that period. Data for the most recent 5 weeks (shown with dashed line) are typically less than 90% complete, with lower levels of completeness in more recent weeks. Death counts are updated as additional deaths are received and coded.
SOURCE: NCHS, National Vital Statistics System. Estimates are based on provisional data.

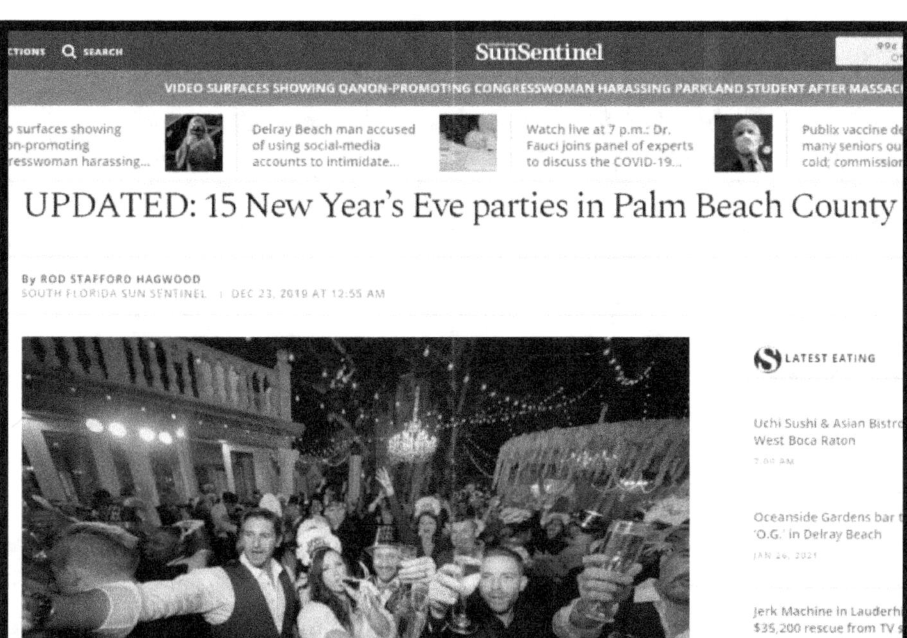

o surfaces showing
on-promoting
resswoman harassing...

Delray Beach man accused
of using social-media
accounts to intimidate...

Watch live at 7 p.m.: Dr.
Fauci joins panel of experts
to discuss the COVID-19...

Publix vaccine de
many seniors ou
cold; commission

UPDATED: 15 New Year's Eve parties in Palm Beach County

By ROD STAFFORD HAGWOOD
SOUTH FLORIDA SUN SENTINEL | DEC 23, 2019 AT 12:55 AM

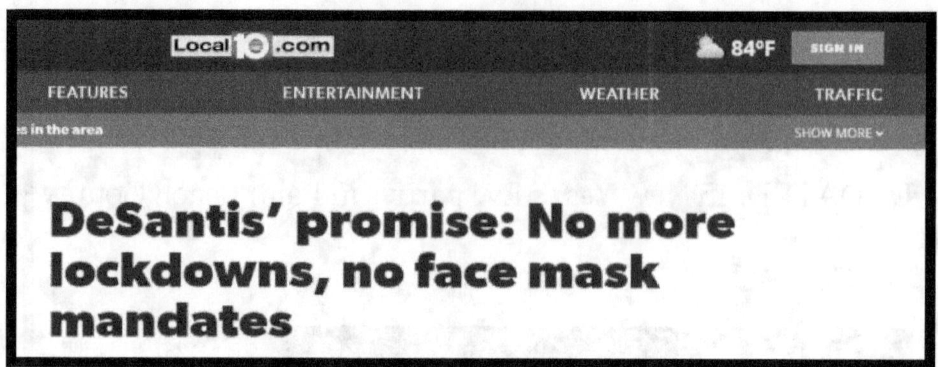

DeSantis' promise: No more lockdowns, no face mask mandates

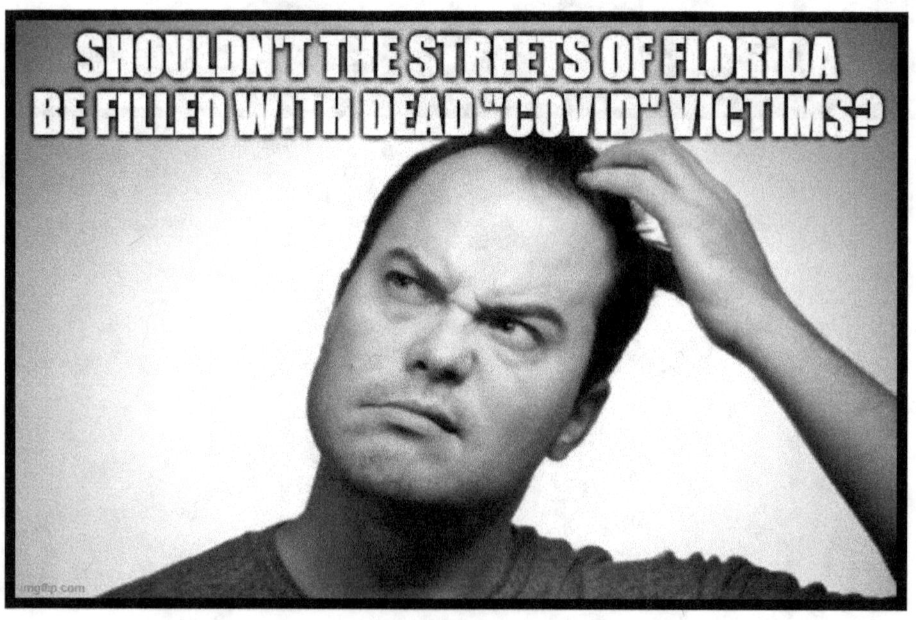

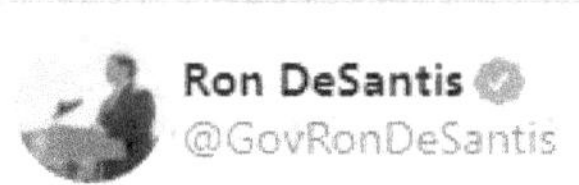

CDC recently updated estimated infection fatality rates for COVID. Here are the updated survival rates by age group:

0-19: 99.997%
20-49: 99.98%
50-69: 99.5%
70+: 94.6%

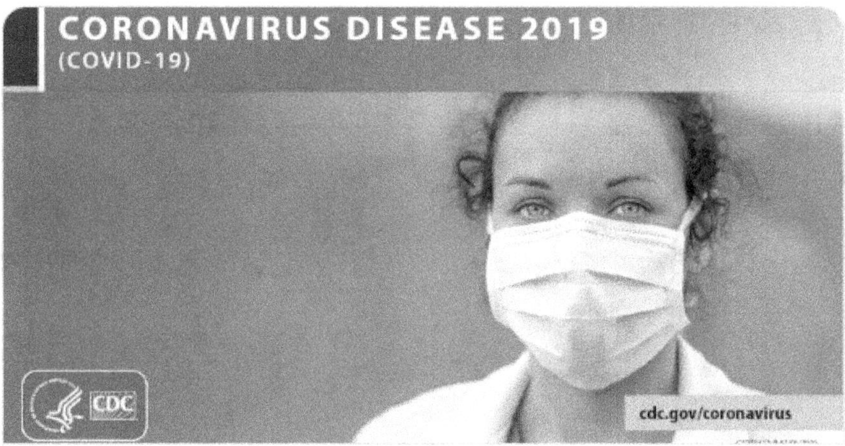

Healthcare Workers
COVID-19 guidance, tools, and resources for healthcare workers.
🔗 cdc.gov

11:44 AM · Sep 23, 2020

 7.3K   ⚡ See the latest COVID-19 information on Twitter

<u>PRESENTED ANOTHER WAY:</u>

Parameter	Scenario 1	Scenario 2	Scenario 3	Scenario 4	Scenario 5: Current Best Estimate
R_0*	2.0		4.0		2.5
Infection Fatality Ratio[+]	0-19 years: 0.00002 20-49 years: 0.00007 50-69 years: 0.0025 70+ years: 0.028		0-19 years: 0.0001 20-49 years: 0.0003 50-69 years: 0.010 70+ years: 0.093		0-19 years: 0.00003 20-49 years: 0.0002 50-69 years: 0.005 70+ years: 0.054

<u>https://www.cdc.gov/coronavirus/2019-ncov/hcp/planning-scenarios.html</u>

REGARDLESS HOW YOU LOOK AT IT, THE TRUTH IS THAT "CASE NUMBERS" DO NOT MATTER, BECAUSE "FATALITY RATES" ARE NEAR ZERO.

WHAT IS THE THREAT OF AN ASYMPTOMATIC PERSON SUPPOSEDLY TESTING POSITIVE FOR "COVID," IF THEY DID NOT EVEN KNEW THEY HAD IT AND THE THREAT OF DEATH IS NEAR ZERO?

WHAT IS THE THREAT?

THE AVERAGE AGE OF VICTIMS WHO DIED OF "COVID" IS ABOUT 75 YEARS OLD.

THE AVERAGE AGE OF DEATH FOR AMERICANS OVERALL IS ABOUT 78 YEARS OLD.

DO NOT YOU SEE WHAT IS HAPPENING?

WE ARE DRIVING PEOPLE TO SUICIDE, TO BANKRUPTCY, TO DRUG OVERDOSE, AND DENIAL OF THEIR CONSTITUTIONAL RIGHTS BECAUSE AN ARBITRARY RATE OF "CASES" INCREASES?

WHAT IS THE THREAT?

THE THREAT OF DEATH IS OBVIOUSLY NOT THE CONCERN.

WHAT IS THE THREAT?

THE THREAT THAT AMERICAN CITIZENS MIGHT BE FREE TO LIVE THEIR LIVES

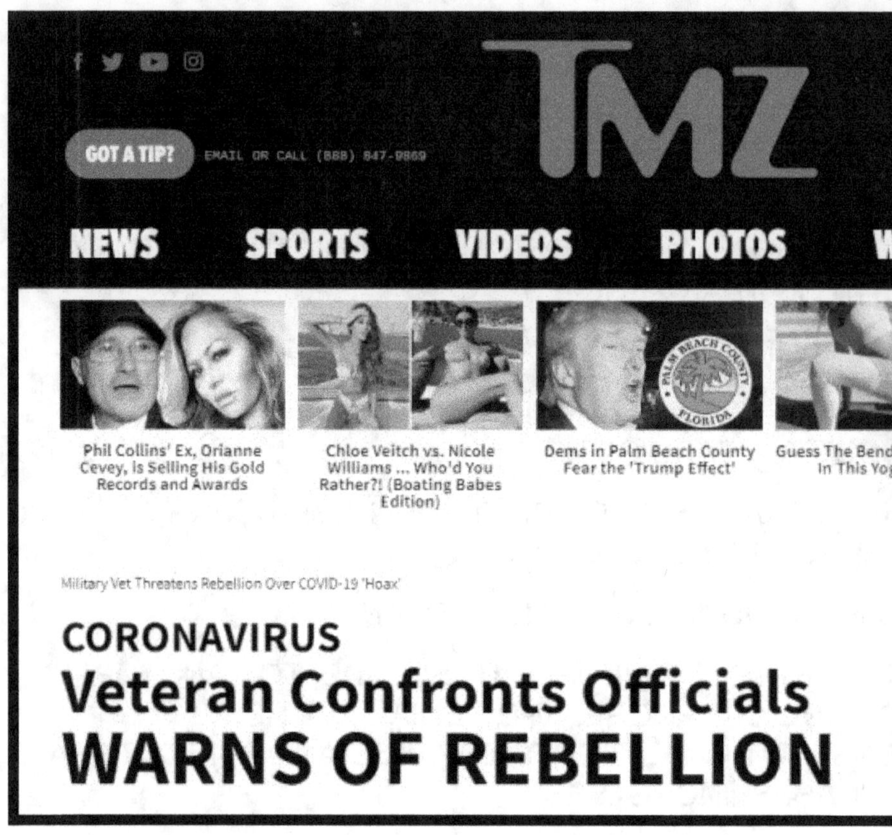

"He angrily said it's not gonna' be pretty if restrictions aren't lifted. The reason for his rage? Zapata says he's had 6 friends, all vets, commit suicide during the pandemic because they lost their jobs."

COVID-19 Survival Rates

- Age 0-19: 99.997%
- Age 20-49: 99.98%
- Age 50-69: 99.5%
- Age 70+: 94.6%

TEACHERS ADVOCATING SCHOOL CLOSURES DO NOT CARE ABOUT THE HARM CAUSED TO CHILDREN.

TEACHERS WOULD RATHER SPIN AROUND IN THEIR LIVING ROOMS INSTEAD OF GO TO WORK LIKE NORMAL ADULTS.

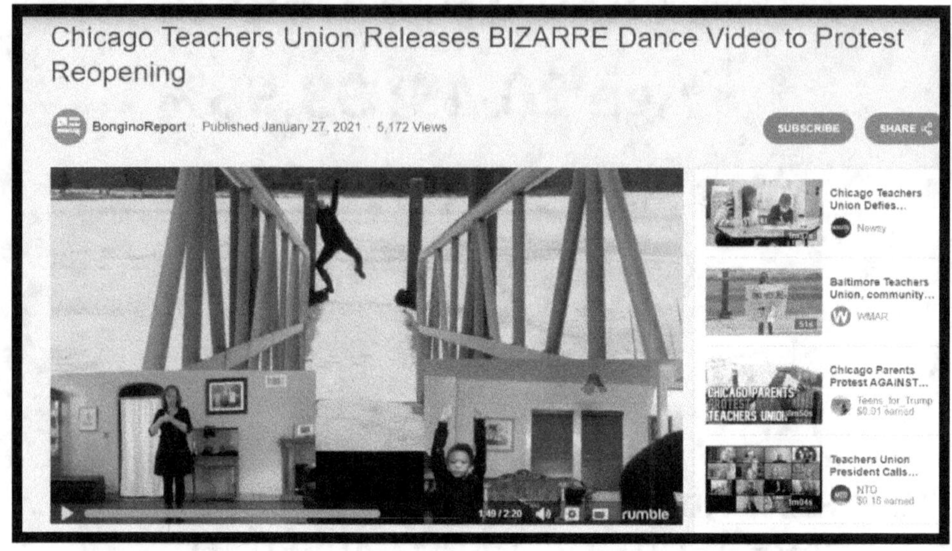

HOW MANY CHILDREN ARE DYING FROM "COVID?"

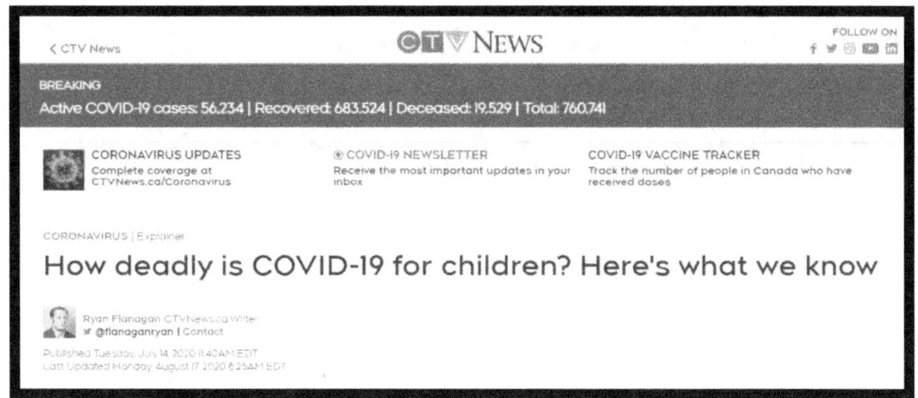

"In Canada, the death rate is about **one per 10,000 infected**," Dr. Stephen Freedman, a Calgary-based pediatric emergency medicine physician and researcher, told CTVNews.ca

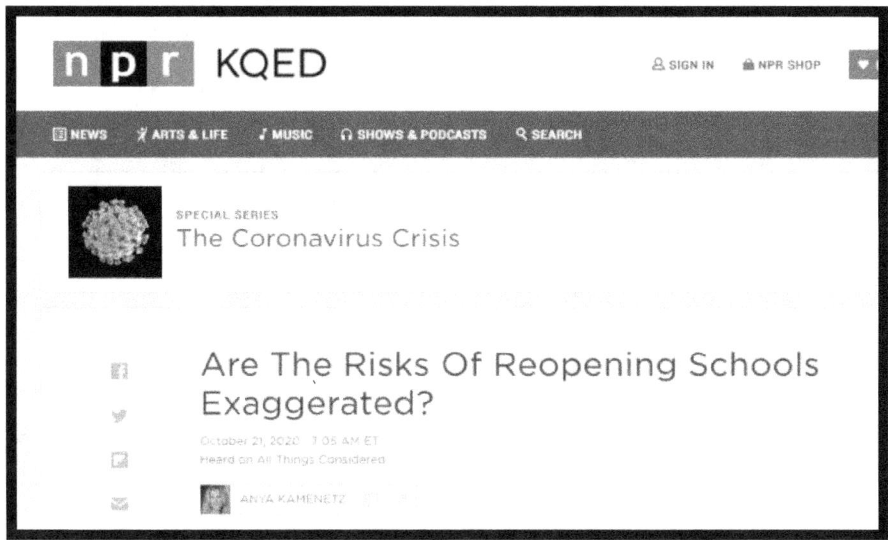

"… two new international studies show **no consistent relationship between in-**

person K-12 schooling and the spread of the coronavirus. And a third study from the United States shows no elevated risk to childcare workers who stayed on the job…"

**(BUT IT IS NOT THE SAFETY OF THE *CHILDREN*
THAT ANYONE CARES ABOUT, IS IT?)**

The New York Times

Teens in Covid Isolation: 'I Felt Like I Was Suffocating'

Remote learning, lockdowns and pandemic uncertainty have increased anxiety and depression among adolescents, and heightened concerns about their mental health.

"Remote learning, lockdowns and pandemic uncertainty have increased anxiety and depression among adolescents, and heightened concerns about their mental health."

"One of the most dangerous trends of our times is making the truth socially unacceptable, or even illegal, with 'hate speech' laws."

– Thomas Sowell

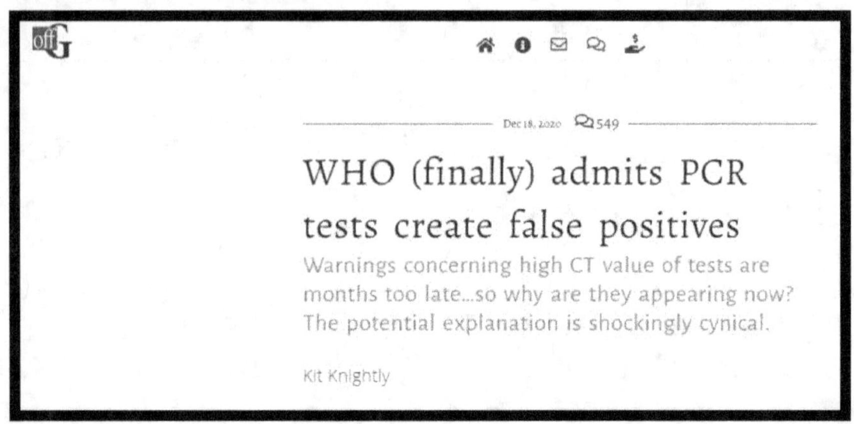

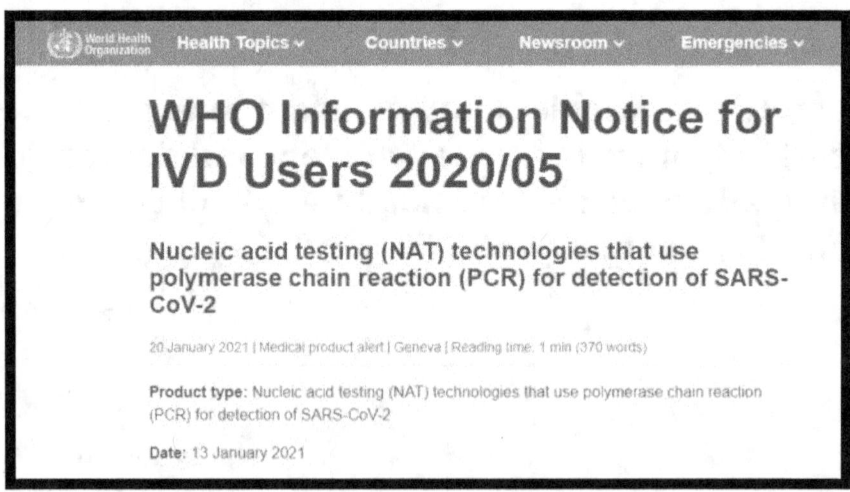

revolver

Right On Cue: As Biden Takes Office, Media and Tyrannical Dems Drop Lockdown Sham

January 20, 2021 (21h ago)   💬 135

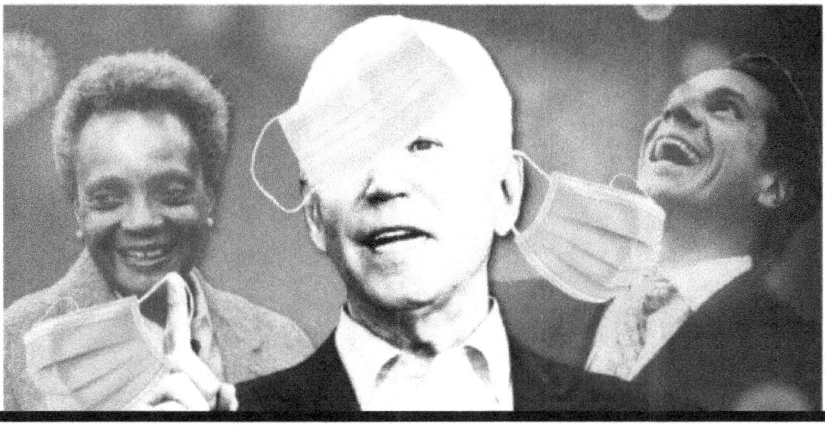

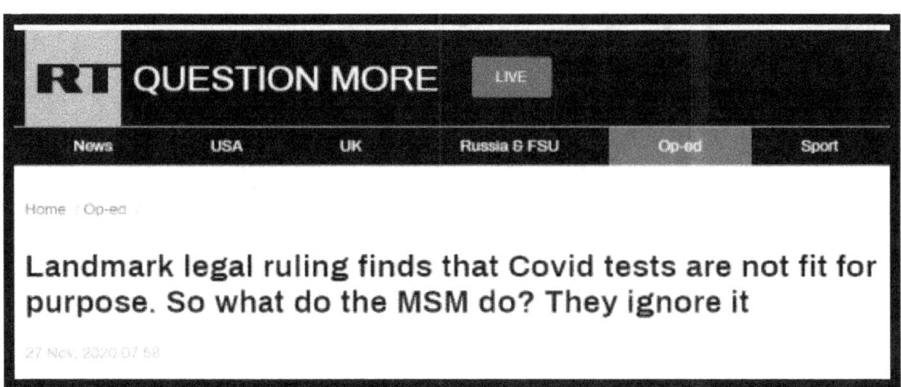

RT QUESTION MORE   LIVE

News   USA   UK   Russia & FSU   Op-ed   Sport

Home / Op-ed

Landmark legal ruling finds that Covid tests are not fit for purpose. So what do the MSM do? They ignore it

27 Nov, 2020 07:58

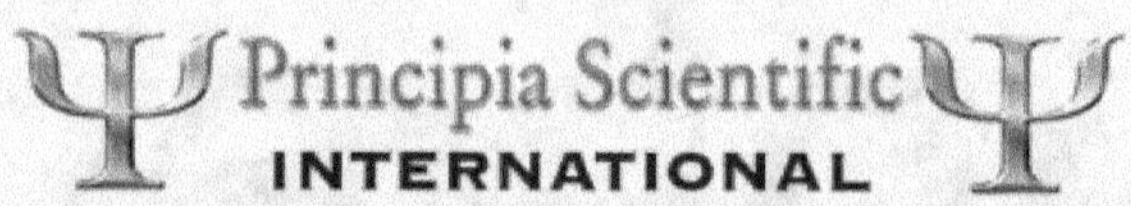

WHO Finally Admits COVID19 PCR Test Has A 'Problem'

Published on December 17, 2020

Written by John O'Sullivan

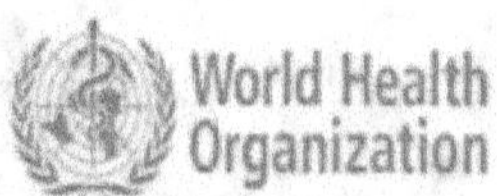

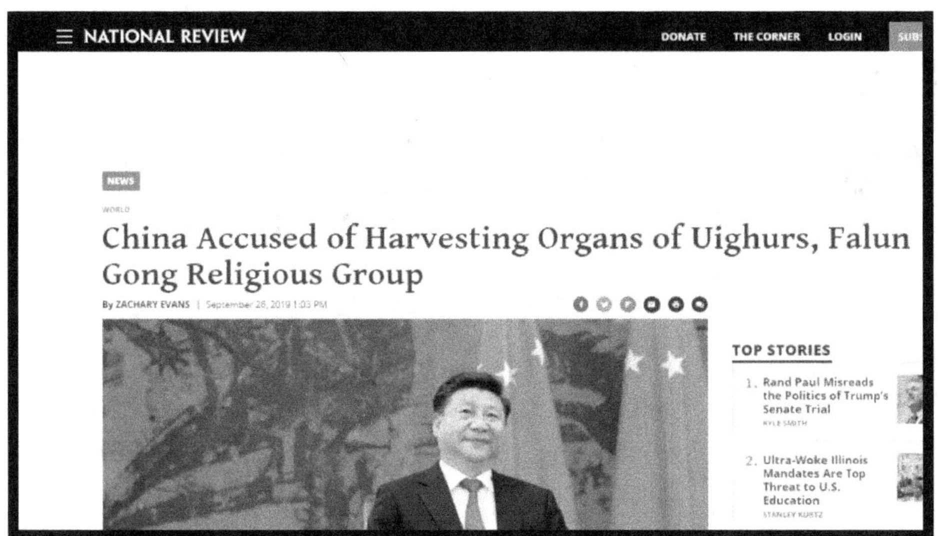
NATIONAL REVIEW
DONATE   THE CORNER   LOGIN   SUBS
NEWS
WORLD
China Accused of Harvesting Organs of Uighurs, Falun Gong Religious Group
By ZACHARY EVANS | September 28, 2019 1:03 PM
TOP STORIES
1. Rand Paul Misreads the Politics of Trump's Senate Trial
KYLE SMITH
2. Ultra-Woke Illinois Mandates Are Top Threat to U.S. Education
STANLEY KURTZ

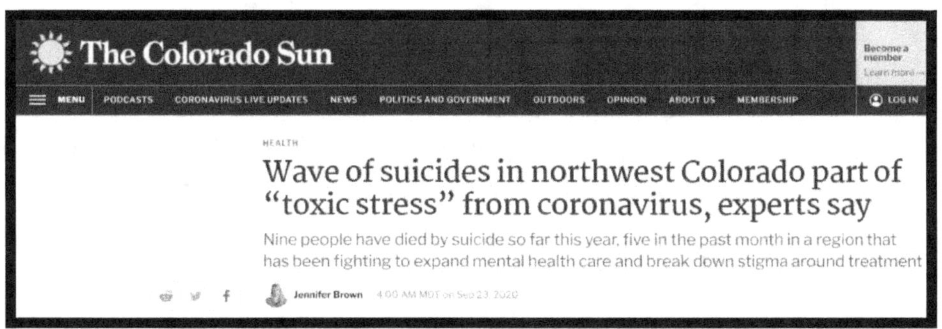
The Colorado Sun
Become a member
Learn more
MENU   PODCASTS   CORONAVIRUS LIVE UPDATES   NEWS   POLITICS AND GOVERNMENT   OUTDOORS   OPINION   ABOUT US   MEMBERSHIP   LOG IN
HEALTH
Wave of suicides in northwest Colorado part of "toxic stress" from coronavirus, experts say
Nine people have died by suicide so far this year, five in the past month in a region that has been fighting to expand mental health care and break down stigma around treatment
Jennifer Brown   4:00 AM MDT on Sep 23, 2020

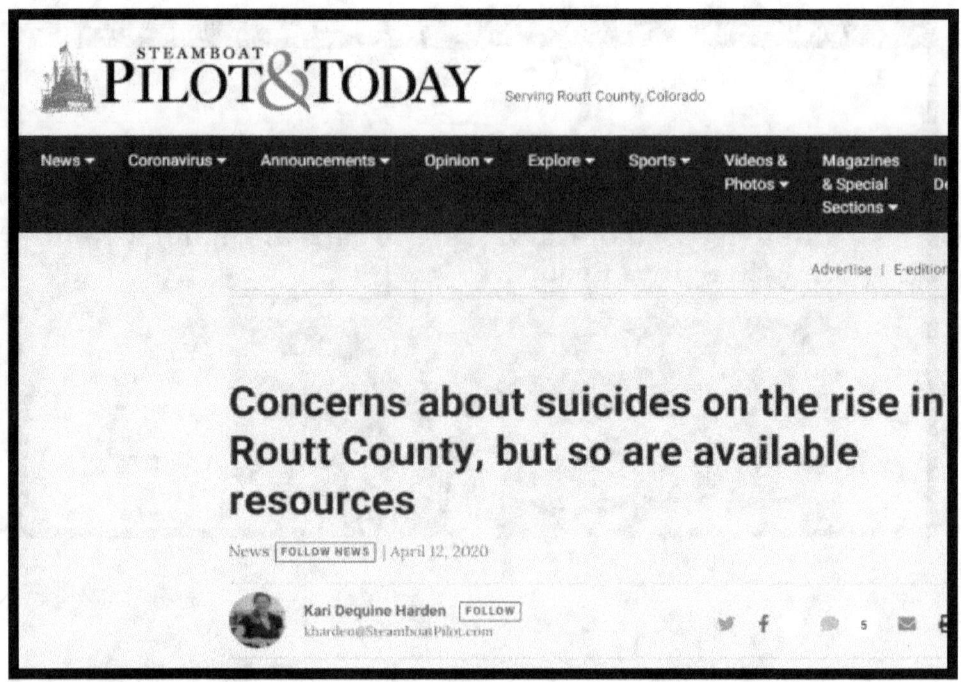

Look at the difference between California and Florida – There is no question about it, the "lockdowns" and "COVID" restrictions ARE CAUSING MORE "INFECTIONS!"

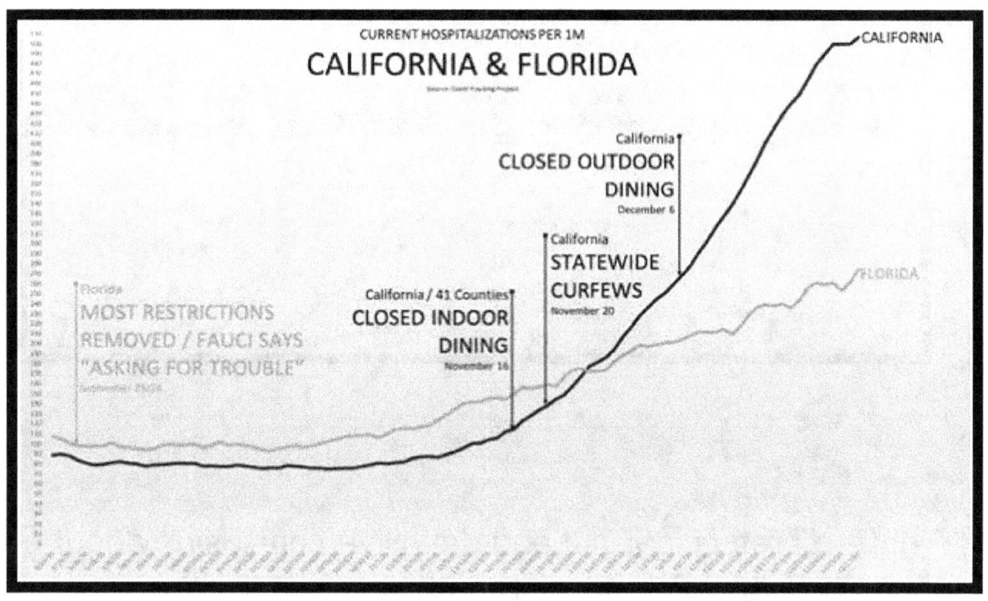

I have already shown you the scientific evidence that "masks" are responsible for CAUSING infections, not preventing them from being spread:

"Moisture retention, reuse of cloth masks and poor filtration may result in increased risk of infection."

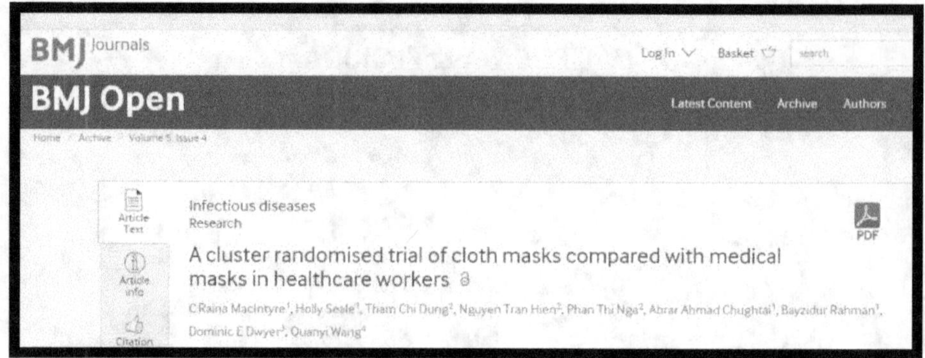

https://bmjopen.bmj.com/content/5/4/e006577

That's a pretty clear-cut and definitive conclusion about the use of "masks" — I will repeat:

"Moisture retention, reuse of cloth masks and poor filtration may result in <u>increased risk of infection.</u>"

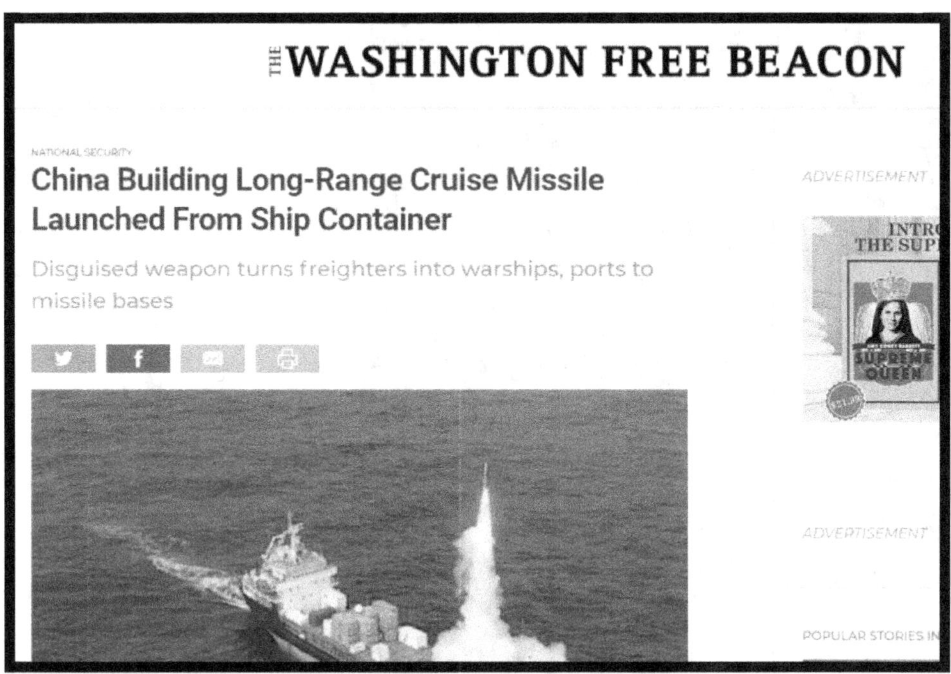

This is not a "parody" or "conspiracy theory" – This is real – China has controlled several of U.S. ports for many years benefitting from the corrupt U.S. politicians that had sold us out prior to the last-minute rescue by the military and the Trump Administration.

Q Clearance Patriot

Anonymous 1 Nov 2017 - 8:56:16 PM

Q Clearance Patriot

My fellow Americans, over the course of the next several days you will undoubtedly realize that we are taking back our great country (the land of the free) from the evil tyrants that wish to do us harm and destroy the last remaining refuge of shining light. On POTUS' order, we have initiated certain fail-safes that shall safeguard the public from the primary fallout which is slated to occur 11.3 upon the arrest announcement of Mr. Podesta (actionable 11.4). Confirmation (to the public) of what is occurring will then be revealed and will not be openly accepted. Public riots are being organized in serious numbers in an effort to prevent the arrest and capture of more senior public officials. On POTUS' order, a state of temporary military control will be actioned and special ops carried out. False leaks have been made to retain several within the confines of the United States to prevent extradition and special operator necessity. Rest assured, the safety and well-being of every man, woman, and child of this country is being exhausted in full. However, the atmosphere within the country will unfortunately be divided as so many have fallen for the corrupt and evil narrative that has long been broadcast. We will be initiating the Emergency Broadcast System (EMS) during this time in an effort to provide a direct message (avoiding the fake news) to all citizens. Organizations and/or people that wish to do us harm during this time will be met with swift fury – certain laws have been pre-lifted to provide our great military the necessary authority to handle and conduct these operations (at home and abroad).

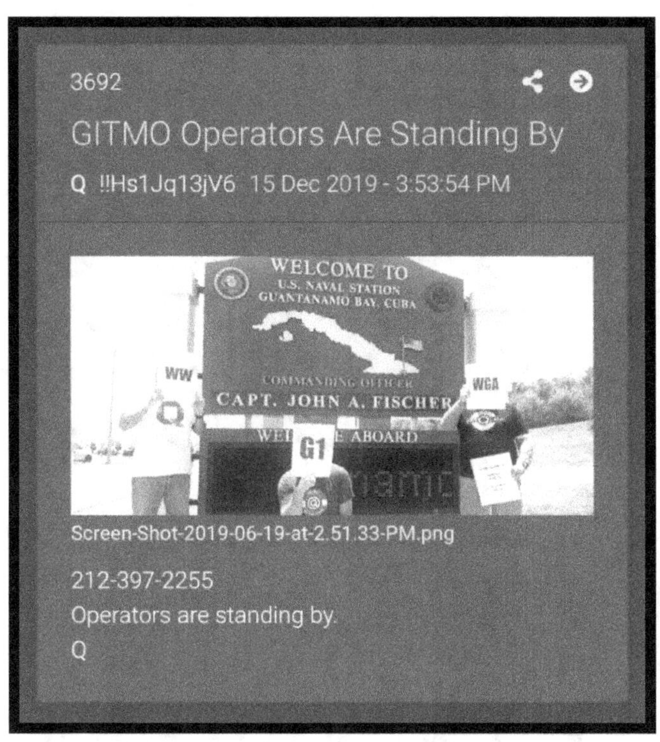

3692

GITMO Operators Are Standing By

Q !!Hs1Jq13jV6 15 Dec 2019 - 3:53:54 PM

Screen-Shot-2019-06-19-at-2.51.33-PM.png

212-397-2255
Operators are standing by.
Q

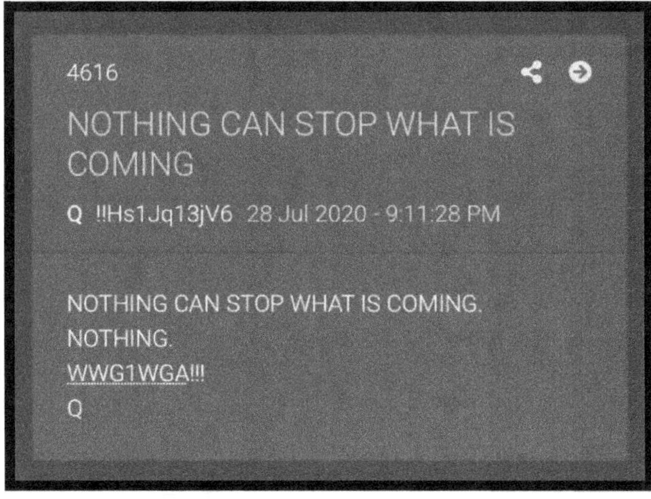

4616

NOTHING CAN STOP WHAT IS COMING

Q !!Hs1Jq13jV6 28 Jul 2020 - 9:11:28 PM

NOTHING CAN STOP WHAT IS COMING.
NOTHING.
WWG1WGA!!!
Q

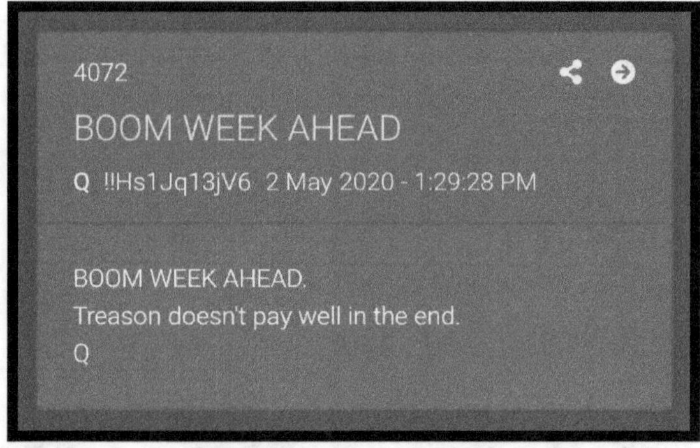

4072

BOOM WEEK AHEAD

Q !!Hs1Jq13jV6 2 May 2020 - 1:29:28 PM

BOOM WEEK AHEAD.
Treason doesn't pay well in the end.
Q

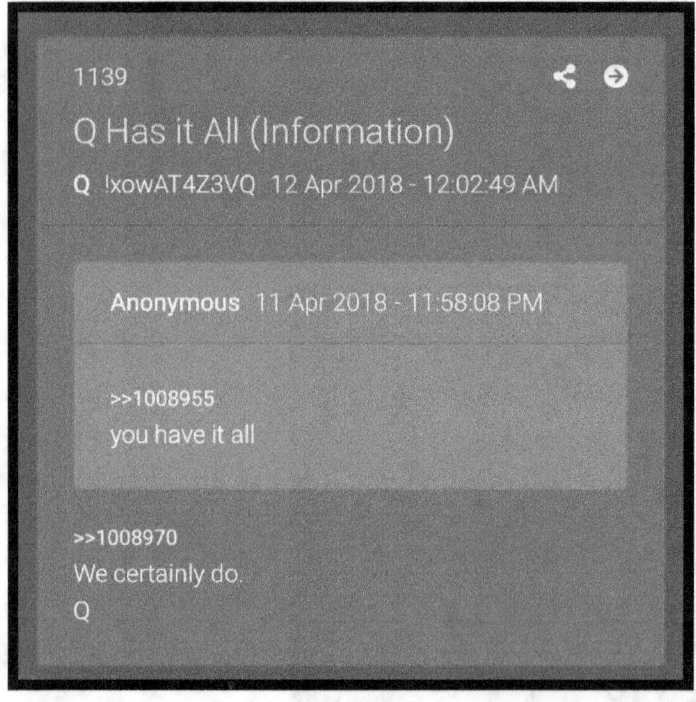

1139

Q Has it All (Information)

Q !xowAT4Z3VQ 12 Apr 2018 - 12:02:49 AM

Anonymous 11 Apr 2018 - 11:58:08 PM

>>1008955
you have it all

>>1008970
We certainly do.
Q

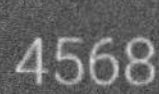

4568

Virginia Roberts with Prince Andrew and Ghislaine Maxwell

Q !!Hs1Jq13jV6 2 Jul 2020 - 4:25:22 PM

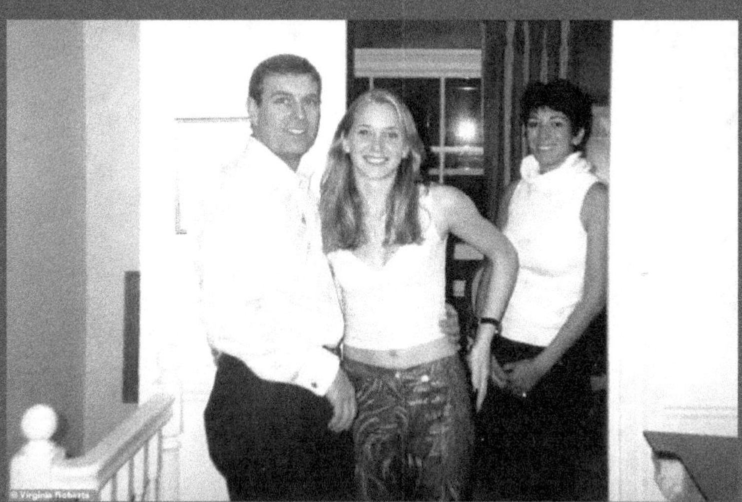

Eb7QXABU8AAr1f8.jpg

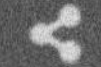 

Obama with AK47 Photos Coming

Q !xowAT4Z3VQ 6 Apr 2018 - 1:17:40 PM

Anonymous 6 Apr 2018 - 1:13:13 PM

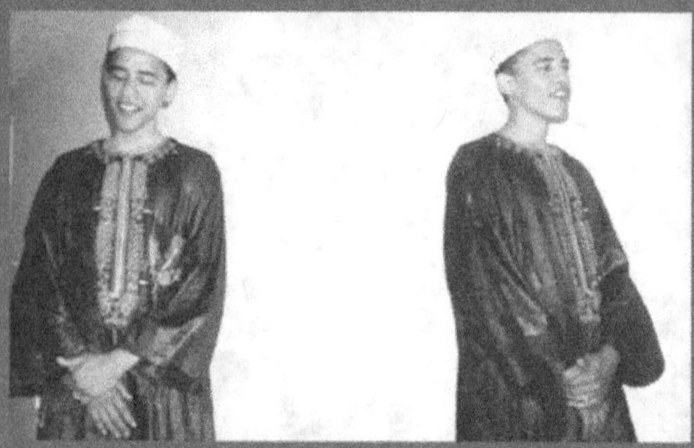

bb10045197285864d9ffe1af03605d08eab2abf1c5
d111b154f1bd2db9044250.jpg

Christian ? Christian Ring ?

>>922075
Pics will surface of Hussein holding AK47 in tribal
attire.
One of many.
Net shut down.
Q

4567

Redrop: Hillary Clinton and Foundation Crime Against Children

Q !!Hs1Jq13jV6 2 Jul 2020 - 4:25:08 PM

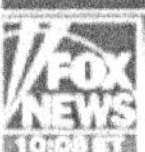

faedd3131d4bddf46bca54b0d9350f6a.jpg

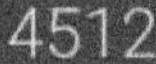 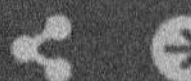

Meme: Obama and Biden Treason Charges

Q !!Hs1Jq13jV6 24 Jun 2020 - 11:32:07 AM

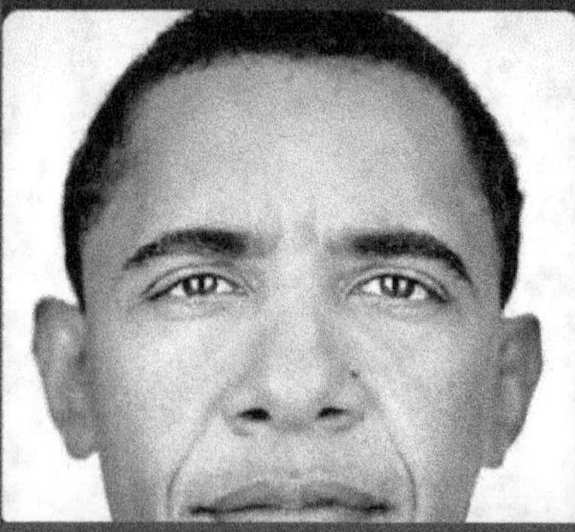

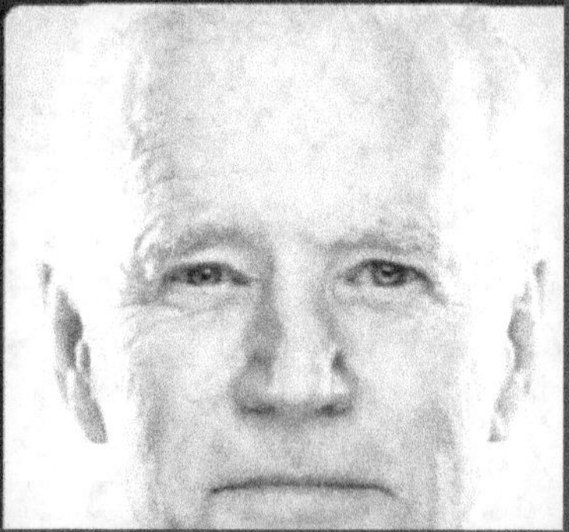

EbSzsRXX0AgVohh.jpg

3901

Redrop: Patriot vs Traitor

Q !!Hs1Jq13jV6 26 Mar 2020 - 11:15:55 AM

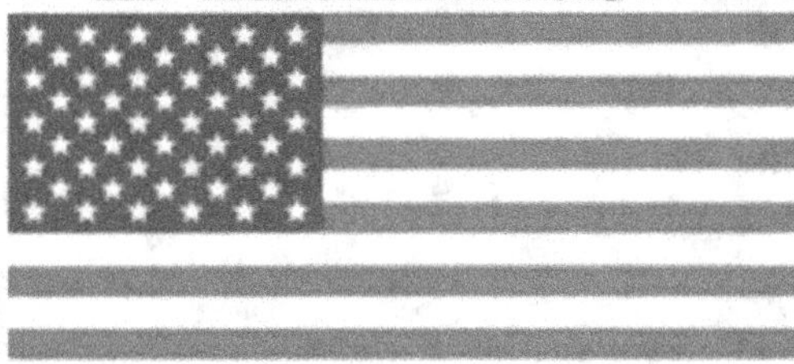

File (hide): a7ffb193423f0a5⋯.png (2.65 KB, 310x163, 310 163, [2] png)

[–] ▶ Q !UW.yye1fxo 02/21/18 (Wed) 20:20:23 No.452 🔒
[2]
Patriot
1. a person who loves, supports, and defends his or
her country and its interests with devotion.
2. a person who regards himself or herself as a
defender, especially of individual rights, against
presumed interference by the federal government.

Traitor
1. a person who betrays another, a cause, or any trust.
2. a person who commits treason by betraying his or her country.
Q

DWsc6pDU8AAW9h1.jpg

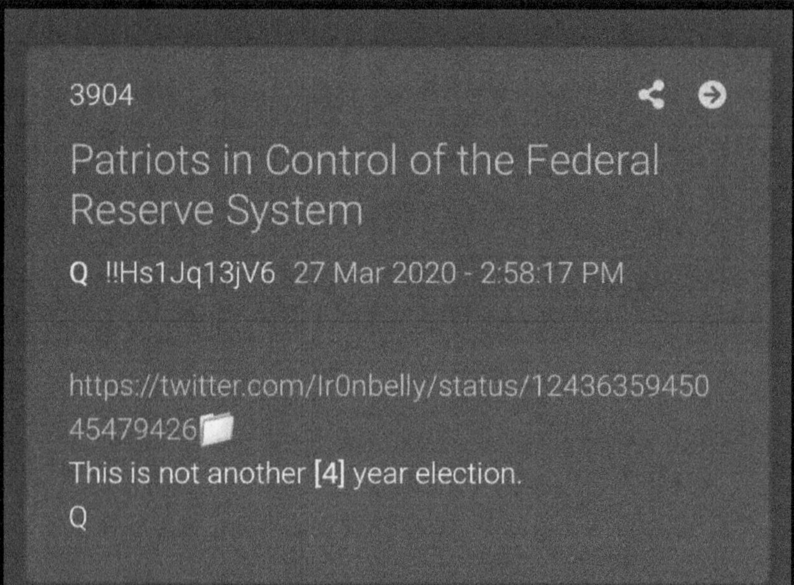
3904

Patriots in Control of the Federal Reserve System

Q !!Hs1Jq13jV6   27 Mar 2020 - 2:58:17 PM

https://twitter.com/lr0nbelly/status/12436359450
45479426
This is not another [4] year election.
Q

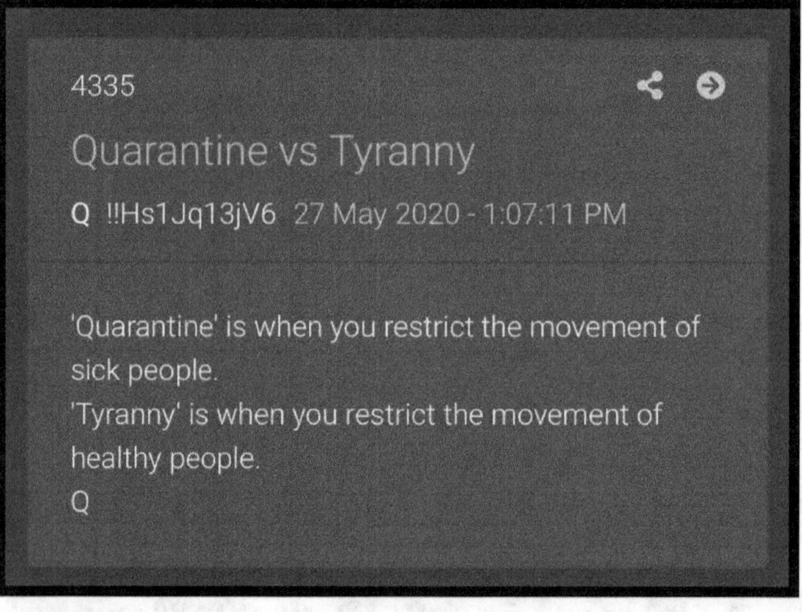
4335

Quarantine vs Tyranny

Q !!Hs1Jq13jV6   27 May 2020 - 1:07:11 PM

'Quarantine' is when you restrict the movement of
sick people.
'Tyranny' is when you restrict the movement of
healthy people.
Q

By the way, "Qanon" people are not "domestic terrorists" – That's the criminals projecting their own guilt

"Qanon" people are true God-loving and freedom-loving patriots:

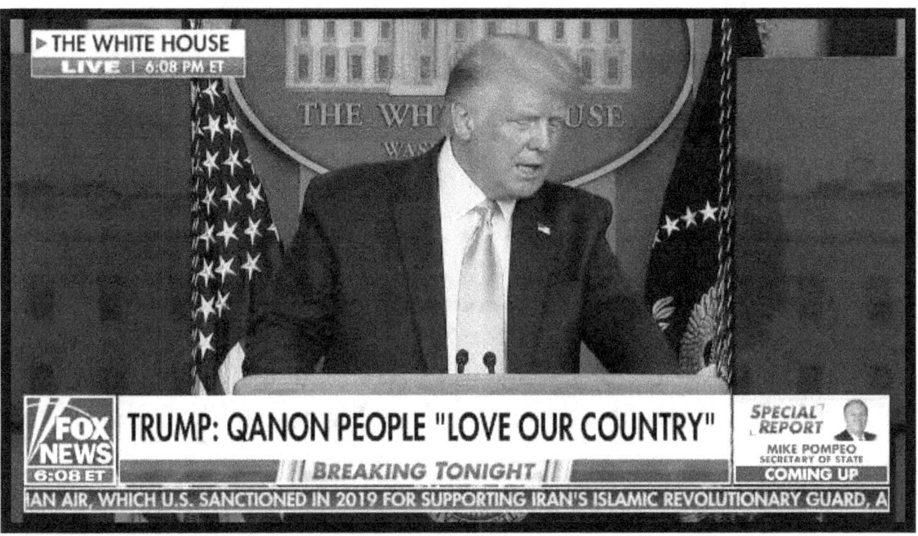

George Floyd Died of Health Complications from a Fentanyl Overdose -- He Was Not Murdered By Minneapolis Police

By Shipwreckedcrew | Aug 27, 2020 3:30 PM ET

"...Derek Chauvin did not cut off George Floyd's oxygen supply.

"Derek Chauvin's knee caused no trauma to George Floyd's airway.

"...the medical cause of George Floyd's death was cardiopulmonary arrest due to pulmonary edema resulting from acute Fentanyl toxicity."

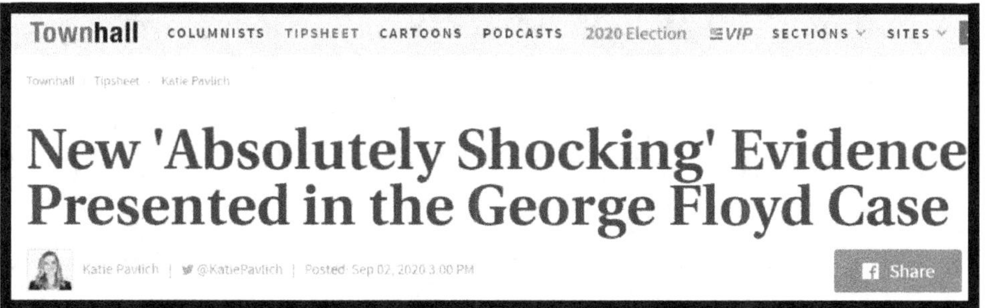

New 'Absolutely Shocking' Evidence Presented in the George Floyd Case

"Attorneys for former Minneapolis Police Officer Derek Chauvin are requesting the dismissal of murder and manslaughter charges against him for the death of George Floyd. They're using the police training manual as justification.

"According to the Minneapolis Police Department training manual, officers are shown how to subdue violent or resisting suspects by placing their knee on the neck."

For a "virus" that over 99% of people survive, that you have to get a "test" just to find out if you have it – The "tests" are fake and I have already provided you with the evidence of the Austrian lawmaker publicly testing a glass of cola "positive" for "COVID" – Here is more:

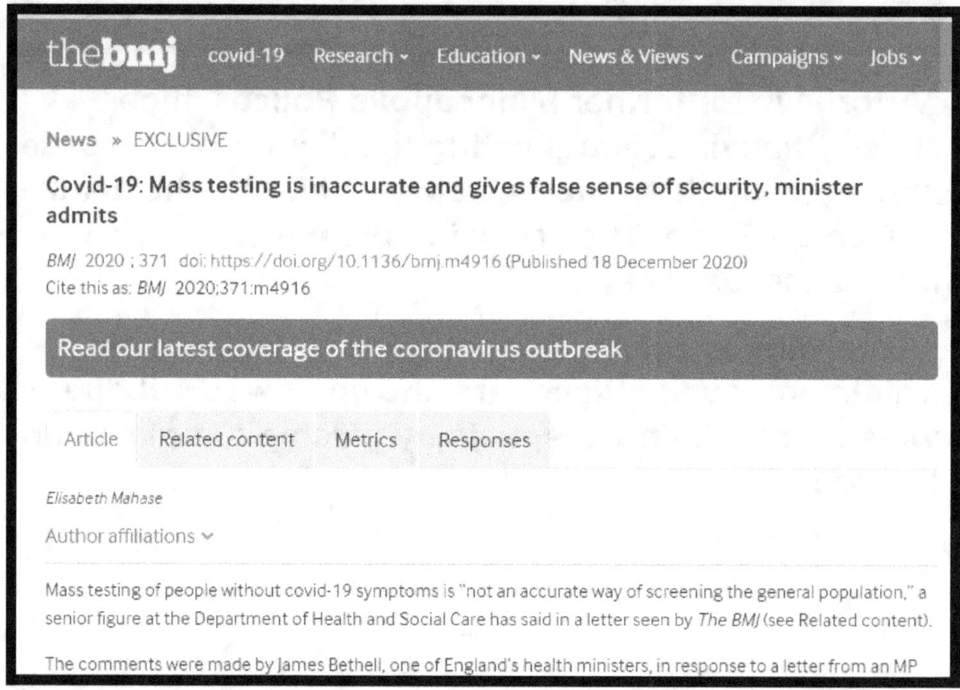

"The comments were made by James Bethell, one of England's health ministers, in response to a letter from an MP raising concerns about blanket polymerase chain reaction (PCR) testing on behalf of a constituent.

"In his letter Bethell stated that 'swab testing people with no symptoms is not an accurate way of screening the general population, as there is a real risk of giving false reassurance.' He added, 'Widespread asymptomatic testing could undermine the value of testing, as there is a risk of giving misleading results. **<u>Rather, only people with covid-19 symptoms should get tested.</u>**'"

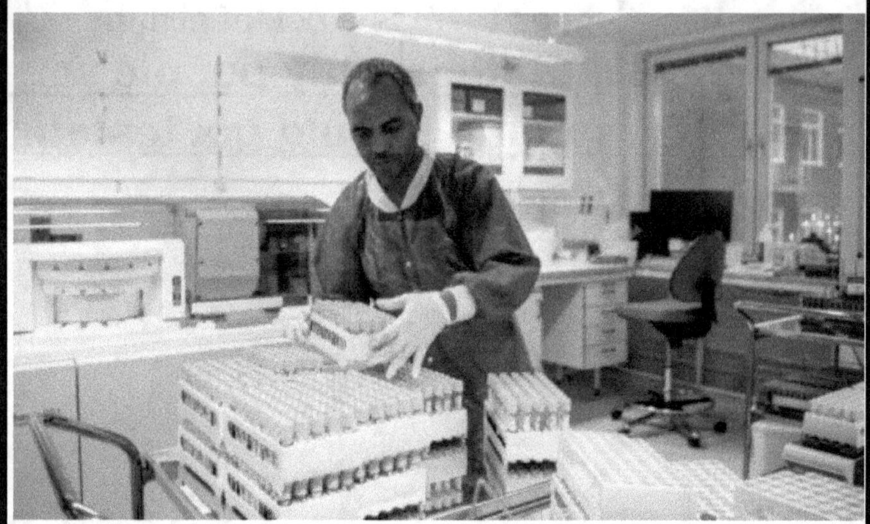

A member of staff at the laboratory of Karolinska hospital operates a machine used in the PCR testing process for people who think they may be suffering from COVID-19, in Solna, near Stockholm, on Dec. 7, 2020. (Jonathan Nackstrand/AFP via Getty Images)

PUBLIC HEALTH INFORMATION PREMIUM

Test to Detect CCP Virus Flawed, Scientists Say

Fragments of dead virus can thwart the diagnostic tool churning out the numbers that dominate headlines

BY MEILING LEE | January 6, 2021 Updated: January 7, 2021

A Å   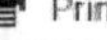 Print

Trump says he's mobilizing military to distribute potential coronavirus vaccine

Kaelan Deese · 5/14/2020

President Trump said Thursday he would prepare the U.S. military to disburse COVID-19 vaccines when they are ready.

Business Standard

You are here: Home » International » News » Others

World is at war with hidden army of Covid-19, but we will win: Donald Trump

Trump referred to the fight against the COVID-19 as a "war" again at a meeting with CEOs of the tourism industry.

Topics
Coronavirus | Donald Trump | Donald Trump administration

Press Trust of India | Washington
Last Updated at March 18, 2020 07:02 IST

The missing flu riddle: 'Influenza has been renamed COVID,' maverick epidemiologist says

As influenza levels continue cratering, some cite COVID measures — even as COVID rates have multiplied nearly sevenfold since the spring in spite of enhanced mitigation policies.

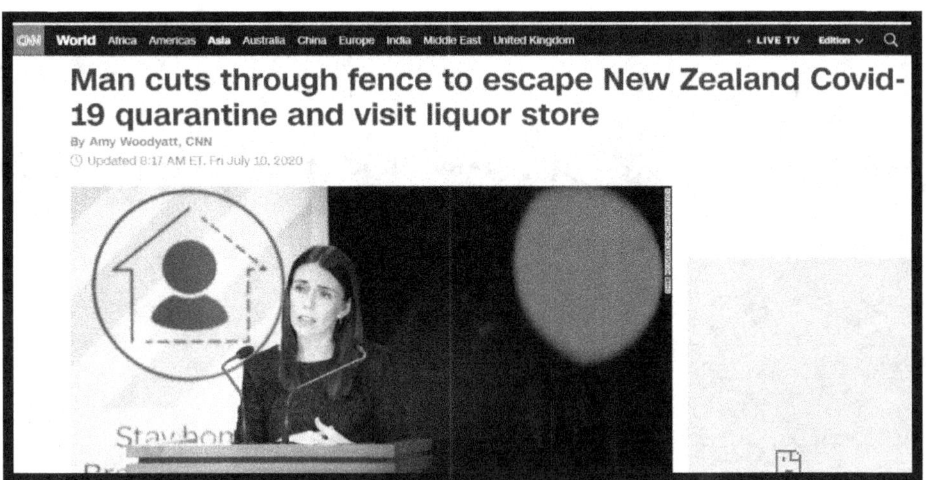

CNN World Africa Americas Asia Australia China Europe India Middle East United Kingdom • LIVE TV Edition Q

Man cuts through fence to escape New Zealand Covid-19 quarantine and visit liquor store

By Amy Woodyatt, CNN
Updated 8:17 AM ET, Fri July 10, 2020

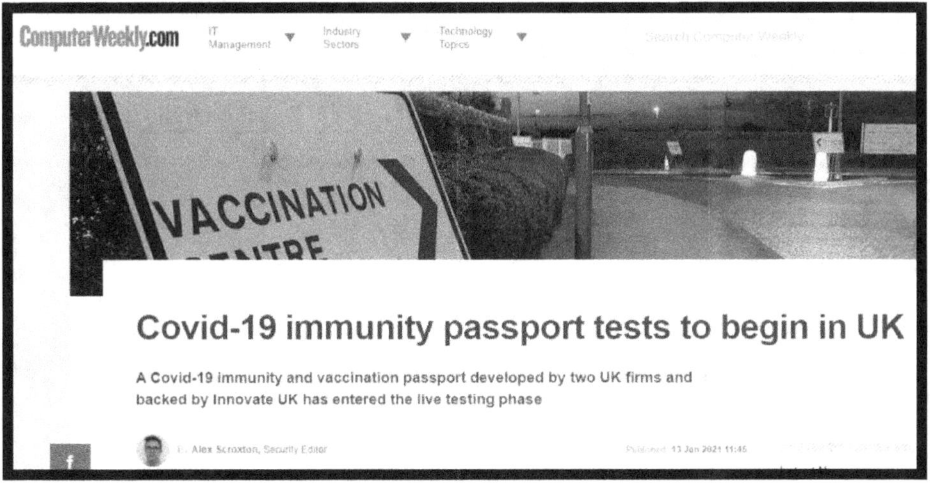

ComputerWeekly.com   IT Management   Industry Sectors   Technology Topics   Search Computer Weekly

VACCINATION CENTRE

Covid-19 immunity passport tests to begin in UK

A Covid-19 immunity and vaccination passport developed by two UK firms and backed by Innovate UK has entered the live testing phase

Alex Scroxton, Security Editor   Published: 13 Jan 2021 11:45

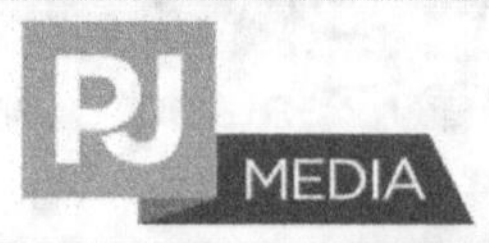

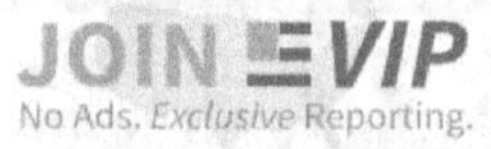

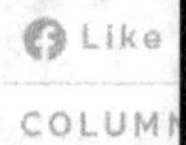

NEWS & POLITICS   COLUMNS   ELECTION 2020   CULTURE   VIP

NEWS & POLITICS

Tables Turned: Detroit Sues Black Lives Matter Group for 'Civil Conspiracy' to Riot and Attack Police

BY TYLER O'NEIL DEC 22, 2020 6:45 PM ET

Oh, you better believe that it's political:

WJ THE WESTERN JOURNAL

News

NEWS

Convicted Terrorist Released by Bill Clinton Now Sits on Board of BLM's Fundraising Organization

<u>First Amendment:</u>

Congress shall make no law respecting an establishment of religion, or prohibiting the free exercise thereof; or abridging the freedom of speech, or of the press; or the right of the people peaceably to assemble, and to petition the Government for a redress of grievances.

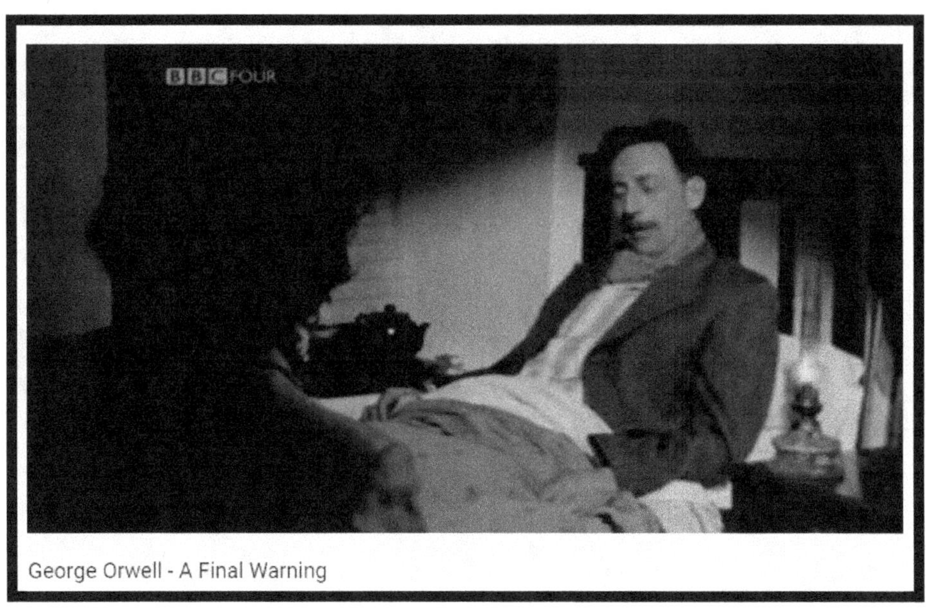

George Orwell - A Final Warning

"**"If you want a picture of the future, imagine a boot stamping on a human face — forever."**

— George Orwell

"In recent years, the proliferation of digital devices and internet-based communications has created significant vulnerabilities and magnified the scope and intensity of the threat of foreign interference, as illustrated in the 2017 Intelligence Community Assessment. I hereby declare a national emergency to deal with this threat."

George Soros's Foundation Pours $220 Million Into Racial Equality Push

Mr. Soros's group will invest $150 million in grants for Black-led racial justice groups, and another $70 million toward local grants for criminal justice reform and civic engagement opportunities.

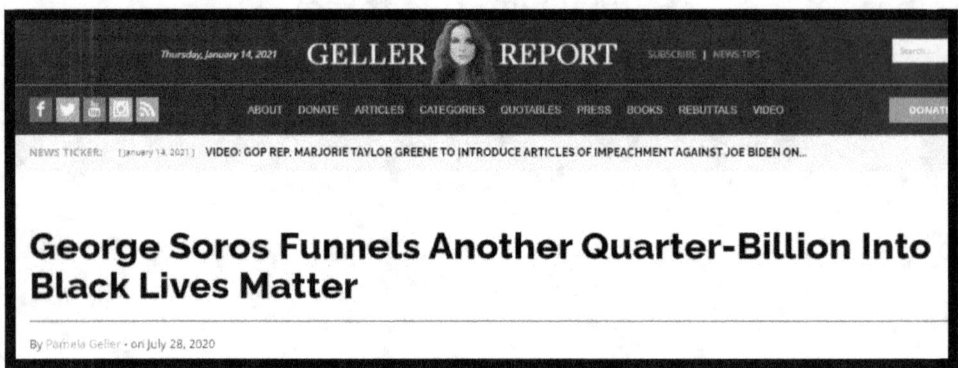

George Soros Funnels Another Quarter-Billion Into Black Lives Matter

By Pamela Geller • on July 28, 2020

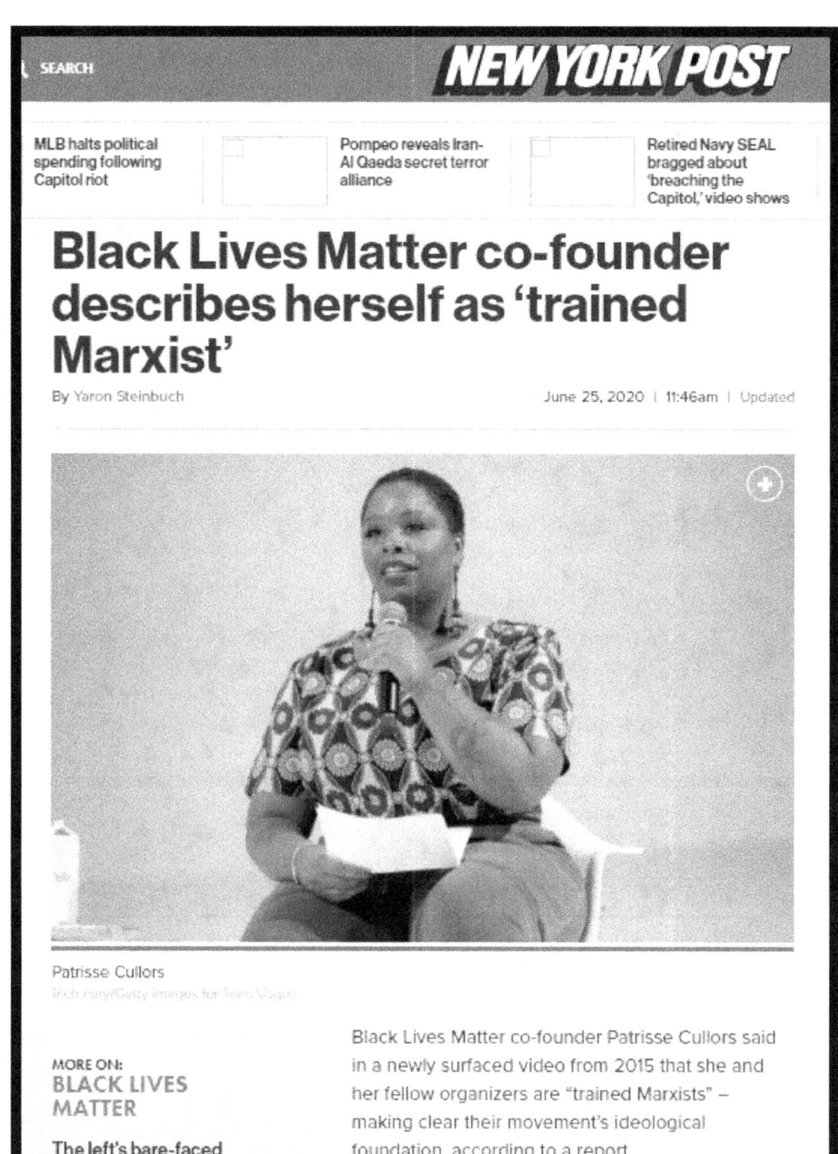

OF COURSE "BLACK LIVES MATTER" IS A POLITICAL ORGANIZATION!

Just look at the timing – This staged and inflated "George Floyd" narrative suddenly sprung up just as we were approaching the most consequential Presidential election in the history of The United States:

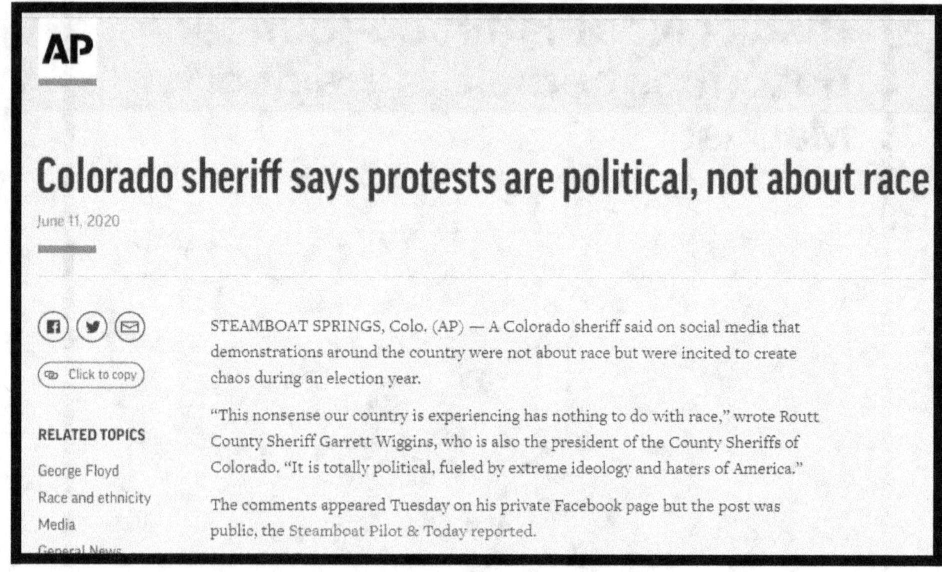

Colorado sheriff says protests are political, not about race

June 11, 2020

STEAMBOAT SPRINGS, Colo. (AP) — A Colorado sheriff said on social media that demonstrations around the country were not about race but were incited to create chaos during an election year.

"This nonsense our country is experiencing has nothing to do with race," wrote Routt County Sheriff Garrett Wiggins, who is also the president of the County Sheriffs of Colorado. "It is totally political, fueled by extreme ideology and haters of America."

The comments appeared Tuesday on his private Facebook page but the post was public, the Steamboat Pilot & Today reported.

RELATED TOPICS

George Floyd

Race and ethnicity

Media

General News

WAKE UP TO WHAT IS HAPPENING!

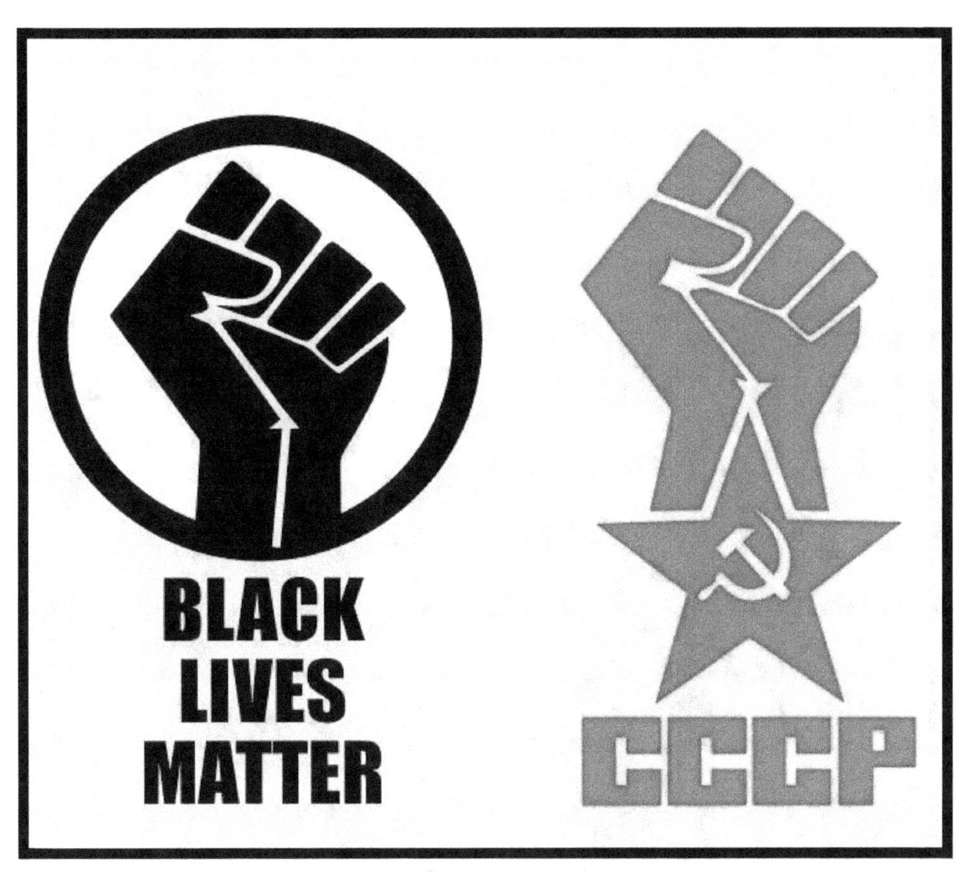

BLACK
LIVES
MATTER
CCCP

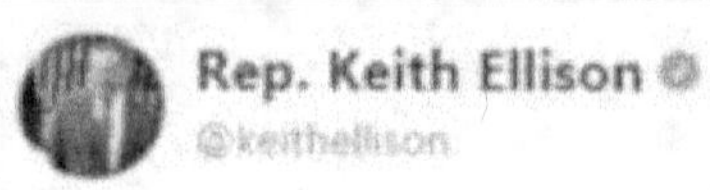

Rep. Keith Ellison
@keithellison
Follow
At @MoonPalaceBooks and I just found the book that strike fear in the heart of @realDonaldTrump 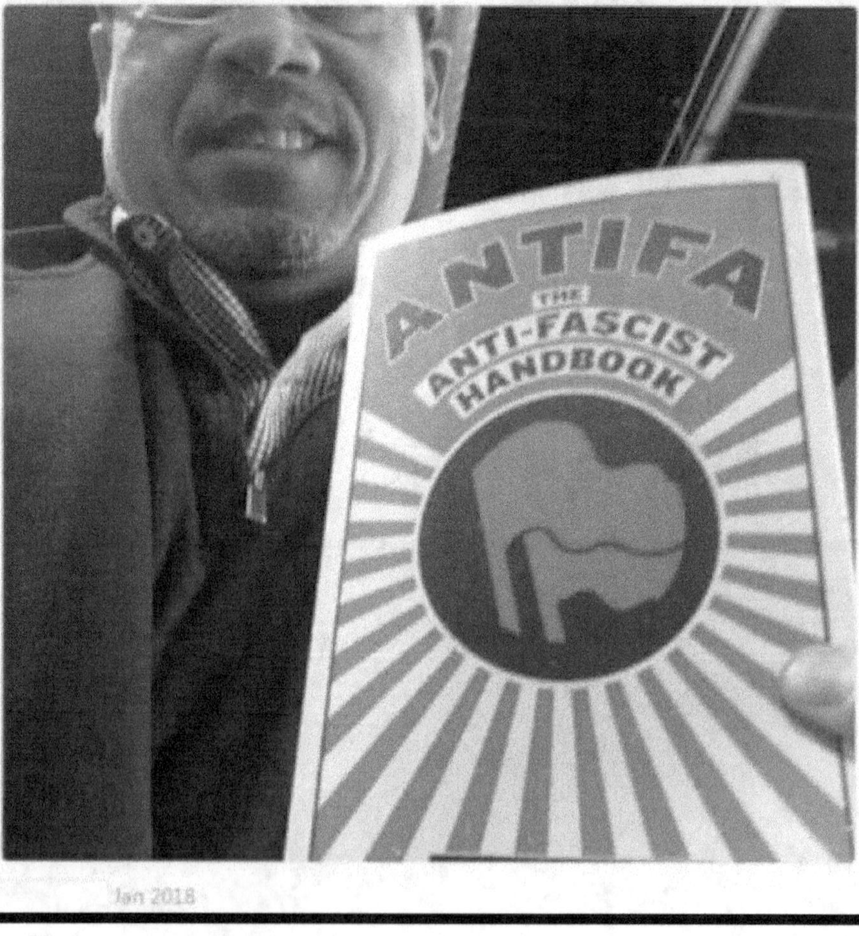
ANTIFA
THE ANTI-FASCIST HANDBOOK
Jan 2018

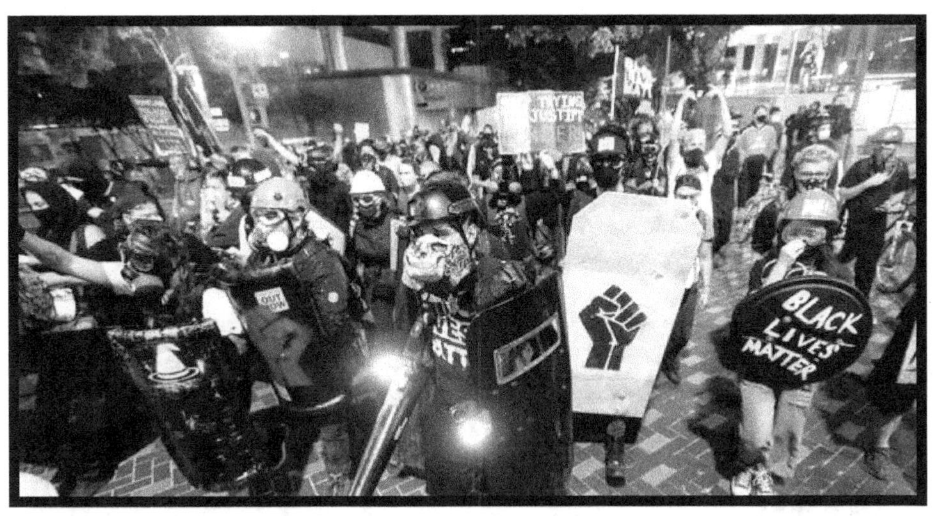
BLACK
LIVES
MATTER
SERVING
JUSTICE

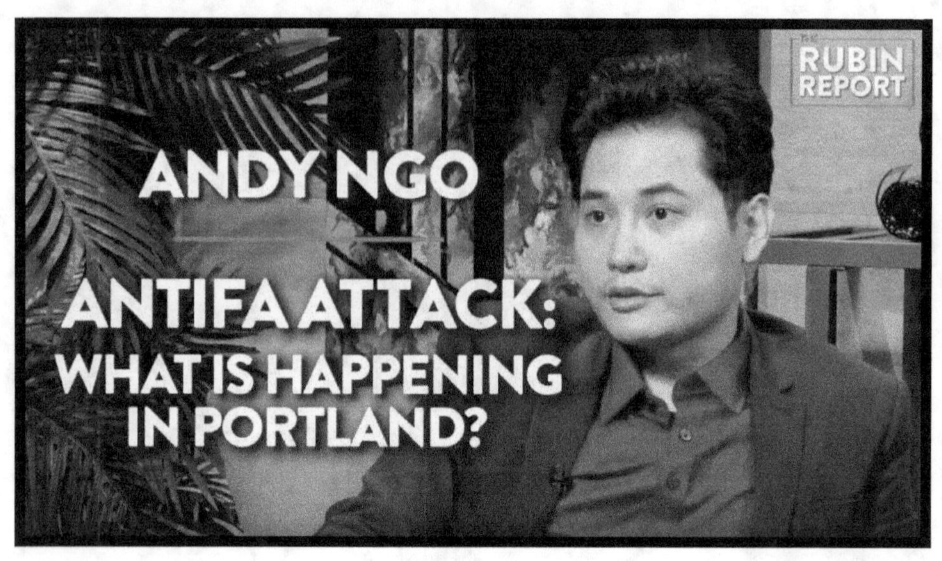

RUBIN REPORT
ANDY NGO
ANTIFA ATTACK:
WHAT IS HAPPENING
IN PORTLAND?

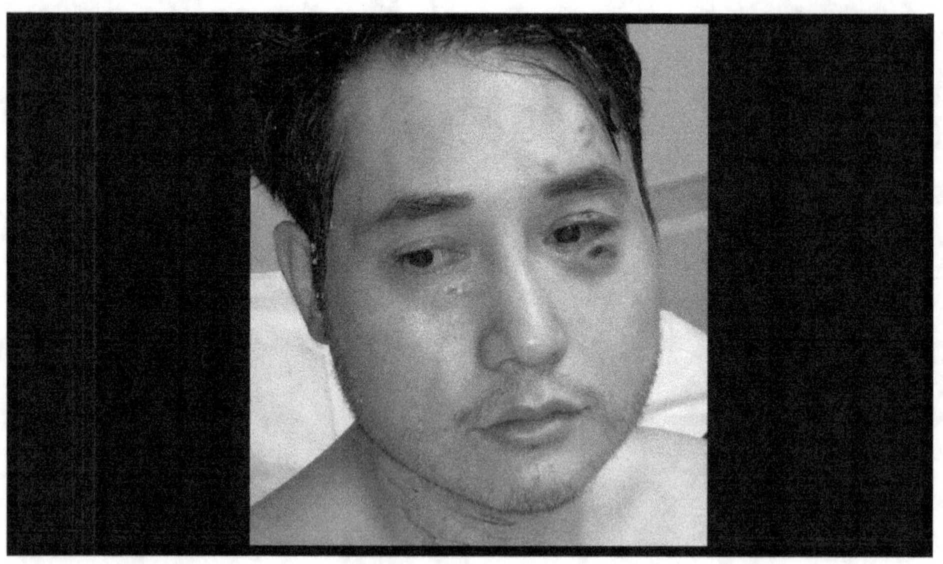

NEW YORK POST

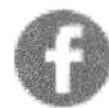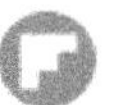

NEWS

Two known Antifa members posed as pro-Trump to infiltrate Capitol riot: sources

By Larry Celona

January 7, 2021 | 12:40am | Updated

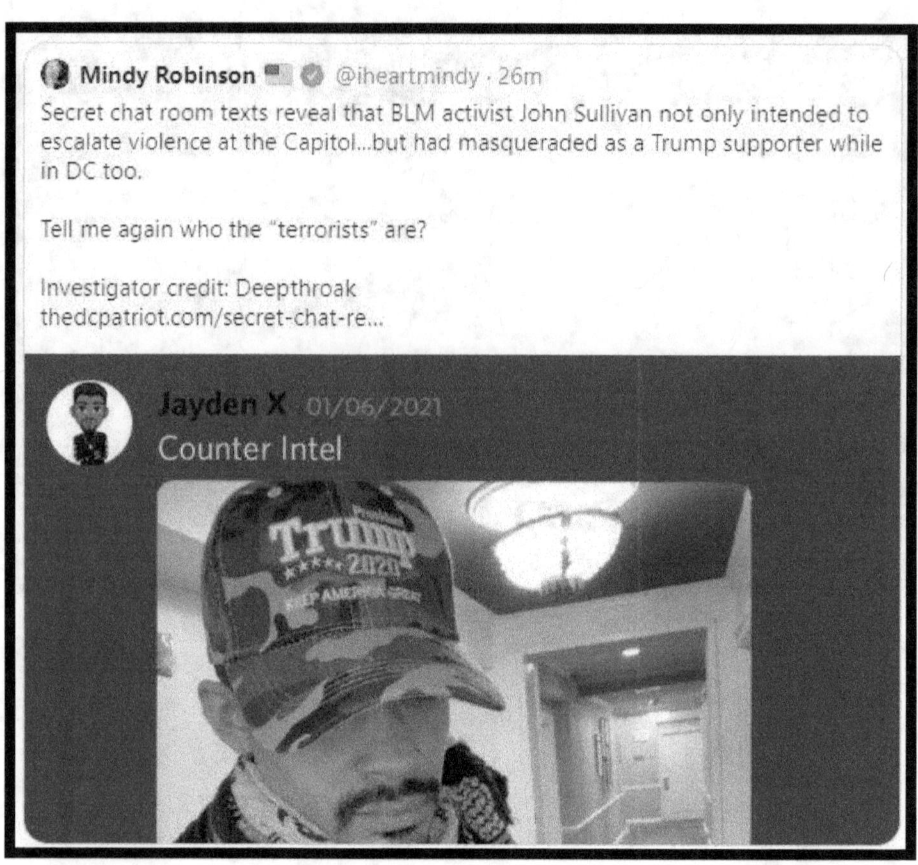

SO-CALLED "CAPITAL HILL RIOT"

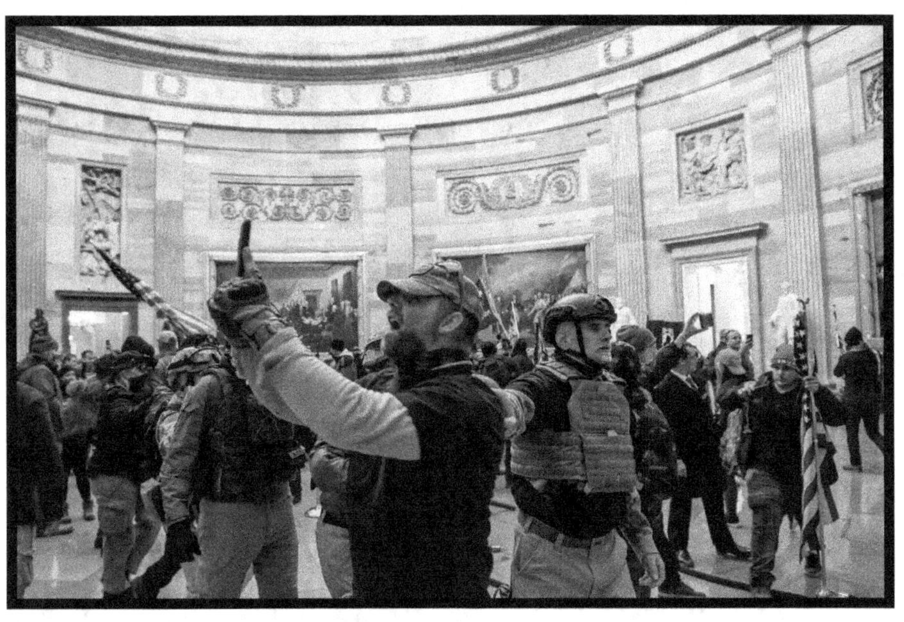

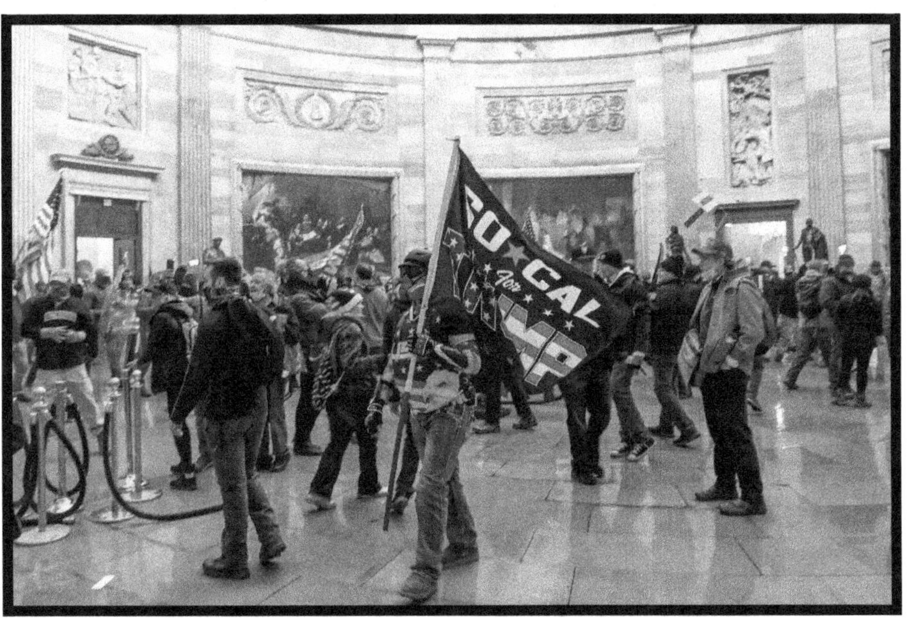

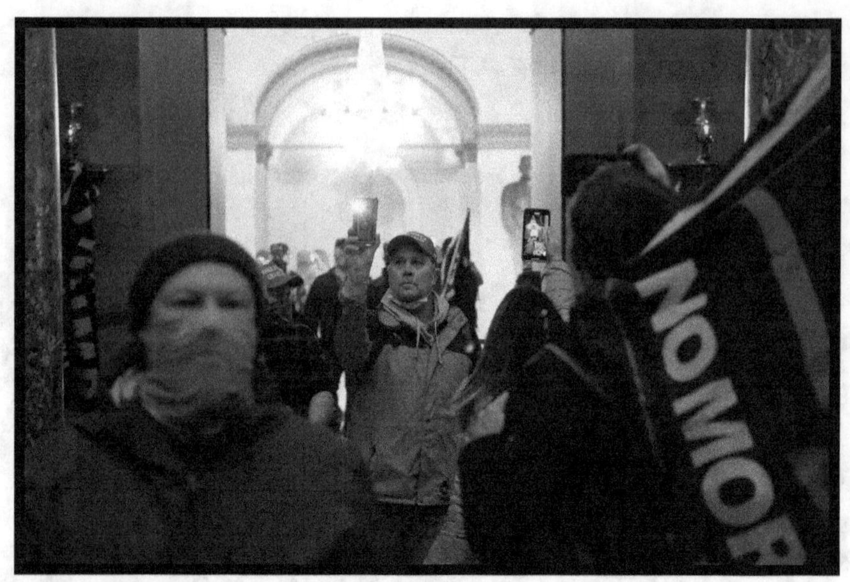

EXCESSIVE FORCE FOR A BUNCH OF PATRIOTS WALKING AROUND TAKING PICTURES?

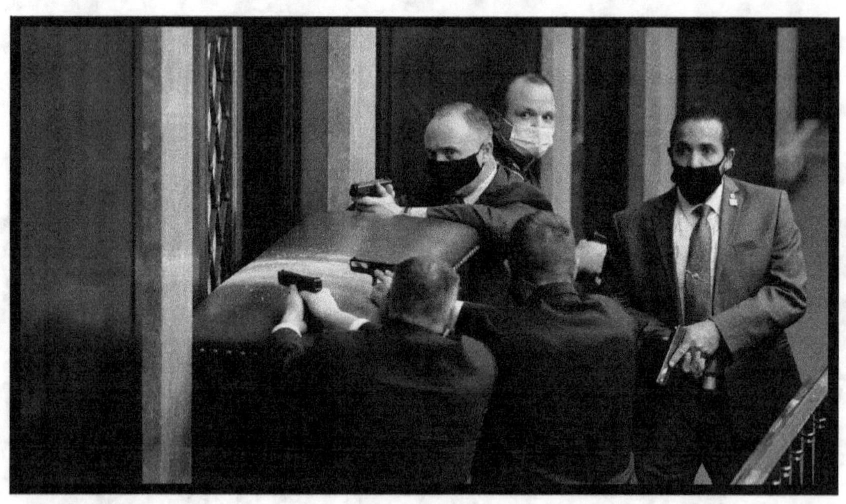

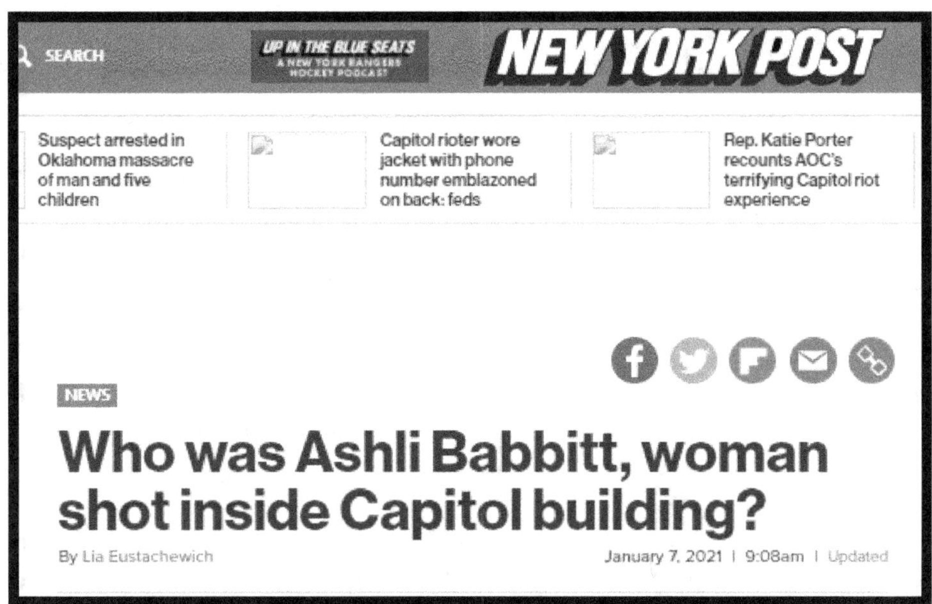

Who was Ashli Babbitt, woman shot inside Capitol building?

By Lia Eustachewich

January 7, 2021 | 9:08am | Updated

"Ashli Babbitt, the Air Force veteran who was fatally shot after breaching the Capitol building Wednesday, was 'never afraid to speak her mind,' according to her ex-husband.

"'I feel absolutely terrible and sick to my stomach about it,' Timothy McEntee, who was married to Babbitt for 14 years, texted the Washington Post after Babbitt's death. 'She was never afraid to speak her mind and in a way this was her way of speaking her mind (going to the rally).'

"Babbitt, who served in the Air Force for 14 years, spent time in Afghanistan and Iraq and was also deployed with the National Guard to Kuwait and Qatar, according to McEntee."

276

NEWS

In some videos, Capitol police appear to let protestors into US Capitol, pose for selfies

Other videos from other parts of the chaotic day show very different interactions between protestors and police.

Sat Jan 9, 2021 - 5:57 am EST

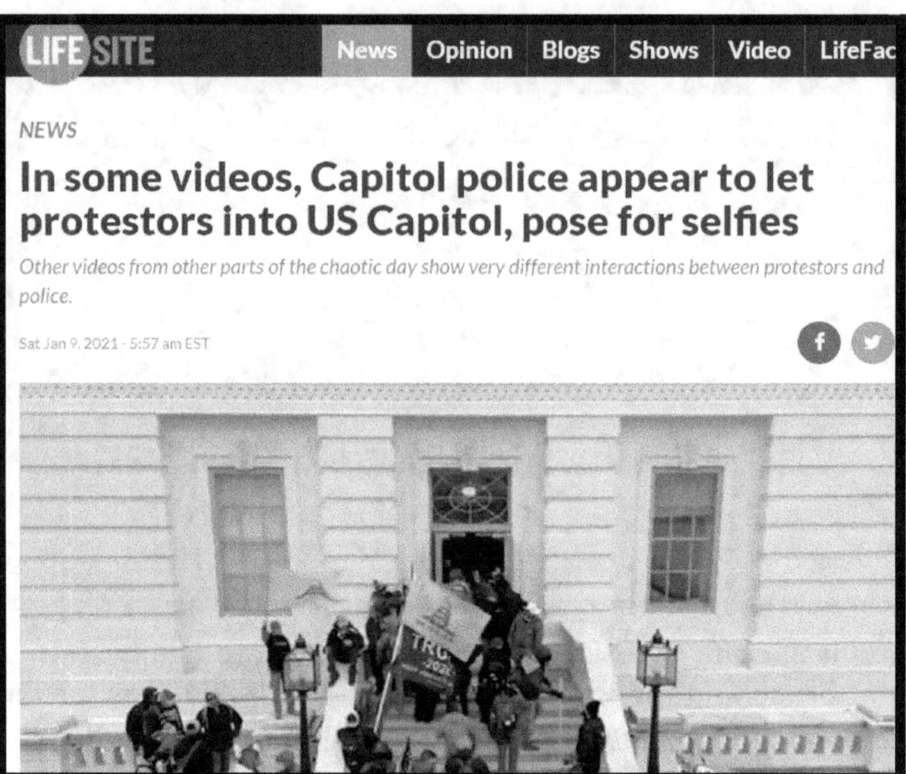

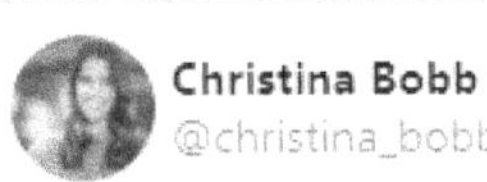

Christina Bobb
@christina_bobb

Capitol police open doors for the protestors. They stand aside and invite them inside.

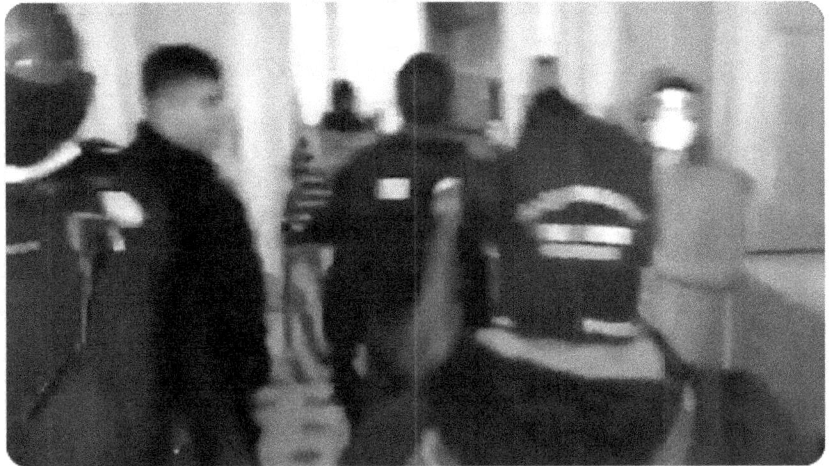

10:29 AM · Jan 8, 2021

♡ 70.8K   💬 52.9K   🔗 Copy link to Tweet

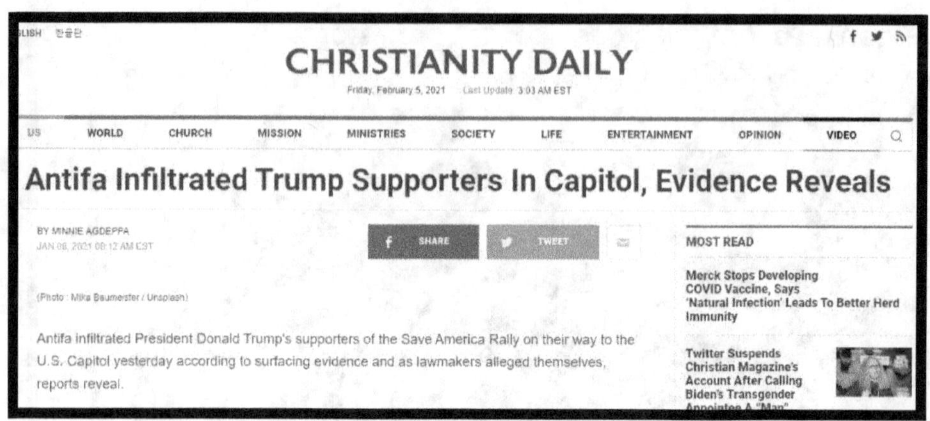

CHRISTIANITY DAILY

Friday, February 5, 2021   Last Update: 3:03 AM EST

US   WORLD   CHURCH   MISSION   MINISTRIES   SOCIETY   LIFE   ENTERTAINMENT   OPINION   VIDEO

Antifa Infiltrated Trump Supporters In Capitol, Evidence Reveals

BY MINNIE AGDEPPA
JAN 08, 2021 08:12 AM EST

SHARE   TWEET

MOST READ

Merck Stops Developing COVID Vaccine, Says 'Natural Infection' Leads To Better Herd Immunity

Twitter Suspends Christian Magazine's Account After Calling Biden's Transgender Appointee A "Man"

(Photo: Mika Baumeister / Unsplash)

Antifa infiltrated President Donald Trump's supporters of the Save America Rally on their way to the U.S. Capitol yesterday according to surfacing evidence and as lawmakers alleged themselves, reports reveal.

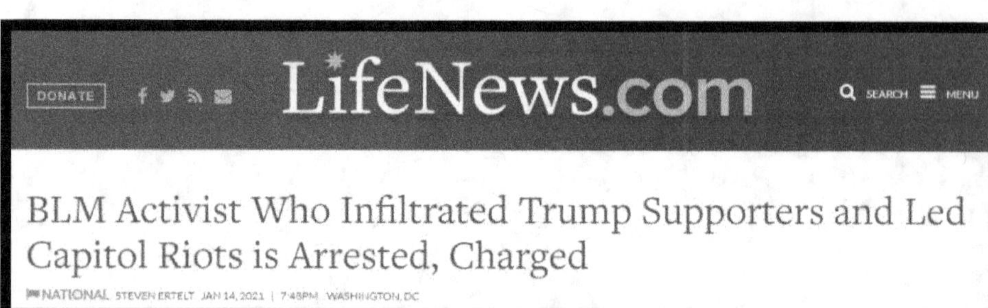

LifeNews.com

DONATE   SEARCH   MENU

BLM Activist Who Infiltrated Trump Supporters and Led Capitol Riots is Arrested, Charged

NATIONAL   STEVEN ERTELT   JAN 14, 2021 | 7:48PM   WASHINGTON, DC

As a professional Researcher, it has been my business to identify information that is factual and significant – Therefore, for the benefit of the community, I share this published information – Please exercise your right to independent thought:

"Masks Not Very Effective at Protecting Wearers, Says New Danish Study"

Reason Magazine, 11/18/2020

"New research published in the *Annals of Internal Medicine* finds that masks do not appear to protect the people wearing them, but are still likely to prevent sick people who wear them from spreading their illness."

This is a "scientific study" – We are supposed to believe in "science," right? Here's more:

"Asymptomatic spread of coronavirus is 'very rare,' WHO says"

CNBC, 06/08/2020

"…the WHO says that while asymptomatic spread can occur, it is 'very rare.'"

Should we listen to "The WHO?"

So if "asymptomatic" people are not contagious, that means that if we do not have symptoms there is no reasonable explanation for legally enforcing American citizens to wear masks over their faces against their will – In fact, it is a Constitutional crime to do so:

Amendment 5

"…nor be deprived of life, liberty, or property, without due process of law;"

And for those who are "contagious?" We will pray for them, but they have a 99% chance of survival according to the "CDC" – Should we listen to the "CDC?"

"CDC Data Shows High Virus Survival Rate: 99%-Plus for Ages 69 and Younger, 94.6% for Older"

<u>Breitbart, 09/25/2020</u>

"The U.S. Centers for Disease and Control and Prevention (CDC) recently updated its estimated Infection Fatality Rate (IFR) parameters to include age-specific data <u>showing the vast majority of people who contract the Chinese coronavirus survives</u>."

These simple examples of recent scientific data conclude that we can likely assume that the best way to respond to this "pandemic" is the same as any other flu season – If you feel sick, then you should probably stay home for a few days until you feel better – And while you are recovering, we will pray for the alleviation of your discomfort, but since there is a 99% survivability rate, we're not going to organize any pity parades for you because, well, we've all been sick before, too.

THE STEAMBOAT SKI AREA SEEMED TO HAVE A FINANCIALLY
SUCCESSFUL WEEKEND - HOW ABOUT "SOCIAL DISTANCING,"
FOLKS?

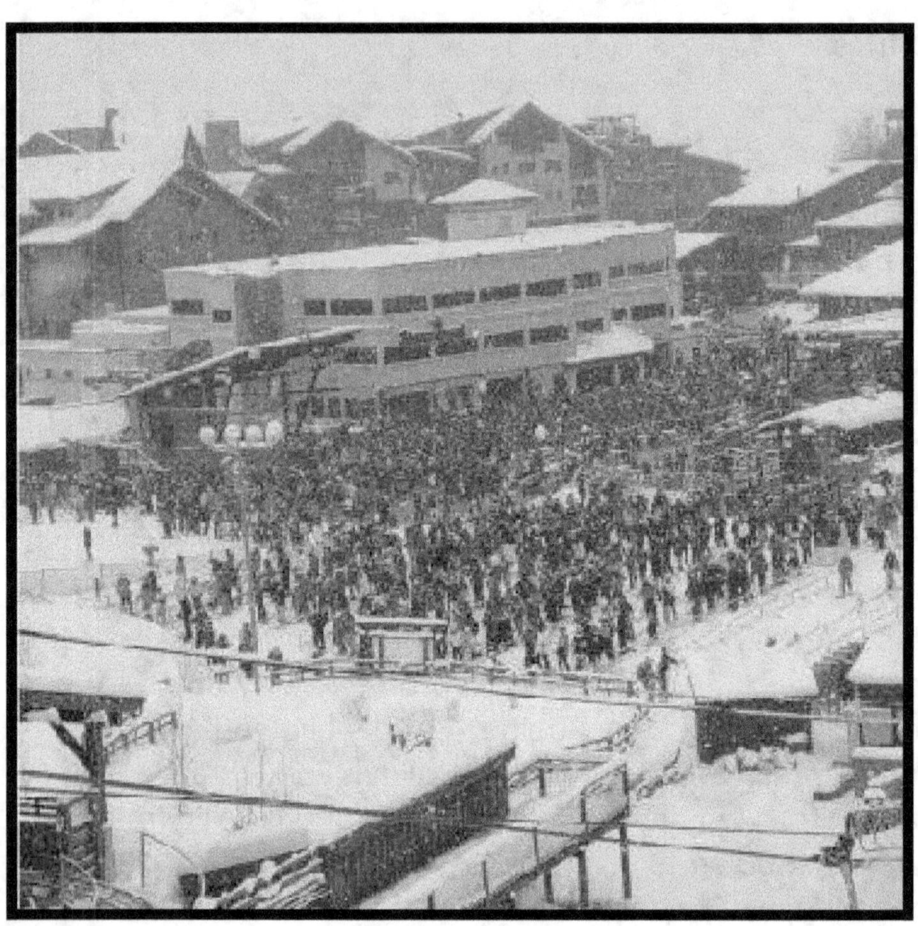

MEANWHILE, LOCAL RESTAURANTS ARE ENDURING THESE
INSANE AND ABUSIVE RESTRICTIONS:

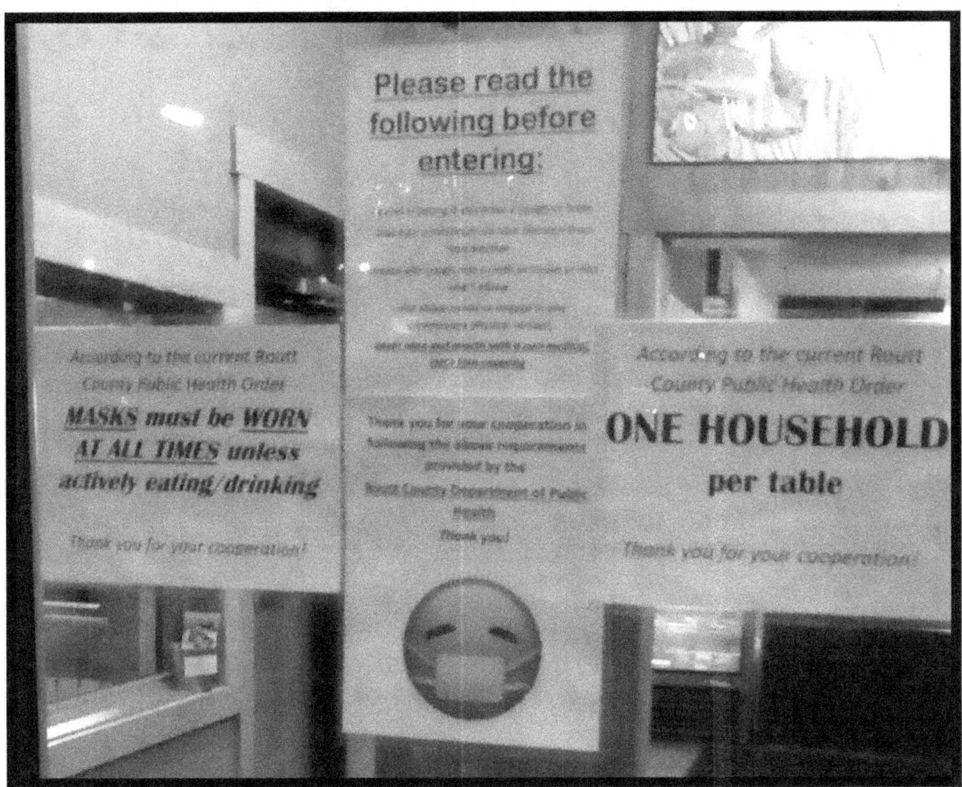

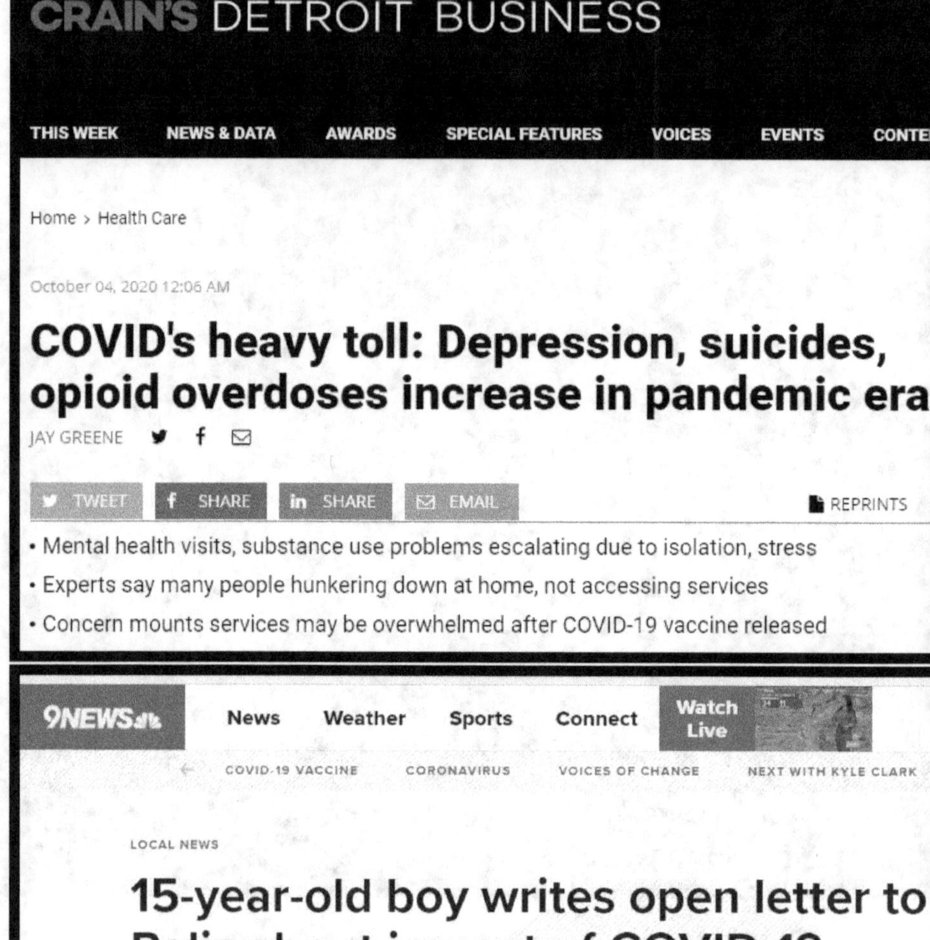

CRAIN'S DETROIT BUSINESS

THIS WEEK   NEWS & DATA   AWARDS   SPECIAL FEATURES   VOICES   EVENTS   CONTEN

Home > Health Care

October 04, 2020 12:06 AM

COVID's heavy toll: Depression, suicides, opioid overdoses increase in pandemic era

JAY GREENE

TWEET   SHARE   SHARE   EMAIL   REPRINTS

• Mental health visits, substance use problems escalating due to isolation, stress
• Experts say many people hunkering down at home, not accessing services
• Concern mounts services may be overwhelmed after COVID-19 vaccine released

9NEWS   News   Weather   Sports   Connect   Watch Live

COVID-19 VACCINE   CORONAVIRUS   VOICES OF CHANGE   NEXT WITH KYLE CLARK

LOCAL NEWS

15-year-old boy writes open letter to Polis about impact of COVID-19 restrictions on teen mental health

Kaden Piel said he wants to raise awareness about how taking away sports and activities can contribute to feelings of isolation.

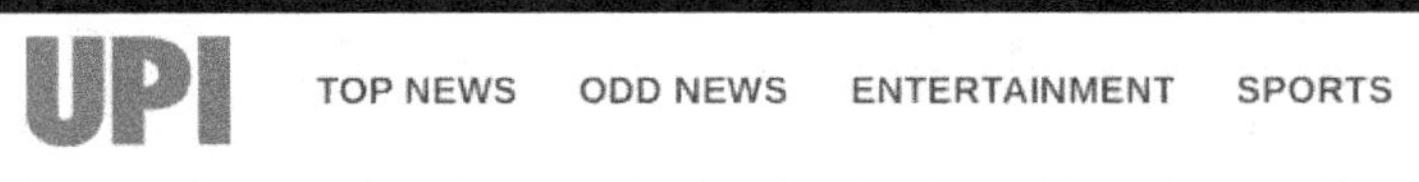

TOP NEWS   ODD NEWS   ENTERTAINMENT   SPORTS   PHOTOS   MORE

TRENDING   Four jackpots   Claudia Conway   Mars probe   Zoom cat   Frozen pants   'Skinniest house'

HEALTH NEWS   FEB. 3, 2021 / 11:03 AM

CDC: ER visits for drug overdoses, suicide attempts rise during pandemic

By Brian P. Dunleavy

2019 General Excellence - 1st Place
Washington Newspaper Association

The Leader

Wednesday, February 10, 2021

NEWS ▾   ARTS & ENTERTAINMENT   SPORTS   CALENDAR ▾   OPINION ▾   OBITUARIES ▾   CLASSIFIEDS ▾   SUBMIT NEWS ▾   SUBSCR

⚠ You have **4 free items** remaining before a subscription is required.   Subscribe now! | Log in

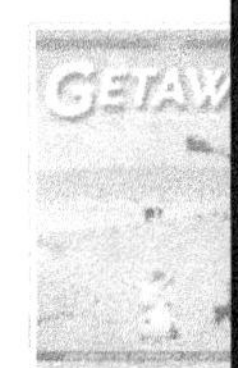

New suicide review team proposed after CDC report finds rising levels of mental-health-related visits for children | 2021 Legislative Session

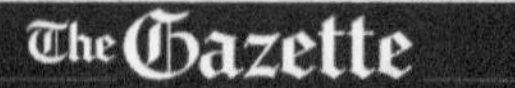

Remote learning, not COVID, is killing kids

Jimmy Sengenberger   Jan 29, 2021

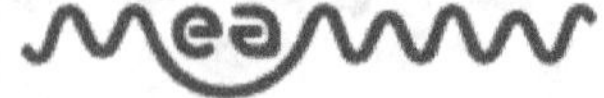

HOME / NEWS / HEALTH

Spike in student suicides forces LA school district to reopen for in-person learning amid rising Covid-19 cases

The Clark County School District in Nevada has seen 18 suicides in nine months since it closed schools in March 2020 as compared to 9 in 2019

By Mihika Basu

Published on : 20:03 PST, Jan 27, 2021

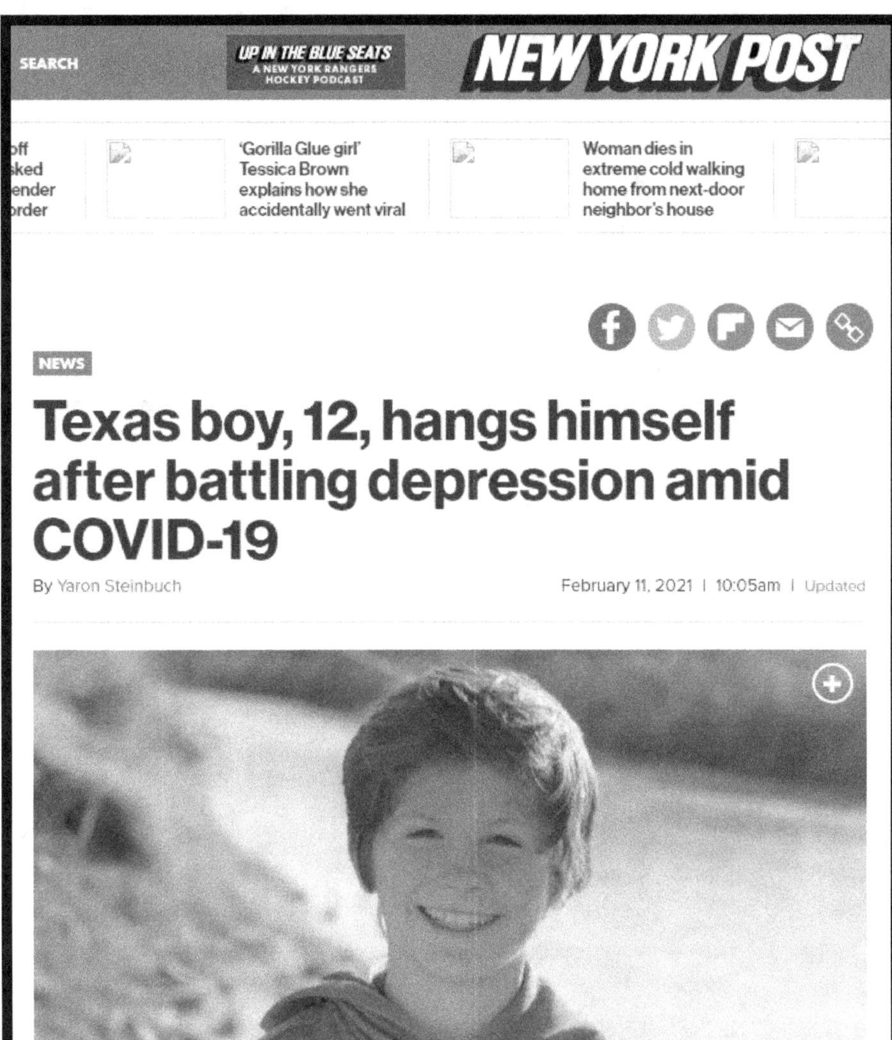

Texas boy, 12, hangs himself after battling depression amid COVID-19

By Yaron Steinbuch

February 11, 2021 | 10:05am | Updated

Parameter	Scenario 1	Scenario 2	Scenario 3	Scenario 4	Scenario 5: Current Best Estimate
R_0*	2.0		4.0		2.5
Infection Fatality Ratio[†]	0-19 years: 0.00002 20-49 years: 0.00007 50-69 years: 0.0025 70+ years: 0.028		0-19 years: 0.0001 20-49 years: 0.0003 50-69 years: 0.010 70+ years: 0.093		0-19 years: 0.00003 20-49 years: 0.0002 50-69 years: 0.005 70+ years: 0.054

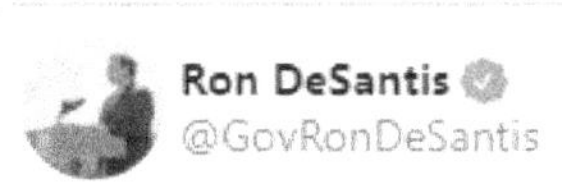

Ron DeSantis ✓
@GovRonDeSantis

CDC recently updated estimated infection fatality rates for COVID. Here are the updated survival rates by age group:

0-19: 99.997%
20-49: 99.98%
50-69: 99.5%
70+: 94.6%

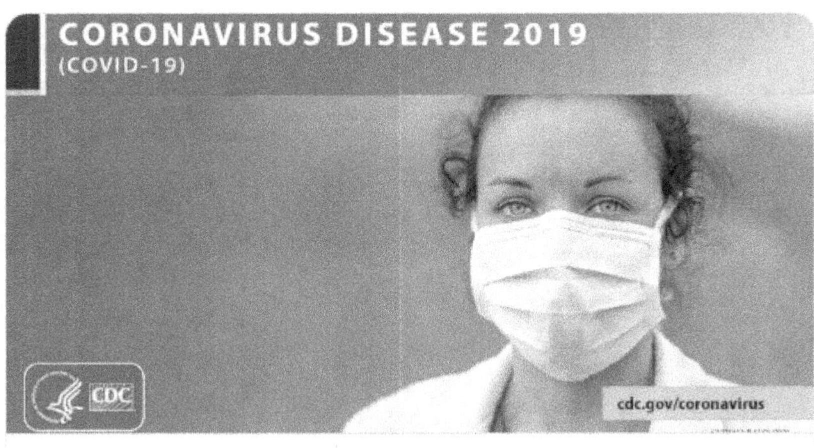

Healthcare Workers
COVID-19 guidance, tools, and resources for healthcare workers.
🔗 cdc.gov

11:44 AM · Sep 23, 2020

 7.3K   ⚡ See the latest COVID-19 information on Twitter